AF795758

Challenging Cases in Rheumatology and Diseases of the Immune System

Massoud Mahmoudi
Editor

Challenging Cases in Rheumatology and Diseases of the Immune System

Springer

Editor
Massoud Mahmoudi
Associate Clinical Professor
Department of Medicine
Division of General Internal Medicine
University of California San Francisco
San Francisco, CA, USA

Adjunct Associate Professor
Department of Medicine
San Francisco College of Osteopathic Medicine
Touro University
Vallejo, CA, USA

Adjunct Associate Professor
School of Osteopathic Medicine
University of Medicine and Dentistry of New Jersey
Stratford, NJ, USA

ISBN 978-1-4614-5087-0 ISBN 978-1-4614-5088-7 (eBook)
DOI 10.1007/978-1-4614-5088-7
Springer New York Heidelberg Dordrecht London

Library of Congress Control Number: 2012951612

© Springer Science+Business Media, LLC 2013
This work is subject to copyright. All rights are reserved by the Publisher, whether the whole or part of the material is concerned, specifically the rights of translation, reprinting, reuse of illustrations, recitation, broadcasting, reproduction on microfilms or in any other physical way, and transmission or information storage and retrieval, electronic adaptation, computer software, or by similar or dissimilar methodology now known or hereafter developed. Exempted from this legal reservation are brief excerpts in connection with reviews or scholarly analysis or material supplied specifically for the purpose of being entered and executed on a computer system, for exclusive use by the purchaser of the work. Duplication of this publication or parts thereof is permitted only under the provisions of the Copyright Law of the Publisher's location, in its current version, and permission for use must always be obtained from Springer. Permissions for use may be obtained through RightsLink at the Copyright Clearance Center. Violations are liable to prosecution under the respective Copyright Law.
The use of general descriptive names, registered names, trademarks, service marks, etc. in this publication does not imply, even in the absence of a specific statement, that such names are exempt from the relevant protective laws and regulations and therefore free for general use.
While the advice and information in this book are believed to be true and accurate at the date of publication, neither the authors nor the editors nor the publisher can accept any legal responsibility for any errors or omissions that may be made. The publisher makes no warranty, express or implied, with respect to the material contained herein.

Printed on acid-free paper

Springer is part of Springer Science+Business Media (www.springer.com)

To the memory of my father,
Mohammad H. Mahmoudi, and to
my mother, Zohreh, my wife, Lily,
and my sons, Sam and Sina, for their
continuous support and encouragement.

Preface

Allow me to present *Challenging Cases in Rheumatology and Diseases of the Immune System*. This book, like our three preceding titles, *Challenging Cases in Allergy and Immunology* (2009), *Challenging Cases in Allergic and Immunologic Diseases of the Skin* (2010), and *Challenging Cases in Pulmonology* (2011), presents the topic in a case-based study format.

Rheumatology is a branch of medicine concerned with the abnormalities and diseases of the musculoskeletal system: joints, muscles, and connective tissues. Immunology is a branch of medicine concerned with the abnormalities and diseases of our immune system. Immune diseases are either due to the deficiency of the immune system leading to "immunodeficiency" or due to the failure of recognizing the "self" from "non-self" and attacking the own system, leading to " autoimmune disease" or due to hypersensitivity diseases such as allergic rhinitis.

Rheumatic and immunologic diseases are closely related because the underlying etiology of certain rheumatic diseases is the abnormality of the immune system. Understanding the immune system is the key factor in recognizing the abnormalities in rheumatic diseases. Therefore, clinical immunologists and rheumatologist may occasionally see and treat similar conditions. In fact, some specialists are dually trained in Allergy/Immunology and Rheumatology.

What makes these two branches of medicine different is their uniqueness. Rheumatologists, for example, evaluate and treat rheumatoid arthritis, osteoarthritis, and fibromyalgia, to name a few. Allergists and clinical immunologists treat hypersensitivities such as allergic rhinitis, allergic asthma, and immunological diseases such as immunodeficiencies, among others. Both specialties, however, deal with autoimmune diseases. As the population ages in the twenty-first century, the role of rheumatology and immunology becomes more apparent and appreciated.

Approaching a patient with multiple rheumatic diseases is not an easy task. In fact, our immune system is perhaps the most complicated system of the human body; this is due to the presence and interactions of a myriad of cells and chemical mediators that participate in complex pathways such as the inflammatory response and others to defend the body and respond to pathogens. In addition, our immune system protects us against further exposure to the harmful substances.

I have had the pleasure of gathering over 30 distinguished contributors to produce such an exciting collection. This book consists of 6 parts and 16 chapters, and each chapter presents 2 cases. Our faithful readers are familiar with the style of this series that is an abstract, followed by case presentation, working diagnosis, data, final diagnosis, and discussion. In addition, for reviewing the subject and stimulating the thought process, we have added five to ten multiple choice questions and answers to each chapter.

This book is a collective effort of contributors, the editorial staff, and Springer. I would like to use this opportunity and thank Richard Lansing, Editorial Director for Clinical Medicine at Springer, who has guided and supported me for all the four books in this collection; Andy Kwan, Assistant Editor; Martine Chevry, Editorial Assistant; and Maria Smilios, Developmental Editor who helped and supported us step by step through the entire manuscript; and, finally, the entire editorial and publishing staff at Springer.

I am pleased to announce that we have received numerous positive and encouraging reviews for the previous books, and we hope that the content of this collection, as the previous one's, would exceed the readers' expectation. I will be happy to hear your comments and use them in the future edition of this book. Please contact me at allergycure@sbcglobal.net.

San Francisco, CA, USA Massoud Mahmoudi

Contents

Contributors

Robert Bettiker, MD Section of Infectious Diseases, Temple University Hospital, Philadelphia, PA, USA

Marcy B. Bolster, MD Division of Rheumatology and Immunology, Director, Rheumatology Fellowship Training Program, Medical University of South Carolina, Charleston, SC, USA

David C. Caretto, MD Department of Internal Medicine, University of California San Francisco, San Francisco, CA, USA

Xavier J. Caro, MD, FACP, FACR Northridge Hospital Medical Center, Northridge, CA, USA

Krati Chauhan, MD Division of Rheumatology, Department of Medicine, Mayo Clinic, Rochester, MN, USA

Vaidehi R. Chowdhary, MD Division of Rheumatology, Department of Medicine, Mayo Clinic College of Medicine, Rochester, MN, USA

Gilbert D'Alonzo, DO Professor of Medicine, Department of Pulmonary and Critical Care, Temple University School of Medicine, Philadelphia, PA, USA

Roshan Dhawale, MD, MPH Division of Rheumatology and Clinical Immunology, University of Pittsburgh Medical Center, Pittsburgh, PA, USA

Floranne Ernste, MD Division of Rheumatology, Department of Internal Medicine, Mayo Clinic Rochester, Rochester, MN, USA

Heather Gladue, DO Division of Rheumatology, University of Michigan, Ann Arbor, MI, USA

Leslie C. Grammer, MD Division of Allergy/Immunology, Northwestern Memorial Hospital, Northwestern University, Chicago, IL, USA

Richart W. Harper, MD Division of Pulmonary, Department of Internal Medicine, Critical Care and Sleep Medicine, UC Davis Medical Center, Sacramento, CA, USA

Phil A. Hart, MD Division of Gastroenterology, Department of Medicine, Mayo Clinic College of Medicine, Rochester, MN, USA

Corey M. Hatfield, DO Division of Rheumatology, Medical University of South Carolina, Charleston, SC, USA

Paul Hoffman, MD Division of Pulmonary, Critical Care and Sleep Medicine, Department of Internal Medicine, UC Davis Medical Center and UC Davis Asthma Network (UCAN), Sacramento, CA, USA

Pim Jetanalin, MD Department of Rheumatology, University of California, San Diego, La Jolla, CA, USA

Toral A. Kamdar, MD Division of Allergy/Immunology, Northwestern Memorial Hospital, Northwestern Memorial Hospital, Chicago, IL, USA

Tanaz A. Kermani, MD MS Division of Rheumatology, University of California Los Angeles, Santa Monica, CA, USA

Susan J. Lee, MD Department of Rheumatology, University of California, San Diego, La Jolla, CA, USA

San Diego Veterans Affairs Medical Center, La Jolla, CA, USA

Massoud Mahmoudi, DO, PhD, RM (NRM), FACOI, FAOCAI, FACP, FCCP, FAAAAI Associate Clinical Professor, Division of General Internal Medicine, Department of Medicine, University of California San Francisco, San Francisco, CA, USA

Adjunct Associate Professor, Department of Medicine, San Francisco College of Osteopathic Medicine, Touro University, Vallejo, CA, USA

Adjunct Associate Professor, School of Osteopathic Medicine, University of Medicine and Dentistry of New Jersey, Stratford, NJ, USA

Rafik Samuel, MD Section of Infectious Diseases, Temple University Hospital, Philadelphia, PA, USA

Elena Schiopu, MD Division of Rheumatology, Scleroderma Program, University of Michigan, Ann Arbor, MI, USA

Michael Schivo, MD, MAS Division of Pulmonary, Critical Care and Sleep Medicine, Department of Internal Medicine, UC Davis Medical Center and UC Davis Asthma Network (UCAN), Sacramento, CA, USA

Christian M. Sebat, DO Division of Pulmonary, Department of Internal Medicine, Critical Care and Sleep Medicine, UC Davis Medical Center, Sacramento, CA, USA

Mather VA Medical Center, Northern California Health Care System (NCHCS), Mather, CA, USA

Kartik V. Shenoy, MD Department of Pulmonary and Critical Care, Temple University School of Medicine, Philadelphia, PA, USA

Jennifer Sloane, MD Department of Rheumatology, Thomas Jefferson University Hospital, Philadelphia, PA, USA

Banafsheh Soltani, MD Section of Infectious Diseases, Temple University Hospital, Philadelphia, PA, USA

Uma Thanarajasingam, MD, PhD Division of Rheumatology, Department of Internal Medicine, Mayo Clinic Rochester, Rochester, MN, USA

Anna Tumyan, MD Department of Internal Medicine, SIU School of Medicine, Division of Rheumatology, Springfield, IL, USA

Diana Vradii, MD Rheumatology Section, Boston University School of Medicine, Boston, MA, USA

Kenneth J. Warrington Division of Rheumatology, Mayo Clinic, Rochester, MN, USA

Amy M. Wasserman, MD Rheumatology Section, Boston University School of Medicine, Boston, MA, USA

Part I
Arthritis

Chapter 1
Rheumatoid Arthritis

Diana Vradii and Amy M. Wasserman

Abstract Rheumatoid arthritis is one of the most frequently diagnosed systemic inflammatory arthritis. Initial presentation and severity of disease may vary by individual. Here we present two clinical cases of rheumatoid arthritis.

Keywords Rheumatoid arthritis • Inflammatory arthritis • Inflammatory markers • Joint pain

Case 1

Our patient is a 43-year-old African-American woman who was referred to Rheumatology clinic for new-onset joint pain and swelling.

She initially presented with 4 weeks of pain and swelling in both wrists, hands, feet, and ankles. Patient described her pain as dull, constant with gradual worsening over a period of 4 weeks. She also noted profound fatigue and some weight loss. The patient reported having morning stiffness that lasted about 2 hours. She was unable to comfortably hold a cup of coffee or button her shirt. Due to swelling in both feet she had difficulty wearing shoes.

Past medical history: Hypertension, obesity, and hyperlipidemia.

Medications: Hydrochlorothiazide, aspirin daily and ibuprofen as needed.

Allergies: Metronidazole.

D. Vradii, M.D. (✉) • A.M. Wasserman, M.D.
Rheumatology Section, Boston University School of Medicine, 72 East Concord Street, Evans 501, Boston, MA 02118-2526, USA
e-mail: diana.vradii@bmc.org; amywass@bu.edu

M. Mahmoudi (ed.), *Challenging Cases in Rheumatology and Diseases of the Immune System*, DOI 10.1007/978-1-4614-5088-7_1,
© Springer Science+Business Media, LLC 2013

Family history: Mother has rheumatoid arthritis and brother with undefined joint pain.

Social history: She is single. Denied drinking alcohol, using illicit drugs, and a history of intravenous drug abuse. She admitted to smoking 2–3 cigarettes a day for 10 years. She uses an intrauterine device for contraception and works as an accountant.

Review of systems: She complained of fatigue, anorexia, weight loss, joint pain, and swelling. The patient denied symptoms of dry eyes or dry mouth. She had no rash, fever, or preceding infection prior to onset of joint symptoms. She denied discoloration of her fingers in response to cold or other symptoms concerning for Raynaud's phenomenon. No shortness of breath, chest pain, nausea, vomiting, or diarrhea. She has had no pregnancies or miscarriages. The rest of review of systems was unremarkable.

Physical examination: She was pleasant, and in no acute distress. Obese, with body mass index of 49. Vitals: BP: 162/92 mmHg, pulse: 98 beats per minute (regular), temperature 98.7°F, oxygen saturation 97% on room air. Head and neck: The examination showed no scleral lesions, ocular erythema, facial rash, alopecia, gouty tophi on pinnae, or lymphadenopathy. Cardiovascular system: Regular rate and rhythm, no murmurs, rubs, or gallops. Lung exam: Auscultation revealed clear breath sounds bilaterally. Abdomen: Obese, no hepatosplenomegaly. Musculoskeletal exam: There was synovitis and tenderness in 5th proximal interphalangeal joint (PIP) on the left, as well as tenderness and swelling in bilateral metacarpophalangeal joints (MCPs) and wrist joints. Range of motion was limited by pain. No tenderness or swelling in elbows or shoulders with full range of motion in these joints. No erythema was noted; however both wrists felt warm. No nodules, tophi, or deformities. Lower extremities with good range of motion in hips and knees. Bilateral knees were without swelling, deformities, warmth, or erythema. Popliteal fossa without fullness. Ankle exam revealed swelling posteroinferior to the medial malleolus and over the dorsum of midfoot. Flexion and extension were preserved, but painful. She had tenderness on palpation of metatarsophalangeal (MTP) joints bilaterally. Skin: No rash, nodules, or psoriatic plaques. Neurological: Normal sensation and strength; gait was antalgic.

The remainder of her examination was normal.

Impression: Inflammatory symmetric arthritis, associated with symptoms of morning stiffness, fatigue, anorexia, and weight loss.

Plan: She was advised to continue taking nonsteroidal anti-inflammatory medication and to follow up in 2 weeks after further workup was performed.

Data: *The* laboratory results are presented in Table 1.1

Chest X-ray imaging did not show hilar lymphadenopathy or acute cardiopulmonary process.

The radiographic imaging of both hands showed no evidence of joint space narrowing, periarticular osteopenia, or erosive changes (see Fig. 1.1).

Table 1.1 Laboratory data

Test	Patient value	Reference range
WBC (K/UL)	8.6	4.0–11.0
HGB (g/dL)	**11.5 L**	11.8–16
HCT (%)	**35 L**	36.0–37
MCV	94	80–97
Platelet (K/UL)	304	150–400
Albumin (g/dL)	**3.4 L**	3.5–5.0
ALT (U/GL)	25	9.0–67.0
AST (U/GL)	21	13–39
BUN (mg/dL)	15	7–25
Creatinine (mg/dL)	0.66	0.5–1.1
GFR	>60	>60
ESR (mm/h)	92	0–20
CRP Cardio (mg/dL)	**17.7 H**	0–5
Rheumatoid factor (IU/mL)	**262 H**	<30
HEP B surface AB	Nonreactive	Nonreactive
HEP B surface AG	Nonreactive	Nonreactive
HEP C antibody	Nonreactive	Nonreactive
CCP Ab (Units)	**>250 H**	0–20
Parvovirus B19 IgG	**5.18 H**	0.89
Parvovirus B19 IgM	0.09	0.89

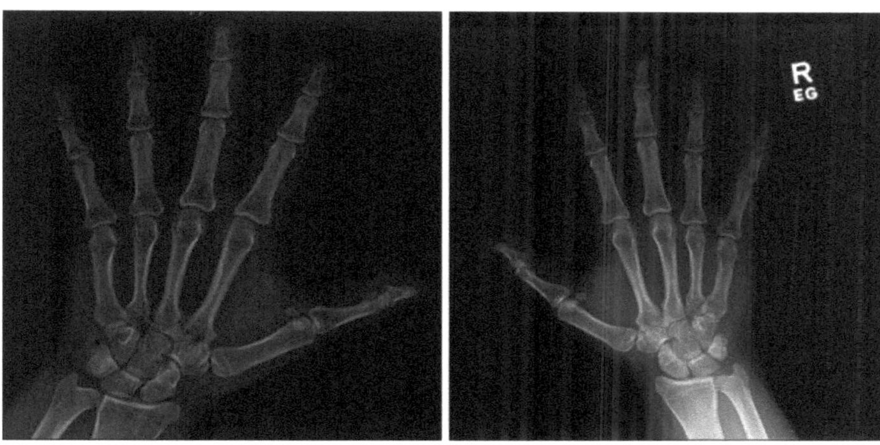

Fig. 1.1 The radiographic imaging of both hands showed no evidence of joint space narrowing, periarticular osteopenia, or erosive changes

With Presented Data What Is Your Diagnosis and Why?

42-year-old African-American woman presented with 4 weeks of symmetric polyarthralgias, joint swelling, anorexia, weight loss, and fatigue. She is found to have synovitis on exam, elevated inflammatory markers, and high-titer positive rheumatoid factor (RF) and anti-cyclic citrullinated (CCP) antibodies. She also has anemia and elevated Parvovirus IgG antibody titer.

Differential diagnosis

Parvovirus B19: This infection in adults can present as symmetric inflammatory polyarthritis resembling rheumatoid arthritis; however symptoms typically resolve in less than 6 weeks. This patient had exposure to parvovirus in the past, as evidenced by elevated IgG level, but no recent infection since IgM was negative.

Crystal arthropathy: Gout and pseudogout typically present with acute flares of joint swelling and pain that resolve over 1–2 weeks' time. This patient had longer duration of symptoms and she does not have typical risk factors of renal insufficiency, alcohol use, or diabetes.

Hepatitis B and C: Both hepatitis B and C infection can cause inflammatory arthritis. The immune complex associated with this chronic infection may result in a positive rheumatoid factor. This patient had nonreactive antibodies to hepatitis B and C.

Systemic lupus erythematosus (SLE): SLE may be distinguished from RA when associated systemic symptoms are present such as photosensitivity, malar or discoid rashes, oral ulcers, serositis, nephritis, or hematologic abnormalities. However, SLE with primarily articular involvement can easily be confused with RA. Antinuclear antibody (ANA) may be positive in patients with SLE or RA.

Palindromic rheumatism: This is another clinical syndrome that can mimic RA. Patients usually experience sudden attacks of inflammatory arthritis and in a distribution similar to RA that last for a number of days before remitting spontaneously.

Psoriatic arthritis: No skin or nail lesions suggestive of psoriasis were found on this patient.

Sarcoidosis: This patient's chest imaging did not suggest sarcoidosis. She did not have skin lesions consistent with erythema nodosum, which may be associated with sarcoidosis.

Seronegative spondyloarthropathy: This patient did not have inflammatory back symptoms, history of inflammatory bowel or inflammatory eye disease that may be associated with spondyloarthropathy.

Our patient had a unique presentation of early rheumatoid arthritis, with synovitis on exam, high-titer rheumatoid factor, anti-citrullinated peptide antibody (CCP), and elevated inflammatory markers.

Follow up Patient followed up 2 weeks after initial evaluation. During that time she was taking NSAIDS daily without much relief of symptoms. She continued to have swelling in both ankles, pain in wrists, ankles, and knees. At that time she was given low-dose prednisone and was started on methotrexate. 2 weeks later she presented to us with significant improvement in symptoms and decrease in inflammatory markers. 6 weeks later (or 14 weeks after initial presentation) patient was in complete clinical remission, with zero tender or swollen joints. She discontinued prednisone and continued on methotrexate monotherapy.

Case 2

30-year-old woman presented with joint pain in both hands, wrists, elbows, and ankles. She had been having intermittent symptoms over 3 years and had been taking ibuprofen with some relief of the symptoms. Six months prior to this presentation she reports having constant joint pain and swelling with impairment in function and daily activities. She also complained of fatigue and decreased appetite. On further questioning she had morning stiffness lasting about 2–3 hours. She denied rash, fevers, chest pain, oral ulcers, photophobia, eye pain, or vision changes.

Past medical history: She had no other medical conditions, denied having any drug or food allergies, and never had surgeries or hospital admissions.

Family history is significant for diabetes in mother, denied having first-degree relatives with rheumatoid arthritis, SLE, or other joint disease.

Social history: She is Hispanic, single, and has a 9-year-old healthy child. She denied smoking, drinking alcohol, or recreational drug use. She is not currently sexually active, however used to use Depo-Provera for contraception in the past.

On review of systems: She denied photosensitivity, eye pain, color changes in fingers and toes, mouth ulcers, dryness in eyes or mouth, chest pain, or difficulty breathing. She had mild epigastric discomfort with Ibuprofen, denied bleeding disorders, diarrhea, or constipation. No history of psoriasis, gout, or skin conditions. She denied night sweats, chills, or weight loss.

On physical exam she was well appearing, vital signs within normal limits. Head and neck exam: No butterfly rash, no mouth ulcers, no lymphadenopathy. Eye exam revealed erythematous injection of the conjunctiva bilaterally. Visual acuity testing showed intact vision and penlight examination revealed pupils equal, reactive to light and accommodation, no discharge. Cardiovascular and pulmonary examination was normal. Abdominal exam was positive for mild mid-epigastric tenderness. No hepatosplenomegaly. Musculoskeletal exam with swelling and tenderness in 4th and 5th MCP and PIP joints bilaterally, tenderness without swelling in 2nd, 3rd MCPs and PIPs bilaterally. Both wrist and elbow joints were tender to palpation with appreciable warmth. Shoulders without pain and had full

Table 1.2 Preliminary laboratory data

Test	Patient value	Reference range
WBC (K/UL)	6.3	4.0–11.0
HGB (g/dL)	**11.7 L**	11.8–16
HCT (%)	**35.5 L**	36.0–37
MCV	86	80–97
Platelet (K/UL)	262	150–400
ALT (U/GL)	20	9.0–67.0
AST (U/GL)	22	13–39
BUN (mg/dL)	10	7–25
Creatinine (mg/dL)	0.64	0.5–1.1
GFR	>60	>60
ESR (mm/h)	12	0–20
CRP cardio (mg/dL)	**29 H**	0–5
Rheumatoid factor (IU/mL)	**32 H**	<30
HEP B surface AB	Nonreactive	Nonreactive
HEP B surface AG	Nonreactive	Nonreactive
HEP C antibody	Nonreactive	Nonreactive

range of motion. Lower extremity exam showed no pain with range of motion in the hips, knees, and ankles. These joints were without effusions or warmth. She had tenderness on palpation of MTP joints with positive MTP squeeze test. Skin: No rash, psoriatic plaques, nodules, tophi. Neurologic examination showed normal strength and sensation. The remainder of her examination was normal. Preliminary laboratory data are presented in Table 1.2.

With Presented Data and Laboratory Findings What Is Your Working Diagnosis and Plan?

A 30-year-old woman who presented with 3 years of progressive joint symptoms, associated with morning stiffness and fatigue. She has inflammatory arthritis on exam and ocular findings. In addition, basic laboratory testing revealed mild anemia, elevated CRP and normal renal and liver function tests. This clinical presentation was highly suspicious for rheumatoid arthritis.

What Laboratory Studies Would Support Your Diagnosis of RA?

Active RA is associated with a variety of hematological abnormalities. Acute-phase responses such as elevated erythrocyte sedimentation rate, C-reactive protein, platelet count, and serum ferritin can be seen in many patients. Anemia of chronic disease may be present as well. Extra-articular manifestations of RA are

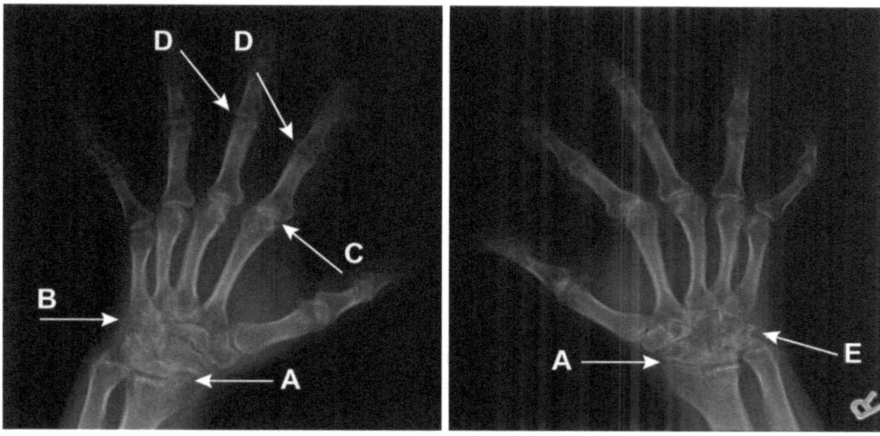

Fig. 1.2 X-rays of the hands in this case showed significant narrowing of the radiocarpal joints bilaterally (A), with narrowing of carpal (B) and metacarpal–phalangeal joints (C). Narrowing of the second and third PIP joints (D). Erosions seen within carpal bones (E). No evidence of subluxation

noted almost exclusively in seropositive RA patients, those with positive RF and/or CCP antibodies. Individuals with seropositive RA may also be at more risk for erosive disease.

Workup in our patient revealed mild anemia, normal renal and hepatic function, ESR 12 mm/h, CRP 29 mg/L, RF 32 IU/ml, and CCP>250. The remainder of the workup was normal which included Hepatitis B and C serology, HIV, SSA, SSB, and ANA antibodies. Her skin testing for latent tuberculosis was negative and baseline CXR was unrevealing. Radiological changes due to RA may appear within first years of disease in majority patients. Periarticular erosions are characteristic of RA; juxta-articular osteopenia and early joint space narrowing are less specific but may be present as well.

XRAYS of the hands are depicted in Fig. 1.2.

With Presented Data What Is Your Final Diagnosis?

This patient had a symmetric inflammatory arthritis associated with constitutional symptoms and ocular findings. She was found to have low positive RF, high positive anti-CCP antibody, and elevated inflammatory markers. She also had joint space narrowing and carpal bone erosions on radiographic imaging of her hands. Seropositive RA (those patients with positive RF and/or CCP) may have a worse prognosis, with greater possibility of erosive disease and extra-articular manifestations. Presence of radiological changes may indicate a longer untreated disease.

This patient has active seropositive erosive rheumatoid arthritis with possible extra-articular manifestations.

Follow-up: DAS28 is a quantitative measure of disease activity used to monitor the treatment of rheumatoid arthritis. This score is calculated using a formula that includes the number of tender and swollen joints (28 joints maximum) and ESR or CRP. Our patient was found to have high disease activity by her DAS28 score at initial visit. She was initially started on methotrexate and prednisone. She underwent workup and screening for TB, Hepatitis B and C, and had chest X-ray imaging. When she returned in 6 weeks she continued to have highly active disease and was started on a tumor necrosis factor (TNF) antagonist. On subsequent follow-up she was found to have improving symptoms and decrease in DAS28 score. Our patient was evaluated by Ophthalmology, and felt to have keratoconjunctivitis sicca consistent with secondary Sjogren's as an extra-articular manifestation of her RA.

Discussion

Rheumatoid arthritis is the most common inflammatory arthritis, with a lifetime prevalence of up to 1% worldwide. Onset can occur at any age, but peaks between 30 and 50 years. Use of tobacco, female gender, and family history of the disease are all risk factors for RA [1–3]. A patient with joint pain and with physical exam findings of synovitis should be evaluated for rheumatoid arthritis including testing for RF, anti-CCP antibodies, and inflammatory markers. Early diagnosis of rheumatoid arthritis is critical, so that appropriate treatment can be administered.

Pathophysiology

The pathogenesis of RA is multifactorial. 50% of risk for developing RA is attributed to genetic factors [4]. The first known genetic association in RA was HLA-DR4. Although infections may unmask an autoimmune response, no particular pathogen has been proven to cause RA. An external trigger (infection, trauma) that triggers an autoimmune reaction is theorized to lead to synovial hypertrophy and chronic joint inflammation [5]. Abnormal production of cytokines, chemokines, and other inflammatory mediators (TNF-alpha, IL-1, IL-6, TGF-beta, IL-8, and PDGF) leads to inflammation, exuberant proliferation of synovium (i.e., pannus), and destruction of cartilage, bone, tendons, ligaments, and blood vessels.

Workup and Diagnosis

The workup for RA starts with a detailed history and careful physical exam. Potentially useful laboratory studies include ESR, CRP, CBC, RF, ANA, and anti-CCP Ab. Diagnosis is made using a combination of clinical, laboratory, and imaging

Table 1.3 The 2010 ACR/EULAR classification criteria for Rheumatoid Arthritis. The 2010 ACR/EULAR classification criteria for RA [7]

Target population (who should be tested)	
Patients:	
Who have at least one joint with definite clinical synovitis (swelling)	
Whose synovitis is not better explained by other diseases (e.g., lupus, gout)	
If the above criteria fulfilled, continue to score for classification. A score of ≥6/10 is needed for definite diagnosis of RA	
	Score
A. Joint involvement	
1 large joint	0
2–10 large joints	1
1–3 small joints	2
4–10 small joint	3
>10 joints (at least 1 small joint)	5
B. Serology (at least one test result is needed for classification)	
Negative RF and negative ACPA	0
Low positive RF or low positive ACPA	2
High positive RF or high positive ACPA	3
C. Acute-phase reactants (at least one test result is needed)	
Normal ESR and normal CRP	0
Abnormal ESR or abnormal CRP	1
D. Duration of symptoms	
<6 weeks	0
≥6 weeks	1

features. The ESR and CRP level may be associated with disease activity. RF is not a specific test for RA, as it is also present in other connective tissue disorders, chronic infections, and seen in 1–5% of healthy people. Studies of anti-CCP antibodies suggest a sensitivity and specificity equal to or better than those of RF, especially in early RA [6]. Anti-CCP antibodies can be present for years before articular manifestations, and is highly specific for RA (97% specificity). This specificity makes anti-CCP antibodies useful in differentiating RA from other disorders with articular symptoms. Additionally, the presence of anti-CCP antibodies indicates a potentially more aggressive phenotype of RA.

In 2010, the American College of Rheumatology (ACR) and European League against Rheumatism (EULAR) collaborated to create new rheumatoid arthritis classification criteria to try to diagnose rheumatoid arthritis in earlier state [7]. The new criteria do not include the presence of rheumatoid nodules or radiographic erosive changes, both of which are less likely in early RA. Symmetric arthritis is also not required in the 2010 criteria, allowing for early asymmetric presentation.

According to 2010 ACR/EULAR criteria (see Table 1.3) our first patient had a score of 7 and our second patient had a score of 9, both of which are diagnostic for RA.

Clinical presentation in RA can vary. The second patient had long-standing disease associated with extra-articular manifestations, while the first case had an early presentation.

Extra-articular Manifestations

Although often thought of as a disease of the joints, RA can affect several organs and systems.

Cutaneous: Rheumatoid nodules are usually painless subcutaneous nodules that tend to occur on extensor surfaces and overpressure points. Vasculitic lesions may manifest as palpable purpura or skin ulcerations. In addition palmar erythema and pyoderma gangrenosum have been described.

Ocular: Sicca symptoms frequently accompany secondary Sjogren's syndrome in RA. Both episcleritis and scleritis can occur in patients with RA. If scleral inflammation persists, scleral thinning and scleromalacia perforans can occur. It is important to recognize that early ophthalmological evaluation can prevent irreversible damage.

Pulmonary: Interstitial fibrosis may occur in RA, which can be difficult to distinguish from methotrexate-induced lung disease. Interstitial lung disease may manifest as interstitial pulmonary fibrosis or cryptogenic organizing pneumonia. Rarely pleural effusions can be a first manifestation of RA. Effusions are usually exudative with high protein and very low glucose levels. Rheumatoid nodules in lungs can be solitary or multiple. Caplan's syndrome involves multiple rheumatoid nodules in coal miners.

Cardiac: Coronary artery disease is the leading cause of mortality in RA patients. Asymptomatic pericardial effusions are common. Myocarditis, coronary vasculitis, valvular disease, and conduction defects are occasionally seen.

Gastrointestinal: Hepatomegaly can occur in patients with Felty's syndrome (triad of RA, splenomegaly, and neutropenia).

Renal: Kidneys are usually not affected directly by RA. Secondary involvement due to medications or associated diseases (Sjogren's, renal tubule acidosis) can occur.

Neurologic: Carpal tunnel syndrome and mononeuritis multiplex are both manifestations reported in RA patients. Peripheral myopathy may rarely occur.

Safety Considerations

Prior to initiation of treatment with biologic agents (especially anti-TNF therapy), patients should be screened for latent tuberculosis infection. Hepatitis

B and C infections should be screened for as well. Once started on immunosuppressive therapy, patients should be regularly monitored for side effects and efficacy of medication. Patients with RA should be screened for risk factors for cardiovascular disease and osteoporosis and managed appropriately. According to Advisory Committee on Immunization Practices (ACIP) 2011 guidelines, patients who have primary or secondary altered immunocompetence may receive all inactivated vaccines [8]. Live, attenuated viral and bacterial vaccines are contraindicated in those who are significantly immunosuppressed (the ACIP specifically identified those who are receiving TNF alpha antagonists or prednisone ≥20 mg/day for greater than 2 weeks).

Treatment: Once diagnosis of RA is established, pharmacologic and non-pharmacologic therapies are available for treatment. Medication-based therapies include NSAIDs, corticosteroids, and disease-modifying antirheumatic drugs (DMARDs). Several recent guidelines have addressed the management of RA, but patient preferences also play a major role. The goals of therapy are to improve quality of life and control articular and extra-articular manifestations of the disease. NSAIDs and steroids are ideally used for short-term management. DMARDs are the mainstay therapy in RA. DMARDs can be divided into biologic and non-biologic DMARDs. Biologic agents include monoclonal antibodies and recombinant receptors to block cytokines that promote the inflammatory cascade responsible for RA symptoms. Methotrexate is recommended as the first-line treatment in all patients with active RA, unless contraindicated or not tolerated. Leflunomide may be used as an alternative to methotrexate, although gastrointestinal side effects can be greater. Sulfasalazine or Hydroxychloroquine are recommended as monotherapy in patients with low disease activity or without poor prognostic features (seronegative, nonerosive disease). Combination therapy with two DMARDs is more effective, but side effects may also be greater. If the disease is not well controlled with a non-biologic DMARD, then initiation of a biologic DMARD is indicated. TNF inhibitors have been the most studied of all the biologic DMARDs, and are suggested as first-choice biologic therapy. If a patient does not respond to anti-TNF therapy, additional biologic therapeutic options can be considered. Biologic agents are typically not used during active infections or malignancy.

Summary and conclusions: Rheumatoid arthritis is a systemic chronic inflammatory disease with hallmark features of symmetric polyarthritis. The presence of both anti-CCP antibodies and rheumatoid factor is highly specific for RA. Optimal care of patients with rheumatoid arthritis requires early treatment to control disease activity. In addition to consultation with a rheumatologist, involvement of other specialists may be needed if extra-articular manifestations are suspected. Clinical course of rheumatoid arthritis may comprise exacerbations and remissions. Approximately 40% of patients become disabled after 10 years, but outcomes are highly variable [7]. The overall life expectancy in patients with RA is slightly less than that of the general population. In those with severe extra-articular disease, such as rheumatoid vasculitis, the mortality rate is much greater. With the introduction of biologic therapy, earlier diagnosis, and treatment of RA, there is potential for improvement in long-term outcomes, including disability and mortality rates.

Questions

1. What joints of the hands are usually spared in Rheumatoid Arthritis?
   (a) DIP
   (b) PIP
   (c) MCP
   (d) Wrist
2. 55-year-old woman with rheumatoid arthritis on Methotrexate. She had Etanercept added to her regimen 1 year ago and low-dose prednisone started 6 months ago. She also takes folic acid supplement. Three weeks ago she is diagnosed with melanoma. She had surgical excision of the lesion with clear surgical margins. What is the most appropriate step in modifying her treatment regimen?
   (a) Start Hydroxychloroquine
   (b) Stop Etanercept
   (c) Do not make any changes
   (d) Stop all medications
3. What is the first choice of imaging in initial evaluation of a patient with suspected RA?
   (a) Ultrasound
   (b) PET CT
   (c) Plain X-rays
   (d) MRI
4. What is the first-line DMARD treatment recommended in RA (considering there are no contraindications)?
   (a) Leflunomide
   (b) Sulfasalazine
   (c) Methotrexate
   (d) Hydroxychloroquine
5. What laboratory value is usually NOT affected in RA?
   (a) CRP
   (b) Platelet number
   (c) ESR
   (d) Urine microalbumin
6. Which finding is NOT a component of Felty's syndrome?
   (a) Anemia
   (b) Thrombocytopenia
   (c) Leukopenia
   (d) Splenomegaly

7. Which eye manifestation is NOT commonly seen in Rheumatoid Arthritis?
   (a) Keratoconjunctivitis
   (b) Uveitis
   (c) Scleritis
   (d) Episcleritis
8. What is used to monitor RA disease activity in daily clinical practice?
   (a) Plain radiographs
   (b) MRI
   (c) DAS28
   (d) ACR70
9. Which extra-articular manifestation can occur in RA?
   (a) Scleritis
   (b) Palpable purpura
   (c) Interstitial pulmonary fibrosis
   (d) All of the above
10. What radiologic findings may be seen in RA?
   (a) Periarticular erosions
   (b) Osteopenia
   (c) Joint narrowing
   (d) All of the above

Correct answers: 1(a), 2(b), 3(c), 4(c), 5(d), 6(b), 7(b), 8(c), 9(d), 10(d).

References

1. Ahlmén M, Svensson B, Albertsson K, Forslind K, Hafström I. Influence of gender on assessments of disease activity and function in early rheumatoid arthritis in relation to radiographic joint damage. Ann Rheum Dis. 2010;69(1):230–3.
2. Areskoug-Josefsson K, Oberg U. A literature review of the sexual health of women with rheumatoid arthritis. Musculoskeletal Care. 2009;7(4):219–26.
3. Carlens C, Hergens MP, Grunewald J, Ekbom A, Eklund A, Hoglund CO, et al. Smoking, use of moist snuff, and risk of chronic inflammatory diseases. Am J Respir Crit Care Med. 2010;181(11):1217–22.
4. Orozco G, Barton A. Update on the genetic risk factors for rheumatoid arthritis. Expert Rev Clin Immunol. 2010;6:61–75.
5. Lipsky PE. Harrison's principles of internal medicine. In: Isselbacher KJ, Braunwald E, Fauci AS, et al., editors. Rheumatoid arthritis. 16th ed. New York, NY: McGraw-Hill; 2005. p. 1968–9.
6. Silveira IG, Burlingame RW, von Muhlen CA, Bender AL, Staub HL. Anti-CCP antibodies have more diagnostic impact than rheumatoid factor in a population tested for RF. Clin Rheumatol. 2007;26:1883–9.
7. Alehata D, Neogi T, Silman AJ, Funovits J, Felson DT, Bingham CO, et al. 2010 rheumatoid arthritis classification criteria: an American College of Rheumatology/European Union League Against Rheumatism collaborative initiative. Ann Rheum Dis. 2010;69:1580–8.
8. Mok CC, et al. Management of rheumatoid arthritis: consensus recommendations from the Hong Kong Society of Rheumatology. Clin Rheumatol. 2011;30(3):303–12.

Chapter 2
Osteoarthritis

David C. Caretto and Massoud Mahmoudi

Abstract Osteoarthritis is the most common musculoskeletal disease of joint dysfunction, which, with progression of disease, leads to loss of joint function and disability. The symptoms of osteoarthritis, specifically joint pain, are a common presenting complaint to primary care and rheumatology clinics. Osteoarthritis is a clinical diagnosis whose management requires a multidisciplinary approach to make use of the wide range of appropriate therapies. Here, we present two challenging cases of joint pain and osteoarthritis.

Keywords Osteoarthritis • Joint pain • Osteophytes • Inflammatory arthritis

Case 1

This patient is a 58-year-old African-American man with a history of peptic ulcer disease and gastrointestinal bleeding (GIB) who presents to arthritis clinic with progressive bilateral knee pain. He characterizes his pain as an ache, right greater then left, located in the joint, behind his kneecap, and worse at the end of the day or after

D.C. Caretto, M.D. (✉)
Department of Internal Medicine, University of California San Francisco,
San Francisco, CA, USA
e-mail: dccaretto@gmail.com

M. Mahmoudi, D.O., Ph.D., RM (NRM), FACOI, FAOCAI, FACP, FCCP, FAAAAI
Department of Medicine, Division of General Internal Medicine, University of California
San Francisco, San Francisco, CA, USA

Department of Medicine, San Francisco College of Osteopathic Medicine, Touro University,
Vallejo, CA, USA

School of Osteopathic Medicine, University of Medicine and Dentistry of New Jersey,
Stratford, NJ, USA
e-mail: allergycure@sbcglobal.net

M. Mahmoudi (ed.), *Challenging Cases in Rheumatology and Diseases of the Immune System*, DOI 10.1007/978-1-4614-5088-7_2,
© Springer Science+Business Media, LLC 2013

walking 50–100 ft. He reports that he feels his knee "popping" when he steps off curbs or going down stairs. He treats his pain with hydrocodone/acetaminophen (5/500 mg) tablets because nonsteroidal anti-inflammatory drugs (NSAIDs) are contraindicated due to his history of peptic ulcer disease complicated by GIB. He denies morning stiffness or locking of the joints. He denies acute swelling, redness, or pain. He denies constitutional symptoms or unexplained weight loss.

Of note, patient reports chronic right shoulder pain that has progressively worsened during the past 4–6 weeks. Patient states that he may have "overused his shoulder" when cleaning the house two months ago. He reports right shoulder weakness and pain when carrying objects. He reports a history of a right mid-clavicular fracture sustained in a fall 30 years ago.

Past medical history: Patient's past medical history is significant for peptic ulcer disease with a remote gastrointestinal (GI) bleed treated with partial gastrectomy 35 years ago, now with recent diagnosis of angioectasias on GI capsule study. He has chronic back pain secondary to L3–L4 disc herniation sustained 13 years ago during a fall. He had a laparoscopic hernia repair 3 years ago.

Medications/allergies: His medications include omeprazole 40 mg twice daily, lisinopril 40 mg daily, ferrous sulfate 325 mg twice daily, alendronate 70 mg once weekly, tramadol 50 mg three times daily, and hydrocodone/acetaminophen (5/500 mg) tablets, 1–2 tablets every 6 h for breakthrough pain. He has no known drug allergies.

Family history: There is no family history of osteoarthritis, rheumatoid arthritis, gout, or other immune-mediated diseases. Family history is significant for hypertension. There is no family history of coronary artery disease or diabetes mellitus.

Social and occupational history: The patient is married and lives with his wife and brother. He previously was a kitchen supervisor for the state prison system for many years, but is now disabled. He states that he only smoked cigarettes for one summer when he was 21, but has not smoked since. He has been sober from alcohol for 25 years. He last used inhaled cocaine over 25 years ago. He states that his ability to exercise is limited by his knee and back pain, but enjoys gardening and hiking a small stream near his house.

Review of systems: Patient reports occasional insomnia, decreased vision, and hearing loss over the past year. He reports occasional nocturia approximately 3×/week. He denies any fevers, chills, sweats, or unexplained weight loss. He denies morning stiffness, new myalgias, or arthralgias. He reports 3 days of diarrhea last week that has since resolved.

Physical exam: Vitals: Wt: 228 lbs, BMI: 33.7, Temp: 36.8, HR: 92 beats/min, RR 20 breaths/min, BP: 156/110 mmHg. He is a pleasant conversationalist in no apparent distress. His pupils are equal and reactive to light, extraocular movements are intact, moist mucus membranes, anicteric sclera, and normal cephalic, atraumatic head. His heart was regular rate and rhythm with no rubs, gallops, or murmurs. His pulses were equal and intact in all four extremities with no lower extremity edema. His lungs were clear to auscultation in all lung fields, with good inspiratory effort, and normal breath sounds. His abdomen was soft,

Table 2.1 Case 1 diagnostic studies

Test	Result	Reference range
Sodium	137	135–145 mEq/L
Potassium	4.1	3.5–5.0 mEq/L
Chloride	104	95–105 mEq/L
Bicarbonate	25	23–27 mmol/L
Calcium	8.7	8.5–10.5 mg/dL
Magnesium	2.2	1.7–2.3 mg/dL
BUN	24 H	8–22 mg/dL
Creatinine	Cr 1.1	0.4–1.2 mg/dL
White blood cell count	7.8	$4.0–10 \times 10^3/mm^3$
Hemoglobin	13.1 L	13.5–18 g/dL
Platelets	227	$150–400 \times 10^3/mm^3$
SPEP	Negative	3.3–19.4 mg/L
UPEP	Negative	0–5 mg/L

SPEP serum protein electrophoresis, *UPEP* urine protein electrophoresis
H denotes higher than normal and L denotes lower than normal values

non-tender, non-distended, with bowel sounds present. His neurological exam was within normal limits, except for his use of a cane when ambulating.

Examination of his right shoulder was significant for tenderness to palpation at the acromioclavicular joint and long head of biceps. Patient exhibited full range of motion, but reported pain with shoulder abduction. He had a positive right shoulder impingement sign. Both knees were cool without effusions, non-tender, with full active and passive range of motion present with mild crepitus on the right. The McMurray's test, anterior drawer, and Lachman tests were all negative. There was no midline joint tenderness or tenderness of the medial or lateral aspects of his right and left knees.

Diagnostic Studies

Our initial data are presented in Table 2.1.

An X-ray of bilateral acromioclavicular (AC) joint (Fig. 2.1) revealed mild right shoulder separation with degenerative changes.

With the Presented Data, What Is Your Working Diagnosis?

Impression

1. Subacute to chronic noninflammatory bilateral knee pain. The presenting symptoms could be secondary to malalignment, osteoarthritis, trauma, inflammatory disease, or systemic processes.
2. Chronic noninflammatory unilateral shoulder pain in the setting of a remote history of trauma.

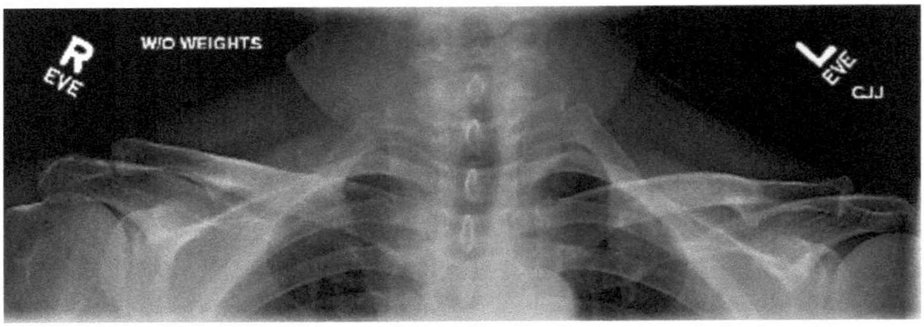

Fig. 2.1 Mild degenerative changes seen in right AC joint

Plan

Knee Pain: Bilateral knee X-rays with three views, including sunrise view, to evaluate for degenerative changes. Increase hydrocodone/acetaminophen dose for pain management given the inability to use NSAIDs to control inflammation due to history of GIB and angioectasias. Recommend weight reduction, referral to physical therapy for quadriceps, and gluteus medius-strengthening exercises. Right knee intra-articular injection of 20 mg corticosteroids.
Right AC joint osteoarthritis: Continue physical therapy for deltoid strengthening exercises. Refer patient to orthopedic surgery for shoulder replacement evaluation. Perform right AC joint intra-articular injection of 20 mg corticosteroids.

Differential Diagnosis

1. Osteoarthritis (OA): Chronic onset, characterized by morning stiffness that lasts less than 30 min, buckling with use, pain that worsens with use, and progressive loss of function. A clinical diagnosis, osteoarthritis is confirmed on X-ray with the presence of joint space narrowing and osteophytes.
2. Prepatellar Bursitis: Pain located at the front of the knee, associated with trauma, pressure, or kneeling. Also known as "housemaid's knee." Generally acute presentation, but can be chronic with repetitive irritation or inflammation of the knee bursa.
3. Patellofemoral syndrome: A diagnosis of exclusion, the pain in this condition is poorly localized to the anterior portion of the knee. Symptoms are exacerbated by prolonged sitting, such as driving long distances, running, or when ascending or descending stairs.
4. Rheumatoid arthritis (RA): Typically, the morning stiffness associated with RA lasts greater than 30 min and involves multiple joints in the peripheral skeleton. Warm, swollen, and tender joints characterize joint involvement in rheumatoid arthritis.
5. Hemochromotosis: First presentation of arthritis pain in hemochromotosis is localized to metacarpophalangeal joints (MCPs), but can also involve bilateral knees. This disease presents with a subacute to chronic duration with minimal inflammation and increased severity with age.

6. Calcium pyrophosphate dihydrate (CPPD) deposition disease: The knee is a commonly affected joint with bilateral involvement being a greater presentation vs. unilateral involvement. Symptoms are indistinguishable from osteoarthritis; however, the diagnosis is made by characteristic calcium deposition seen on X-rays.

Workup

Iron, Ferritin, Total Iron Binding Capacity (TIBC), Transferrin Saturation (Ferritin/TIBC), Erythrocyte Sedimentation Rate (ESR), C-reactive protein (CRP), Rheumatoid Factor, and Cyclic Citrullinated Peptide antibody (anti-CCP) tested and all were within normal limits.

A three-view X-ray of bilateral knees revealed bones that appeared normal with no acute abnormalities or significant osteoarthritic changes.

What Is Your Diagnosis and Why?

This is a 58-year-old man with subacute to chronic progression of bilateral knee pain, localized to the anterior knee compartments, worse with walking and stepping off curbs and associated with a "popping sensation" of his kneecap. He denies any signs of inflammation in his knees, previous trauma to his knees, or family history of osteoarthritis, gout, or rheumatoid arthritis.

1. Rheumatoid arthritis: Less likely due to lack of characteristic morning stiffness or inflammatory symptoms of the knee. There is no involvement of other classic joints such as the MCPs and the ankle. ESR and CRP serologies are normal and rheumatoid factor is negative.
2. Hemochromotosis: A diagnosis that should be considered in older men who present with arthritis symptoms, less likely in this patient due to no other findings suggestive of increase iron depositions (bronzing of skin, increased confusion, diabetes mellitus). His iron serologies are normal and his Ferritin/TIBC ratio is less than 45 %.
3. Prepateller Bursitis: Less likely due to lack of trauma to the anterior compartment of the knee or repetitive kneeling. Time course of presentation is not acute to suggest prepateller bursitis. There was no swelling or tenderness to palpation of patella on exam to suggest periarticular process.
4. CPPD deposition disease: Although the time of symptom onset and description of pain are suggestive of CPPD, his calcium crystal pyrophosphate levels are negative and there was no evidence of calcium deposition on X-ray.
5. Osteoarthritis: High pretest probability for osteoarthritis given the patient's age, his description of symptoms, the presence of crepitus on exam, and progressive

loss of function; however, given the lack of radiological findings on exam other diagnoses should be considered.

Review of the patient's clinical presentation, his history including the sensation of knee "popping" when stepping off curbs, diffuse "achy" pain localized behind his knee cap, and lack of joint space narrowing on X-ray make osteoarthritis less likely and suggest patellofemoral syndrome as an alternative explanation.

Since this patient's presentation in 2011, he has undergone additional imaging of his knees which show mild bilateral patellofemoral narrowing without evidence of degenerative changes. He has committed himself to a rigorous physical therapy routine to increase quadriceps bulk and strength and has noticed an improvement in the stability of his knees when walking and using stairs. He has not needed any further knee joint injections and has been able to decrease his quantity of pain medications. The resolution of his knee laxity and improvement in pain with these interventions confirm the initial diagnosis of patellofemoral syndrome.

Case 2

This is a 61-year-old Caucasian man who presents to primary care clinic with bilateral ankle pain, tenderness to touch of his ankles, and new left index, middle, and ring finger swelling. The patient explains that he has a history of mild chronic bilateral ankle pain, but that this pain has steadily worsened over the past 4–6 months. He reports that the first onset of left finger swelling is less than 3 months ago. He states that he awakens with morning stiffness that improves after 1 h, located in his hands and ankles. He characterizes his joint pain as an ache worse with movement and states that occasionally his ankles appear swollen. However, he has never awoken from sleep with tenderness or pain and denies involvement of his toes, knees, hips, back, shoulders, elbows, or wrists. He states that although the swelling in his fingers will wax and wane, his hand joints have never been red or warm.

Of note, he also reports chronic back stiffness in the morning that resolves after 30 min. He denies fever, chills, night sweats, or unexplained weight loss. Aside from these symptoms, he denies new myalgias, arthralgias, or rashes. He denies headache, changes in vision, eye pain, or eye redness. He denies nausea, vomiting, diarrhea, blood in his stool, or abdominal pain. He denies hematuria, dysuria, or flank pain.

Past medical history: Patient's past medical history is significant for an ascending thoracic aortic aneurysm diagnosed in 2003, and diagnosis of sick sinus syndrome with pacemaker placement in 2007. Additional medical comorbidities include hypertension and hyperlipidemia. His past surgical history includes a Nissen fundoplication in the 1960s to treat gastroesophageal reflux that was refractory to medical management.

Medications/Allergies: His medications include lisinopril 20 mg twice a day, metoprolol 100 mg twice a day, oxycodone 1–2 tabs prn moderate pain, rosuvastatin 20 mg daily, and aspirin 81 mg daily. He has allergies to penicillin which has given him hives, angioedema, and dyspnea.

Family history: His family history is significant for his paternal grandfather who died of myocardial infarction at age 55. His father has sustained three myocardial infarctions, his first at the age of 49. There is no family history of arthritis, rheumatoid arthritis, gout, psoriasis, Crohn's disease, ulcerative colitis, reactive arthritis, Graves' disease, or other autoimmune diseases.

Social and occupational history: This patient lives alone in a rural area near a lake located in the foothills of the Sierra Nevada mountain range. He works as a gold miner and this has been his occupation for 30 years. He is a former heavy smoker with approximately 50 pack-years. He is a former heavy drinker, but has abstained for 15 years. He denies drug use.

Review of Systems: His review of systems is as per history of present illness, no other significant complaints.

Physical exam: Vitals: Wt: 182.8 lbs, BMI: 27.0, Temp: 36.9, HR: 70 beats/min, RR 16 breaths/min, and BP: 144/88 mm Hg. He is a man older than the stated age in no apparent distress. He is alert and oriented with normal mood and affect. His pupils are equal and reactive to light, extraocular movements are intact, moist mucus membranes, anicteric sclera, and normal cephalic, atraumatic head. His heart was regular rate and rhythm with no rubs, gallops, or murmurs. His pulses were equal and intact in all four extremities with no lower extremity edema. His lungs were clear to auscultation in all lung fields, with good inspiratory effort, and normal breath sounds. His abdomen was soft, non-tender, non-distended, with bowel sounds present. His neurological exam was within normal limits and with normal gait. His skin exam exhibits dry skin on his bilateral hands.

His musculoskeletal exam was significant for mild synovitis of his third and fourth bilateral hand proximal interphalangeal joints (PIPs). Full range of active and passive motion, no evidence of tenderness or pain was present on exam. Regarding his bilateral ankles, his joints were cool with no evidence of swelling or tenderness, but pain with flexion, extension, eversion, and aversion full range of motion. The arches of patient's feet are flattened.

With the Presented Data, What Is Your Working Diagnosis?

This is a 61-year-old man with a history of subacute or chronic polyarthralgias involving bilateral ankles and PIPs of his bilateral hands. This patient's age, occupation as a miner, and fattened bases of his soles are suggestive of osteoarthritis; however the presence of morning stiffness that lasts for 1 h, moderate to severe tenderness of ankles on exam, and synovitis on exam are suggestive of inflammatory arthritis as likely explanation. Furthermore, his presentation is complicated by chronic low back pain, raising the possible diagnosis of spondyloarthropathy. Given his constellation of findings on history and exam, our initial working diagnosis is rheumatoid arthritis vs. reactive arthritis presenting with involvement of hands and ankles.

Differential Diagnosis

The differential includes inflammatory etiologies such as rheumatoid arthritis, gout, pseudogout/CPPD, reactive arthritis, psoriatic arthritis, and ankylosing spondylitis. Noninflammatory causes include osteoarthritis. Paraneoplastic syndromes should be considered in this age group, in addition to metabolic causes such as hyperparathyroidism and hemochromotosis.

Plan

Polyarthritis: Diagnostic management will include laboratory studies such as complete blood count (CBC), ESR, CRP, RF, CCP, complements C3 and C4, SPEP/UPEP, thyroid-stimulating hormone (TSH), parathyroid hormone (PTH), iron studies, and liver function tests. Radiological studies will include bilateral hand and ankle X-rays, and CT pelvis to evaluate the pelvic girdle. Treatment of patient's pain will include naproxen 375 mg twice a day with meals for active pain or inflammation.

Workup

Our initial data are presented in Table 2.2.

Bilateral hand X-rays revealed hook osteophytes and degenerative changes of the right 2 and 3 MCPs. Joint space narrowing and mild chondrocalcinosis at left fifth distal interphalangeal joint (DIP), no evidence of erosions (Fig. 2.2).

Bilateral X-ray of the ankles revealed mild joint space narrowing, but otherwise normal with no presence of osteophytes or enthesophytes.

The CT of pelvis revealed right-sided ilial irregularities and degenerative joint disease. Bridging osteophytes are present at the left sacroiliac (SI) joint (Fig. 2.3).

What Is Your Diagnosis and Why?

Rheumatoid arthritis: Patient's history of swelling and pain involving MCPs, PIPs, and ankles was initially concerning for RA; however, laboratory workup was negative for elevated white blood cell count, RF was negative, and other inflammatory serologies such as ESR and CRP were unremarkable. There were no characteristic erosions or swelling seen on X-ray and this patient's symptoms resolved with minimal intervention.

Table 2.2 Case 2 diagnostic studies

Test	Result	Reference range
Sodium	141	135–145 mEq/L
Potassium	3.9	3.5–5.0 mEq/L
Chloride	105	95–105 mEq/L
Bicarbonate	24	23–27 mmol/L
Calcium	9.7	8.5–10.5 mg/dL
Magnesium	1.9	1.7–2.3 mg/dL
BUN	17	8–22 mg/dL
Creatinine	1.2	0.4–1.2 mg/dL
White blood cell count	7.4	$4.0–10\times10^3/mm^3$
Hemoglobin	14.6	13.5–18 g/dL
Platelets	141	$150–400\times10^3/mm^3$
SPEP	Negative	3.3–19.4 mg/L
UPEP	Negative	0–5 mg/L
Iron	120	76–200 μg/dL
Ferritin	90	18–250 ng/mL
TIBC	350	262–474 μg/dL
Transferrin saturation	35 %	$x<45$ %
ESR	5	$x<30$ mm/h
C-reactive protein (CRP)	1	$x<6$ mg/L
Rheumatoid factor (RF)	0	$x<20$ U/mL
CCP antibody	0	$x<20$ IU
Complement C3	80	65–165 mg/dL
Complement C4	15	16–60 mg/dL
Antinuclear antibody (ANA)	1:40	$x>1:40$
HLA-B27	Negative	Positive or negative
TSH	1.21	0.3–3.0 mIU/L
PTH	20	10–55 pg/mL
Total bilirubin	0.4	0.3–1.9 mg/dL
AST	23	$x<40$ IU/L
ALT	21	$x<56$ IU/L
Alkaline phosphatase	29	30–120 IU/L
Albumin	3.9	3.5–5.3 g/dL

HLA-B27 human leukocyte antigen-B27, *AST* aspartate aminotransferase, *ALT* alanine aminotransferase

Gout: Gout typically presents in the first metatarsal, but can also involve knees and elbows. Tophi are typically present on knees and earlobes. Evaluation of synovial fluid is the gold standard for diagnosis. This patient has never presented with a large inflamed toe, denies waking up at night with pain, and denies family history or gout risk factors such as high-protein diet or alcohol consumption.

Pseudogout/CPPD: Pseudogout is another term for CPPD, an inflammatory arthropathy characterized by inflammation secondary to calcium deposition within joint spaces. Oftentimes it can overlap with a diagnosis of osteoarthritis. Less likely in setting of negative CCP and no evidence of calcium deposition on X-ray.

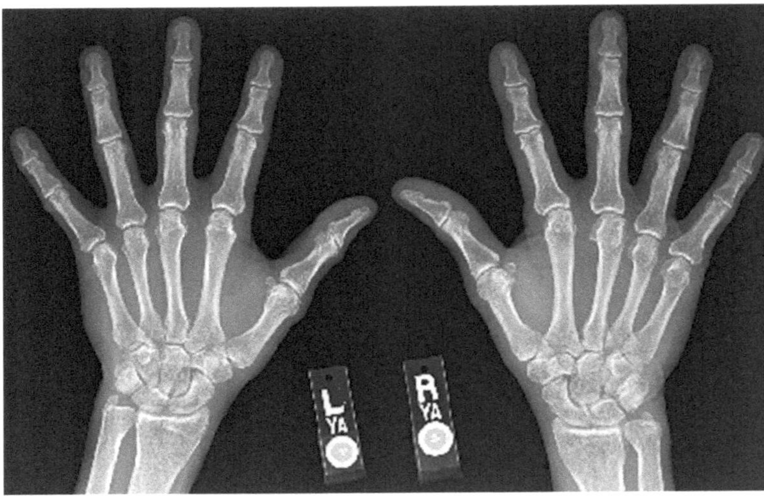

Fig. 2.2 Osteophytes (right second DIP, bilateral fifth DIPs), degenerative joint disease without the presence of erosions (right second, third, and fourth DIPs), and joint space narrowing (bilateral first MCPs and DIPs, bilateral fifth DIPs) are characteristics of osteoarthritis shown in these bilateral hand X-rays

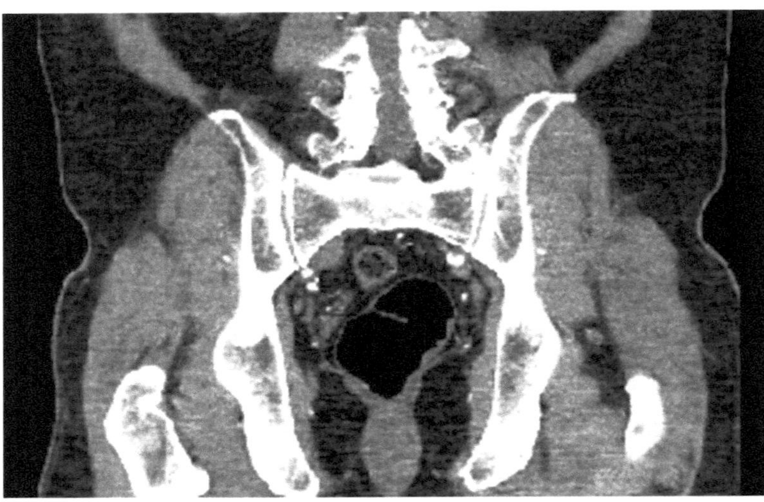

Fig. 2.3 Osteoarthritis of sacral iliac joint with asymmetric degenerative changes on the right side and bridging osteophytes on the left side

Spondyloarthropathy: Reactive arthritis, psoriatic arthritis, ankylosing spondylitis typically present with several features of lower back pain, peripheral arthritis, dactylitis (sausage digit finger), inflammatory bowel disease, conjunctivitis, and enthesitis (inflammation of Achilles or patellar tendons). While this patient exhibits chronic lower back pain and peripheral arthritis, his serologies and imaging are negative for any of the key findings for these diseases.

Paraneoplastic syndromes, *Hyperparathyroidism*, and *Hemochromotosis*: Arthritis can be a presenting symptom of these types of metabolic conditions. These conditions should be considered in patients who present with subacute and progressive symptoms. This patient's age and his 30-year history of occupational exposure are risk factors for these diseases, but his normal iron studies, normal PTH, and negative SPEP/UPEP indicate that metabolic etiologies are unlikely.

Osteoarthritis: Osteoarthritis is clinical diagnosis that is made based on the criteria that includes location of joint pain, age, ESR less than 20 mm/h, and crepitus. Radiographic evidence of osteophytes or joint space narrowing is helpful for supporting the diagnosis and characterizing the degree of joint space damage. However, it is important to consider inflammatory causes of arthritis since overlap between the two conditions can be observed. The diagnosis of osteoarthritis is supported in this patient with the joint space narrowing and osteophytes located in his hands, ankles, and left SI joint. His negative inflammatory serologies including RF, ANA, C3, C4, and HLA-B27 are reassuring that inflammatory arthritis is not complicating this picture.

This patient's presenting findings are suggestive of noninflammatory and inflammatory arthritis. His diagnosis of osteoarthritis can be explained by his age, his occupation of taxing physical labor for decades, and the presence of chondrocalcinosis; these factors all positively correlate with the development of osteoarthritis. Cool joints in the setting of mild joint swelling support this diagnosis. Furthermore, he responded to occasional intermittent NSAID use and his symptoms resolved with minimal intervention.

Discussion

Osteoarthritis is the most common joint disorder worldwide. This form of arthritis is characterized by the loss of joint cartilage, remodeling of involved bone within the joint, and eventual loss of joint function. As of 2005, there are approximately 25 million patients in the United States with osteoarthritis, a figure that is expected to increase to 60 million by 2020 [1].

The pattern of joint involvement in osteoarthritis can be categorized into idiopathic and secondary forms. Idiopathic osteoarthritis can be further divided into localized and generalized distributions. Localized osteoarthritis predominately affects knees, hips, spine, and hands. Less common sites involve the feet, ankles, shoulder, and temporomandibular joints. Generalized osteoarthritis is defined as arthritis involving three or more joint sites. Increased age, female gender, obesity, occupations with high physical labor, and sports with repetitive high-impact exercise are associated with the development of osteoarthritis [2–4]. Secondary osteoarthritis is classified according to specific risk factors or comorbidities that are known to promote osteoarthritis. Previous joint trauma or injury, proprioceptive deficits, or medical conditions such as gout, pseudogout/CPPD, rheumatoid arthritis, and Paget's disease are associated with secondary arthritis [5]. Etiologies for secondary osteoarthritis are shown in Table 2.3.

Table 2.3 Causes of secondary osteoarthritis

Endocrine/metabolic	Inflammatory	Musculoskeletal
Acromegaly	CPPD	Amyloidosis
Diabetes mellitus	Gout	Congenital deformities
Hemochromatosis	Psoriatic arthritis	Connective tissue disease
Hyperparathyroidism	Reactive arthritis	Developmental deformities
Hypothyroidism	Rheumatoid arthritis	Joint trauma/injury
Paget's disease	Septic arthritis	Neuropathy (Charcot joint)
Wilson's disease	Spondyloarthropathies	Osteonecrosis

Pathophysiology

Previously thought to be a disease of advanced age, osteoarthritis is now viewed as a result from abnormal molecular remodeling processes as a reaction to mechanical stress and subsequent inflammation in affected joints [6]. In healthy joints, cartilage is composed of type II collagen, water, and proteoglycans. Chondrocytes continually replace and remodel this composition to maintain the extracellular matrix of healthy cartilage.

The molecular steps leading to osteoarthritis involve increased chondrocyte proliferation and production of extracellular matrix proteins within the joint space as a response to aging and mechanical force [7]. These changes lead to increased catabolic activity and inflammation within the extracellular matrix. This change leads to an imbalance between biochemical, inflammatory, and extracellular matrix repair processes within the joint, culminating in increased catabolic activity that propagates joint space cartilage damage [6–8]. Over time, this abnormal repair process between cartilage remodeling and destruction leads to the clinical features of osteoarthritis.

Clinical Features

Pain is the main presenting symptom of osteoarthritis and the primary reason for patients to seek care with their primary care physician or rheumatologist. This pain is mild to moderate in early stages of the disease and easily treated. As the disease progresses, the pain in affected joints worsens in frequency and severity. Exacerbating factors include pain that is worse with use, improves with rest, and is worse with walking, standing, or with stairs. Other symptoms include morning stiffness that lasts less than 30 min and stiffness after rest or inactivity [8]. In later stages of osteoarthritis, patients report increased instability or buckling when using affected joints. Severe disease is characterized by pain at rest or nocturnal pain [8].

On physical exam, bony enlargement of affected joints, limited range of motion, effusions, and crepitus are signs consistent with osteoarthritis [5, 8]. These signs indicate disruption of articular surfaces, the presence of periarticular inflammation, and osteophyte formation. Patients with moderate to severe knee osteoarthritis commonly have crepitus on exam. Hand osteoarthritis is another common location, resulting in pain and limited motion. Bony enlargements known as Heberden's and Bouchard's nodes are often found at the distal and proximal interphalangeal joints, respectively. Hip osteoarthritis is characterized by pain and limitation of motion. The pain in hip osteoarthritis can radiate to the inguinal region, lumbar spine, or knee.

The primary role in evaluating a patient's first presentation of joint pain is to distinguish between noninflammatory and inflammatory etiologies (Table 2.4). The presence or absence of these findings on history and examination will be helpful in guiding the diagnostic workup.

Workup

Osteoarthritis is a clinical diagnosis based on history and physical exam. In general, individual signs and symptoms have poor sensitivity and specificity for osteoarthritis, but the likelihood of this diagnosis increases when patients present with multiple findings. Although laboratory results in patients with osteoarthritis are usually normal, the goal of the workup is to rule out causes of secondary osteoarthritis and to provide a baseline for future treatment.

These labs would include calcium, phosphorus, magnesium, and TSH to screen for endocrine or metabolic contributions. Creatinine, potassium, and hemoglobin are assessed prior to starting treatment with nonsteriodal anti-inflammatory drugs (NSAIDs). Inflammatory markers such as ESR, CRP, and Rheumatoid Factor (RF) are considered if patient has signs and symptoms of inflammatory arthritis. Synovial fluid analysis is indicated when the patient presents with acute onset of pain or a joint exam that is consistent with an inflammatory process. In osteoarthritis, synovial WBC is less than 2,000 mm^{-3} (normal: $x<2,000$ mm^{-3}) on synovial fluid analysis [5].

X-rays of affected joints are helpful in confirming a diagnosis of osteoarthritis. It is equally important to consider that there is no correlation between severity of radiographic findings and the amount of pain or disability. Characteristic findings are osteophyte formation at the joint margin, asymmetric joint space narrowing decreasing this distance between bones, and occasionally periarticular soft tissue swelling. Bony erosions, not observed in osteoarthritis, are typically associated in rheumatoid arthritis or gout (Table 2.4).

Table 2.4 Inflammatory arthritis vs. osteoarthritis

Features	Inflammatory arthritis	Osteoarthritis
Joint distribution	Hands: MCPs, wrists Axial spine Ankles	Hands: PIPs, DIPs Shoulders and hips Knees
Symptoms	Morning stiffness >30 min Better with use Pain at night	Morning stiffness <30min Worse with use Pain is generally isolated symptom
Joint exam	Warm joint Effusions and/or swelling Tenderness to ROM Multiple joint involvement	Cool joint Bouchard's nodes (PIPs) Heberden's nodes (DIPs) Tenderness to palpation Crepitus Bony prominences
Laboratory findings	RF positive; anti-CPP positive Elevated ESR/CRP Inflammatory synovial fluid (WBC>2,000 cell/cc)	RF negative, anti-CPP negative Normal ESR/CRP Noninflammatory synovial fluid (WBC<2,000 cell/cc)
Radiographic findings	Erosions Soft tissue swelling Uniform joint space narrowing Joint malalignment	No erosions Asymmetrical joint space narrowing Osteophytes

Management/Treatment

Osteoarthritis management requires a continuum of four approaches: patient education and lifestyle changes, physical therapy and muscle strengthening, pharmacological management, and surgical replacement of the joint. The goals of multidisciplinary strategy are to improve symptoms, to maintain joint function, to prevent disability, and to limit potential side effects of therapies. For these reasons, non-pharmacologic therapies are considered a central component and first-line treatment for osteoarthritis [5, 9].

The non-pharmacologic approach begins with patient education about osteoarthritis and strategies to relieve pain and stiffness. This can be accomplished by providing videos, pamphlets, and newsletters from national voluntary health organizations such as the Arthritis Foundation (www.arthritis.org). Patient should be referred to physical therapy for muscle strengthening exercises and development of a fitness program. For instance, in patients with knee osteoarthritis, the beneficial effects of both quadriceps strengthening and aerobic exercise were confirmed in the Fitness Arthritis and Seniors Trial [10]. Aquatic aerobics is one option for patients to undertake moderate non-weight-bearing exercise. The Arthritis Foundation is a valuable resource for linking patients with local disease support groups, self-management programs, and aquatic exercise centers.

Treatment with acetaminophen, a non-opioid analgesic, is considered first-line therapy for osteoarthritic pain. Acetaminophen has been shown to be superior to placebo, but less efficacious than NSAIDs; however, its favorable side-effect profile

Table 2.5 Contraindications to use of nonsteroidal anti-inflammatory drugs (NSAIDs)

Age>65
History of gastrointestinal bleeding
History of peptic ulcer disease
Glucocorticoid use
Warfarin use
Patients with renal disease, congestive heart failure, or cirrhosis

makes acetaminophen the ideal initial medication for osteoarthritis pain [9]. Patients may take up to 4 g/day, but in patients with liver disease or significant alcohol use this dose is limited to 2 g/day. For pain, refractory to acetaminophen, NSAIDs such as ibuprofen or naproxen are appropriate next therapies. Prior to their use, patients should be assessed for GIB risk factors or renal insufficiency (Table 2.5). Selective COX-2 inhibitors, such as celecoxib and etoricoxib, are superior to NSAIDs, but are contraindicated for treatment of osteoarthritis pain due to significant cardiac event risk.

Opioids, such as oxycodone and codeine, are unacceptable for long-term management of osteoarthritis pain due to the risks of tolerance and dependency. Tramadol, a centrally acting analgesic with lower potential for dependency can be used to treat moderate-to-severe pain in patients who have contraindications to NSAIDs including impaired renal function, or in patients who have not responded to previous oral therapy. Tramadol can be dosed at 50 mg orally every 4 h, with an upper limit of 300 mg/day.

Intra-articular glucocorticoid injections can be considered in patients with joint effusions and moderate pain that limit function. Additionally, glucocorticoid injections can be used in addition to systemic therapy or in patients whom NSAIDS are contraindicated. Patients receiving glucocorticoid injections for knee osteoarthritis are twice as likely as controls to have short-term improvement for 4–12 weeks [2, 11]. Intra-articular hyaluronic acid injections provide supplementation of macromolecules important for cartilage maintenance. This intervention may have a benefit on 60 % of patients when compared with intra-articular placebo injections or oral NSAID therapy [2, 8].

Patients with severe symptomatic osteoarthritis characterized by pain that has failed to respond to medical therapy and who have progressive limitation in activities of daily living should be evaluated by orthopedics for potential surgical intervention. Successful outcomes depend upon the chronicity of patient's osteoarthritis, the experience of the surgeon performing procedures, and the patient's preoperative comorbidities, perioperative management, and postoperative rehabilitation.

Alternative therapies for osteoarthritis include glucosamine and chondroitin. Recent studies have shown that there is no difference in symptom improvement compared to placebo and little clinical benefit in using these supplements [12].

Summary and Conclusion

Osteoarthritis is the most common musculoskeletal condition worldwide. Symptoms such as joint pain and joint stiffness can mimic a multitude of other musculoskeletal diseases and can range from mild to severe. Appropriate medical management requires that physicians be able to diagnose osteoarthritis early, recognize factors that may affect the prognosis or complicate the disease, and make effective use of the many available treatments. A multidisciplinary approach is necessary to limit progression of disease, to maintain joint function, and to prevent further disability.

Questions

1. What is the strongest modified risk factor for the development of osteoarthritis?
   (a) Occupation
   (b) Physical activity
   (c) Obesity
   (d) Quadriceps strength
   (e) Tobacco use
2. Alternations in this cell's physiology are primary responsible for initiating a cascade of biochemical, inflammatory, and remodeling processes that lead to osteoarthritis:
   (a) Synovial fibroblasts
   (b) Synovial macrophages
   (c) Osteoclasts
   (d) Osteoblasts
   (e) Chondrocytes
3. Which is the most common physical exam finding in osteoarthritis?
   (a) Joint laxity
   (b) Crepitus
   (c) Pain with passive range of motion
   (d) Malalignment
   (e) Joint stiffness with rest
4. What is not present when evaluating for inflammatory arthritis?
   (a) Warm, tender joints with effusions
   (b) Acute onset of pain
   (c) Positive rheumatoid factor
   (d) Unilateral distribution of joint pain
   (e) Erosions on X-rays

5. A common clinical presentation for osteoarthritis is:

   (a) Joint stiffness that worsens with rest, morning stiffness for less than 60 min, located in bilateral knees.
   (b) Joint pain that improves with rest, morning stiffness for less than 30 min, located in one knee.
   (c) Joint pain that improves with rest, morning stiffness for less than 30 min, located in one wrist.
   (d) Joint pain that worsens with activity, morning stiffness for less than 60 min, located in bilateral ankles.
   (e) Joint pain that improves with activity, morning stiffness for less than 30 min, located in bilateral ankles.

6. What labs would be appropriate for an initial workup of osteoarthritis?

   (a) Calcium, TSH, Creatinine, Potassium, Hemoglobin
   (b) Calcium, TSH, Creatinine, Potassium, Hemoglobin, Rheumatoid Factor
   (c) TSH, Potassium, Hemoglobin, Rheumatoid Factor, ESR/CRP
   (d) Calcium, Potassium, Hemoglobin, Rheumatoid Factor, WBC
   (e) Calcium, TSH, Creatinine, Potassium, Platelets

7. Which of these are not seen on X-rays for osteoarthritis?

   (a) Joint space narrowing
   (b) Subchondral sclerosis
   (c) Subchondral cysts
   (d) Erosions
   (e) Osteophytes

8. Which of the following is considered the differential diagnosis list for first presentation of joint pain?

   (a) Septic arthritis
   (b) Patellofemoral syndrome
   (c) Prepateller bursitis
   (d) Gout
   (e) All of the above

9. What is an appropriate medication for pain management in osteoarthritis?

   (a) Oxycodone
   (b) Toradol
   (c) Tramadol
   (d) Celebrex
   (e) Vicodin

10. All of the following are management recommendations for osteoarthritis except:

   (a) Attempt non-pharmacologic interventions prior to initiating NSAIDs
   (b) Correlate pain with findings on X-rays

(c) Use acetaminophen for breakthrough pain
(d) Consider synovial fluid analysis in patients with effusions and acute pain
(e) Assess for GI risk factors and renal insufficiency prior to starting therapy with NSAIDs.

Answers: 1(c), 2(e), 3(b), 4(d), 5(b), 6(a), 7(d), 8(e), 9(c), 10(b).

References

1. Lawrence RC, Helmick CG, Arnett FC, Deyo RA, Felson DT, Giannini EH, Heyse SP, Hirsch R, Hochberg MC, Hunder GG, Liang MH, Pillemer SR, Steen VD, Wolfe F. Estimates of the prevalence of arthritis and selected musculoskeletal disorders in the United States. Arthritis Rheum. 1998;41(5):778–99.
2. Sinusas K. Osteoarthritis: diagnosis and treatment. Am Fam Physician. 2012;85(1):49–56.
3. Klussmann A, Gebhardt H, Nübling M, Liebers F, Quirós Perea E, Cordier W, von Engelhardt LV, Schubert M, Dávid A, Bouillon B, Rieger MA. Individual and occupational risk factors for knee osteoarthritis: results of a case-control study in Germany. Arthritis Res Ther. 2010;12(3):R88.
4. Buckwalter JA, Martin JA. Sports and osteoarthritis. Curr Opin Rheumatol. 2004; 16(5):634–9.
5. Hunter DJ, Lo GH. The management of osteoarthritis: an overview and call to appropriate conservative treatment. Med Clin North Am. 2009;93(1):127–43. xi.
6. Kapoor M, Martel-Pelletier J, Lajeunesse D, Pelletier JP, Fahmi H. Role of proinflammatory cytokines in the pathophysiology of osteoarthritis. Nat Rev Rheumatol. 2011;7(1):33–42.
7. Goldring MB, Goldring SR. Articular cartilage and subchondral bone in the pathogenesis of osteoarthritis. Ann N Y Acad Sci. 2010;1192:230–7.
8. Manek NJ, Lane NE. Osteoarthritis: current concepts in diagnosis and management. Am Fam Physician. 2000;61(6):1795–804.
9. Hochberg MC, Altman RD, April KT, Benkhalti M, Guyatt G, McGowan J, Towheed T, Welch V, Wells G, Tugwell P. American College of Rheumatology 2012 recommendations for the use of nonpharmacologic and pharmacologic therapies in osteoarthritis of the hand, hip, and knee. Arthritis Care Res. 2012;64(4):455–74.
10. Ettinger Jr WH, Burns R, Messier SP, Applegate W, Rejeski WJ, Morgan T, Shumaker S, Berry MJ, O'Toole M, Monu J, Craven T. A randomized trial comparing aerobic exercise and resistance exercise with a health education program in older adults with knee osteoarthritis. The Fitness Arthritis and Seniors Trial (FAST). JAMA. 1997;277(1):25–31.
11. Arroll B, Goodyear-Smith F. Corticosteroid injections for osteoarthritis of the knee: meta-analysis. BMJ. 2004;328(7444):869.
12. Wandel S, Jüni P, Tendal B, Nüesch E, Villiger PM, Welton NJ, Reichenbach S, Trelle S. Effects of glucosamine, chondroitin, or placebo in patients with osteoarthritis of hip or knee: network meta-analysis. BMJ. 2010;16:341.

Chapter 3
Gout

Pim Jetanalin and Susan J. Lee

Abstract Gout has been recognized for centuries and is currently the most common inflammatory arthritis in men, affecting approximately eight million adults in the United States (Zhu et al. Arthritis Rheum 63(10):3136–41, 2011). Gout is a multifactorial disease characterized by hyperuricemia and monosodium urate monohydrate crystal deposition in the joint and soft tissue. Classically, gout presents as recurrent, acute, monoarticular, or oligoarticular arthritis. The prevalence of gout has increased markedly in the United States in the last two decades due to increased prevalence of associated co-morbidities and longevity. Several new treatments for both acute and chronic gout have been developed in the past decade and they will be reviewed in this chapter using two challenging gout cases.

Keywords Gout treatment • Purine metabolism • Uric acid

Case 1

A 20-year-old male is referred to rheumatology clinic for management of chronic, recurrent gout. His first symptoms started at the age of 13 with severe pain and swelling in his right big toe. Throughout the years, he continued to have intermittent

P. Jetanalin, M.D. (✉)
Department of Rheumatology, University of California, San Diego,
9500 Gilman Drive mailcode 0656, La Jolla, CA 92093, USA
e-mail: pimlin@gmail.com

S.J. Lee, M.D.
Department of Rheumatology, University of California, San Diego,
9500 Gilman Drive mailcode 0656, La Jolla, CA 92093, USA

San Diego Veterans Affairs Medical Center,
La Jolla, CA, USA

M. Mahmoudi (ed.), *Challenging Cases in Rheumatology and Diseases of the Immune System*, DOI 10.1007/978-1-4614-5088-7_3,
© Springer Science+Business Media, LLC 2013

Table 3.1 Laboratory data

Test	Value	Reference range
BUN	25	6–20 mg/dL
Creatinine	1.27	0.51–0.95 mg/dL
Uric acid (current)	7.9	3.4–7.0 mg/dL
(peak and nadir)	16 and 7.4	
AST	34	0–40 U/L
ALT	38	0–41 U/L
Cholesterol	237	0–199 mg/dL
Triglycerides	167	10–170 mg/dL
LDL	193	<160 mg/dL
HDL	45	mg/dL
WBC	7.4	4.0-10.0 × 1,000/mm3 and 140-370 × 1,000/mm^3
Hemoglobin	13.9	13.7–17.5 g/dL
Hematocrit	39.5	40.0–50.0%
Platelet count	276	140–370 1,000/mm^3
Urinalysis	Clear, trace protein, 0–2 WBC, 0–2 RBC, rare bacteria/HPF	Clear, negative protein, 0–2 WBC, 0–2 RBC, none-rare bacteria/HPF

joint pain and swelling in various joints, including his knees, elbows, and fingers. His serum urate level was elevated at 15 mg/dL and knee arthrocentesis revealed negatively birefringent monosodium urate (MSU) crystals. Patient was started on allopurinol, nonsteroidal anti-inflammatory agents, and colchicine but continued to have gout attacks every month, each lasting approximately 2 weeks. His last attack was 2 weeks ago and currently denies any pain. He has been trying to lose weight with exercise but continues to eat red meat and shellfish twice a week. He denies ingesting organ meats and use of alcohol.

His past medical history is significant for obesity, hyperlipidemia, and nephrolithiasis. His family history is notable for chronic kidney disease and early-onset gout (before the age of 20) in his paternal grandmother, father, and older sister. He is a construction worker and smokes ½ pack per day for the past 5 years. He denies use of intravenous drugs.

His current medications are atorvastatin 40 mg daily, allopurinol 600 mg daily, colchicine 0.6 mg twice daily, indomethacin 50 mg as needed, and oxycodone/acetaminophen as needed for pain. He also uses intermittent prednisone taper with last use 3 months ago.

On physical examination, his vital signs are normal. He is obese with a body mass index (BMI) of 30. HEENT examination is unremarkable with clear conjunctiva, moist oral mucosa, and no lymphadenopathy. Lungs are clear to auscultation. His heart rate and rhythm are regular. No rub, gallop, or murmur is noted. Abdomen is obese but soft, nontender, with normo-active bowel sounds. No hepatosplenomegaly. Extremities show no pitting edema. Skin exam is normal with no tophi or psoriasis. Musculoskeletal examination is notable 10° flexion contracture of the right elbow but no active synovitis. Neurological exam is non-focal. The laboratory data are presented in Table 3.1.

With the Presented Data, What Is Your Working Diagnosis?

Patient's clinical history is consistent with gout, confirmed by the presence of MSU crystals in the synovial fluid. However, he continues to have hyperuricemia and frequent gout attacks despite 600 mg of allopurinol daily. It is unknown whether he is a uric acid overproducer or underexcretor but his relatively early onset of gout, history of nephrolithiasis, and strong family history of early-onset gout should raise suspicion for secondary causes of gout such as inborn errors of purine metabolism. His preserved renal function makes it unlikely that he is a urate underexcretor.

Differential Diagnosis (Table 3.2)

Given his preserved renal function, the differential diagnosis should focus on causes of uric acid overproduction. He continues to have significant purine intake in his diet (e.g., red meat, shellfish) further contributing to his hyperuricemia.

Table 3.2 Underlying etiologies of hyperuricemia and gout

Primary hyperuricemia
Uric acid overproduction
Uric acid underexcretion
Secondary hyperuricemia with normal uric acid synthesis but decreased uric acid excretion
HTN
Metabolic syndrome
Chronic kidney disease
Volume depletion
Acidosis
Medications: Thiazides, loop diuretics, low-dose salicylates, niacin, and pyrazinamide
Lead intoxication
Analgesic nephropathy
Polycystic kidney disease
Other familial interstitial nephropathies (i.e., uromodulin-associated disease)
Endocrinopathies (i.e., hyperparathyroidism, hypothyroidism)
Secondary hyperuricemia with increased uric acid synthesis and excretion
Purine over-ingestion
Increased ATP catabolism (i.e., ethanol, tissue ischemia)
Psoriasis
Paget's disease of bone
Hematologic and neoplastic diseases with increased cell turnover
Drugs: Cytotoxic chemotherapy
Rare genetic/metabolic diseases, i.e., PRSs overactivity, deficiency, Gluocse-5-phosphate dehydrogenase deficiency (Von Gierke disease), uromodulin-associated disease

Modified from Terkeltaub R. (2012) Gout and other crystal arthropathies, 1st edition. Philadelphia: Elsevier

PRSs phosphoribosyl pyrophosphate synthetase superactivity, *HPRT deficiency* hypoxanthine–guanine phosphoribosyltransferase

Workup

The workup should focus on secondary causes of hyperuricemia from increased uric acid synthesis. Patient denies alcohol or cytotoxic chemotherapy intake. The skin exam did not reveal any psoriasis or clinical evidence of Paget's disease. His initial labs were unremarkable making underlying hematologic or neoplastic disease unlikely. This leaves purine over-ingestion and/or rare genetic disorder as the likelihood of his underlying hyperuricemia and persistent gout.

1. Calculate Fraction excretion of uric acid (FEua, normal >6%): FEua for this patient = (urine uric acid/plasma uric acid) x (plasma Cr/urine Cr) = 3.4%. FEua may not be accurate when a patient is taking a urate-lowering agent such as allopurinol. Therefore, the patient should be instructed to hold his medication 1 week before the test. Clinicians should be aware that this may precipitate an acute gout attack and may consider initiating prophylactic therapy with colchicine or NSAIDs based on their renal function.
2. Measure 24-h urine uric acid during purine-restricted diet of 1 g purine/kg protein (normal <800 mg/day): 24-h urine uric acid for this patient = 1,265 mg/dL. This test should ideally be performed while on purine-restricted diet. In case of non-purine-restricted diet, this test should be repeated on purine-restricted diet and if the level remains above 670 mg, it suggests hyperuricemia related to underlying metabolic/genetic disorders.
3. Consider renal ultrasound for patients with suspected uromodulin-associated kidney disease (UMOD), particularly medullary cystic kidney disease type 2 (MCKD2). Patient's renal ultrasound was unremarkable with no renal cysts.
4. Consider kidney biopsy in patients with kidney insufficiency to rule out other causes of kidney disease. This was not performed in this patient, as his kidney function was relatively preserved.
5. Consider enzymatic and genetic test for hypoxanthine–guanine phosphoribosyltransferase (HPRT) deficiency and phosphoribosylpyrophosphate synthetase (PRS) superactivity. It is important to counsel the patient about the benefits and drawbacks of genetic testing, allowing them to decide whether he/she wants to pursue the test.

What Is Your Diagnosis and Why?

Final diagnosis for this patient is uromodulin-associated kidney disease. Because there are multiple other family members, including his grandmother, father, and sister suffering from gout, this is unlikely to be an X-linked disorder such as HPRT deficiency. The patient does not have hepatosplenomegaly, recurrent infections, muscle weakness, and/or hypoglycemia, which may be suggestive of underlying glycogen storage disease. Genetic test for uromodulin gene mutation would confirm the diagnosis but our patient refused genetic test. See "Discussion" section below for full explanation. Management issues are further discussed in Case #2.

Discussion

Secondary causes of gout, including inherited or genetic diseases, should be considered in patients who present with gout before the age of 25. Genetic diseases can be divided into three major groups: inborn errors of purine metabolism, inborn errors of glycogen metabolism, and uromodulin-associated kidney disease.

Inborn Errors of Purine Metabolism

Hypoxanthine–Guanine Phosphoribosyltransferase Deficiency

Approximately 90% of free purines produced by the intracellular metabolism are recycled through salvage purine synthesis pathway. This pathway is mediated by three key enzymes: HPRT, adenine-phosphoribosyltransferase (APRT), and adenosine kinase (AK). HPRT breaks down hypoxanthine and guanine back into IMP and GMP, respectively (see Fig. 3.1).

The first clinical case of complete and partial HPRT deficiency was reported in 1964 by Lesch and Nyhan [1] and in 1967 by Kelly and Seegmiller [2], respectively. This partial HPRT deficiency condition is also known as Lesch–Nyhan variants or Kelly–Seegmiller syndrome. HPRT deficiency is inherited in X-linked recessive pattern where female carriers remain largely asymptomatic. Lesch–Nyhan syndrome is rare with an estimated prevalence of 1 in 380,000. The prevalence of Kelly–Seegmiller syndrome is not known, as the disease is milder and underdiagnosed. In both conditions, patients suffer from hyperuricemia-related problems including gouty arthritis, tophi, nephrolithiasis, and renal insufficiency. Cystalluria (urate crytals in urine), typically seen as orange stains or sandy materials on a child's diapers, can be detected as early as first few months of life. Patients with Lesch–Nyhan syndrome also have variable neurological impairment including cognitive impairment, hypotonia, dystonia, and, most characteristically, self-mutilating behaviors. Patients with partial HPRT deficiency lack neurological impairment.
Diagnosis:

1. CBC to look for megaloblastic anemia seen in some patients with this condition.
2. Serum uric acid level >6.8 mg/dL or 400 μmol/L.
3. 24-h urine uric acid excretion >20 mg/kg in children and >800 mg in adults, or urine-to-creatinine ratio >2 is suggestive of uric acid overproduction.
4. HPRT enzyme activity <1.5% of normal in cells from any tissue (e.g., blood, fibroblasts, lymphoblasts) is the gold standard test.
5. Genetic testing by sequence and duplication/deletion analyses of HPRT1. Approximately, 20–24% of female carries who have large deletions in this gene are not detected by sequence analysis alone.
6. Measurement of peripheral blood T-lymphocyte proliferation in the presence of the purine analogue 6-thioguanine in affected male individuals (available for research purposes only).

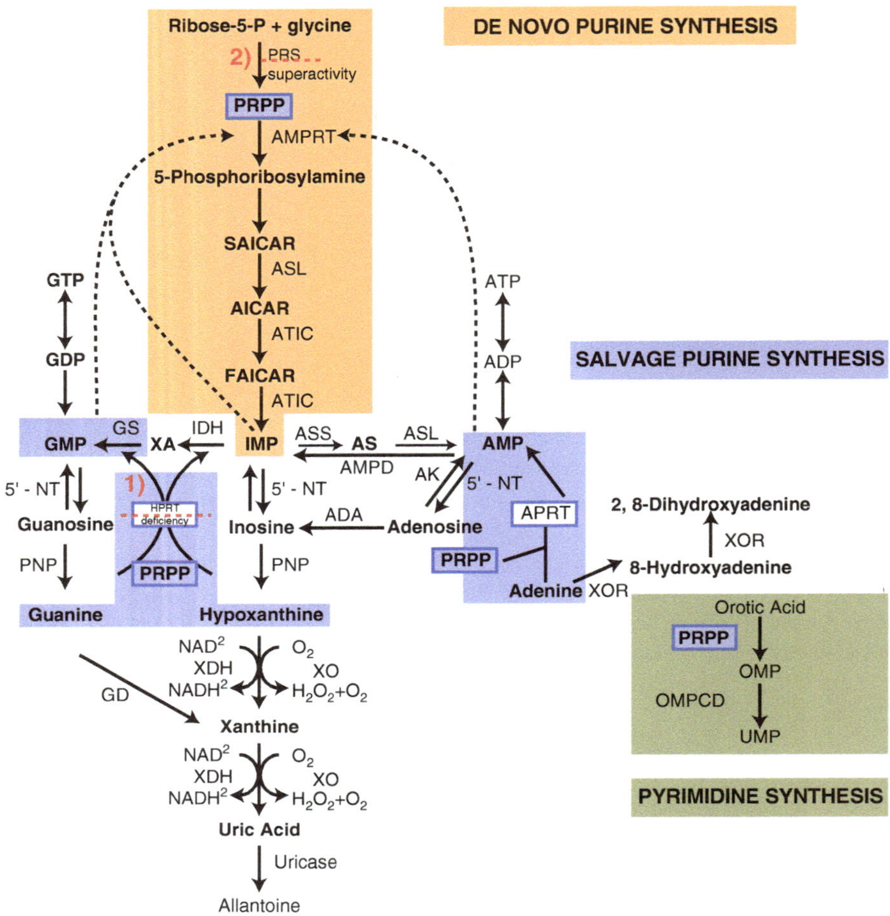

Fig. 3.1 Purine metabolism pathway. Key: 1 = HPRT deficiency (Lesch–Nyhan syndrome/Kelly–Seegmiller); 2 = PRS superactivity. Modified from Terkeltaub R. (2012) Gout and other crystal arthropathies, 1st edition. Philadelphia: Elsevier

Despite the above evaluations, making the correct diagnosis can be challenging in patients who present in the early stage of the disease in which all the classic clinical manifestations may not be present.

Management:

Patients with suspected or established HPRT deficiency should be regularly monitored for serum uric level, urinary uric acid excretion, nephrolithiasis, and neurocognitive/behavioral problems.

Hyperuricemia can be treated with xanthine oxidase inhibitors (allopurinol, febuxostat) while uricosuric agents such as probenecid are contraindicated due to an increased risk of nephrolithiasis. Xanthine oxidase inhibitors inhibit conversion of hypoxanthine and xanthine to uric acid (see Fig. 3.1) *and* can result in accumulation of xanthine and xanthine nephrolithiasis. Thus, when a patient whose uric acid is under control with allopurinol continues to have stones, xanthine nephrolithiasis should be considered. If xanthine stones are proven by stone analysis, allopurinol dose should be reduced. Of note, while xanthine oxidase inhibitors lower serum urate level, they do not improve patient's neurobehavioral and cognitive dysfunction. Due to multiple organ system involvement, multidisciplinary care with rheumatologist, neurologist, psychiatrist, and physical therapist is crucial to the success of treatment.

Phosphoribosylpyrophosphate Synthetase Superactivitiy

PRS is a critical enzyme in de novo purine synthesis pathway, where PRPP, the main substrate in the synthesis of purine, pyridine, and pyrimidine nucleotides is produced (see Fig. 3.1). Mutations in PRPS1 gene result in overactivity of PRS and subsequent hyperuricemia, recurrent uric acid nephrolithiasis, and childhood-onset gout. Some patients suffer from chronic sequelae of recurrent nephrolithiasis including frequent urinary tract infections, hypertension, and renal insufficiency. Patients with a severe phenotype present early in life (infantile–early childhood) and have neurological impairment, most characteristically hypotonia, ataxia, and neurosensory hearing loss. In a milder phenotype, patients present late (late juvenile–early adult) and do not have clinically apparent neurological deficits. The inheritance of this gene is x-linked. The prevalence is unknown due to the rarity of the disease with fewer than 30 cases reported worldwide to date.

Diagnosis:

1. Serum uric acid level >6.8 mg/dL or 400 μmol/L.
2. 24-h urine uric acid excretion >20 mg/kg in children and >800 mg in adults, or urine-to-creatinine ratio >2 is suggestive of uric acid overproduction.
3. Detection of PRS enzyme overactivity in fibroblasts, lymphoblasts, and/or erythrocytes (available for research purposes only).
4. Sequence analysis of PRPS1 gene. Point mutations are found only in patients with the severe phenotypes and account for only 25% of all individuals with this syndrome.

PRS superactivity can be distinguished from HPRT deficiency by certain clinical features: Patients with PRS superactivity lack intellectual disability but suffer from hearing impairment whereas patients with HPRT deficiency have profound mental retardation but do not have hearing problems.

Management:

Patients with PRS superactivity should be monitored for uric acid levels and development of nephrolithiasis. Hyperuricemia should be aggressively treated to prevent complications, e.g., nephrolithiasis, gouty arthritis, and renal insufficiency. These patients should avoid dehydration, uricosuric agents, and high-purine diet. Similar to HPRT deficiency, if patients continue to have recurrent nephrolithiasis despite well-controlled hyperuricemia, this should raise a suspicion of xanthine stones and allopurinol dose should be decreased accordingly.

Inborn Errors of Glycogen Metabolism

Patients with glycogen storage disease (GSD) lack various enzymes in the glycogen metabolism (see Table 3.3). Early-onset hyperuricemia and gout have been reported in GSD type I, III, V, and VII. Patients with GSD type I, also known as Von Gierke's disease or hepatorenal glycogenosis, lack glucose-6-phosphatase (G6Pase), which catalyzes glucose-6-phosphate to glucose and inorganic phosphate in hepatocytes and renal epithelial cells. These patients have impaired glucose production from gluconeogenesis and glycogenolysis and present with severe hypoglycemia, lactic acidosis, ketoacidosis, seizure, triglyceremia, and hyperuricemia. There are two subtypes: Ia and Ib. In addition to clinical features described in type Ia, patients with type Ib have functional defects of neutrophils and monocytes, leading to recurrent bacterial infections, oromucosal ulceration, gingivitis, and periodontal disease. Adult patients may also develop hepatic adenomas. The incidence of GSD type Ia is 1 in 100,000–400,000 births per year among Caucasians and 1 in 20,000 in Ashkenazi Jews. GSD type Ib is even less frequent.

Patients with GSD type III (Cori disease, Forbes disease, Limited dextrinosis, Debranching enzyme disease) have deficiency in glycogen-debranching enzyme, leading to disruption of glycogenolysis and abnormal glycogen accumulation in affected organs, such as liver, muscle, and heart. Clinical manifestations include hypoglycemia, hepatomegaly, short stature, dyslipidemia, and progressive muscle weakness. About 25% of patients also develop hepatic adenomas. The incidence of this disease is approximately 1 in 100,000 births.

GSD type V, also known as McArdle disease, is characterized by deficiency in glycogen phosphorylase (myophosphorylase) enzyme which is required for initiation of glycogenolysis in skeletal muscles. Patients present early in childhood with muscle pain, cramps, and exercise intolerance. In severe cases, myoglobinuria leading to acute renal failure can occur.

GSD type VII, also known as Tarui disease, is defined by phosphofructokinase enzyme deficiency. Clinical and laboratory characteristics are similar to those of type V GSD. This disease is very rare with less than 100 case reports to date.

Diagnosis:

The diagnosis can be confirmed by liver biopsy. GSD Type 1 patients have abundant and uniform distribution of glycogen in enlarged and distended hepatocytes. GSD Type 2 patients have enlarged hepatocytes with abnormal glycogen (limit dextrin with short outer branches). Enzymatic analysis shows deficiency of the branching enzyme in the liver and/or skeletal muscle. Gene mutation analysis can confirm the diagnosis. GSD type V and VII are confirmed with muscle biopsy for enzymatic and gene mutation analyses. GSD type VII shows glycogen accumulation in the subsarcolemmal space.

Management:

Patients with GSD Type I are treated with continuous dietary glucose administration to prevent hypoglycemia. They are advised to restrict dietary fat, fructose, and galactose. If blood chemistry abnormalities persist despite dietary interventions, specific medications (e.g., allopurinol for hyperuricemia, gemfibrozil for hypertriglyceridemia) may be required.

Table 3.3 Glycogen storage diseases that are associated with hyperuricemia

Type	Deficient enzyme	Inheritance	Locus	Classic symptoms
Ia	Glucose-6-phosphatase	AR	17q21	Hypoglycemia, hypertriglyceridemia, lactic acidosis
Ib	Glucose-6-phosphatase transporter	AR	11q23	Similar to those of type Ia and recurrent infections, oromucosal ulceration
III	Glycogen debranching enzyme	AR	1q21	Hypoglycemia, hepatomegaly, dyslipidemia, muscle weakness
V	Muscle glycogen phophorylase	AR	11q13	Muscle cramps, exercise intolerance
VII	Muscle phosphofructokinase	AR	12q13.3	Muscle cramps, exercise intolerance

Patients with GSD type 2 are recommended to eat frequent meals high in carbohydrate and uncooked cornstarch supplements. Patients with GSD Type V and VII should avoid strenuous exercise and consume high-protein diet supplemented with branched chain amino acid (leucine, isoleucine, valine) and vitamin B6. Gene transfer by using an adenovirus vector with recombinant myophosphorylase cDNA has shown to be promising in in vitro studies.

Uromodulin-Associated Kidney Disease

Uromodulin protein is the most abundant urinary protein present in healthy individuals. Mutations in the uromodulin gene result in precipitation of dysfunctional uromodulin proteins within renal tubular cells. The exact prevalence of this disease is unknown, but believed to be rare. It accounts for less than 1% of all end-stage renal disease (ESRD) cases. Although the exact mechanism is not known, two main hypotheses have been proposed:

1. The decreased excretion of abnormal uromodulin protein affects the concentrating ability of the nephron. This change is compensated by enhanced sodium reabsorption in the proximal tubule, leading to secondary increased uric acid reabsorption.
2. The altered uromodulin protein precipitates and accumulates in the tubular cells, resulting in apoptosis and tubular atrophy.

These mutations have been associated with at least three autosomal dominant clinical diseases: familial juvenile hyperuricemic nephropathy (FJHN), MCKD2, and glomerulocystic kidney disease (GCKD) [3]. FJHN is characterized by chronic interstitial nephritis with renal uric acid underexcretion. MCKD2 is characterized by the presence of renal cysts resulting in tubulo-interstitial nephropathy and eventually ESRD. GCKD is a rare form of renal cyst disease characterized by cystic dilatation of Bowman's space. Patients typically present with hyperuricemia, early-onset gout often in teenage years, and chronic kidney disease. Not all patients develop gout but all have a strong family history of gout. These individuals will eventually develop chronic tubulo-interstitial kidney disease with very low or absent proteinuria. Gout typically precedes the onset of chronic kidney disease. This suggests that gout occurs independently, and is not a consequence of CKD. The onset and severity of chronic kidney disease (CKD) vary with some patients developing it early in life while some not until their third or fourth decade of life.

REN-related kidney disease presents similarly to uromodulin-associated disease and is related to mutations in the REN gene. This causes marked reduction in normal renin production and abnormal collection of aberrant renin. Clinical features of this condition include hyperuricemia, mild anemia, mild hypotension, mild hyperkalemia, and susceptibility to acute kidney failure, resembling the effects of angiotensin-converting enzyme inhibitors (ACEI). Hyperuricemia is believed to be related to a compensatory mechanism to hypotension in which there is an increase of uric acid reabsorption in the proximal tubule. Because UMOD mutations are more common than REN mutations, one should consider the diagnosis of UMOD-associated kidney before testing for REN mutation, particularly if the patient has a strong family history of gout.

Diagnosis:

1. Strong family history owing to its autosomal dominant inheritance pattern.
2. Serum uric acid level >6.8 mg/dL or 400 μmol/L.
3. Urinalysis with mild proteinuria (<1 g/24 h) but no cells or active sediments.
4. FE uric acid ≤5%. However, as CKD progresses, FE uric acid will rise and may not be accurate or helpful when estimated GFR <70 mL/min.
5. Renal ultrasound shows normal- to small-sized kidneys and may or may not reveal cysts.
6. Renal biopsy is generally not indicated in this condition due to the cost and risks of procedure relative to its modest benefit. FJHN and MCKD2 show chronic interstitial nephritis and thickening of tubular basement membranes whereas GCKD shows diffuse glomerular cysts with markedly dilated Bowman's space. Other findings are nonspecific and include chronic interstitial nephritis with focal tubular atrophy and interstitial fibrosis with occasional lymphocytic infiltration. Immunostaining, which is not routinely performed, shows intense staining of uromodulin protein confined to a number of tubules with intracellular and intratubular heterogeneity on high power field. Normally, uromodulin protein is evenly distributed in the tubular cells lining the ascending limbs of the loops of Henle and early distal convoluted tubules.
7. Genetic analysis is the gold standard:
   (a) Sequence analysis of coding regions and associated intron boundaries which detects >95% of the cases.
   (b) Sequence analysis of select exons 3,4,5,7 with exons 3,4 being most commonly detected.

Treatment:

There are no specific treatments for these disorders. Although allopurinol is often prescribed for the treatment of hyperuricemia/gout, it has not been shown to prevent the development of renal insufficiency or alter the disease course.

Case 2

A 64-year-old Filipino male is referred to rheumatology clinic for management of chronic tophaceous gout. The patient was diagnosed with gout more than 15 years ago, initially treated with indomethacin. He was also prescribed allopurinol but developed rash. Allopurinol and oxypurinol desensitization was unsuccessfully attempted. He subsequently developed chronic renal insufficiency further preventing the use of NSAIDs. He continues to have gout flares approximately 2–3 times/month with each episode lasting 7–10 days. He has been intermittently treated with

Table 3.4 Laboratory data

Test	Value	Reference range
BUN	37	6–20 mg/dL
Creatinine	2.6	0.51–0.95 mg/dL
Uric and (current)	13.2	3.4–7.0 mg/dL
(peak and nadir)	16 and 8.7	
AST	37	0–40 U/L
ALT	29	0–41 U/L
Hemoglobin A1C	9.2%	<6%
Cholesterol	184	0–199 mg/dL
Triglycerides	155	10–170 mg/dL
LDL	165	<160 mg/dL
HDL	37	mg/dL
WBC	8.9	4.0–10.0 1,000/mm^3
Hemoglobin	10.1	13.7–17.5 g/dL
Hematocrit	33.0	40.0–50.0%
Platelet count	358	140–370 1,000/mm^3
Urinalysis	Clear, 2+ protein, 0–2 WBC, 0–2 RBC, rare bacteria/HPF	Clear, negative protein, 0–2 WBC, 0–2 RBC, none-rare bacteria' HPF

oral corticosteroids. Over the last 10 years, he has noted progressively enlarging masses on his elbows, hands, fingers, knees, and ankles interfering with his daily function.

His past medical history includes diabetes mellitus, hypertension, dyslipidemia, chronic renal insufficiency, atrial fibrillation on anticoagulation therapy, and coronary heart disease (CAD). He denies history of kidney stones and previous lead exposure. His family history is notable for gout in two of his four brothers. He works as a truck driver. He is a former smoker with 20 pack-year history of smoking. He drinks six-pack of beer a day and occasionally hard liquor (2–3 times/month). He denies illegal drug use. His review of system is otherwise unremarkable.

His current medications are lantus insulin in the AM, lispro insulin as needed, HCTZ 25 mg daily, lisinopril 20 mg daily, ASA 81 mg daily, atrovastatin 40 mg daily, and tramadol 100 mg twice daily. He takes prednisone intermittently for gout flares with last use 1 week ago.

On physical examination, his vital signs are normal. He is obese with a BMI of 35. HEENT examination is normal with no oral mucosal lesions or lymphadenopathy. His lungs are clear to auscultation bilaterally. His heart sounds are irregularly irregular. His abdomen is obese, but soft, and not tender. He has 1+ pitting edema up to above his ankles bilaterally. His skin examination reveals multiple tophi varying in size on his bilateral pinna, elbows, fingers/toes, knees, and ankles. Musculoskeletal exam revealed 1+ synovitis of his R elbow, R 2nd and 3rd PIPs, R knee, L ankle, and L midfoot. Laboratory data are shown in Table 3.4.

Imaging

Feet X-ray showed multiple erosions with overhanging edges at the left 2nd and right 5th metatarsophalangeal (MTP) joints and a marginal erosion at the left 1st MTP. Multiple soft tissue tophi were also seen.

Ultrasound of the bilateral feet reveals double contour sign, erosion, and hyperechoic tophaceous material at the left 1st MTP.

With the Presented Data, What Is Your Working Diagnosis and Why?

The clinical history is consistent with tophaceous gout with active synovitis. His diagnosis is confirmed by prior joint aspirate with urate crystals and the chronicity of his disease is confirmed by the presence of tophi and erosions noted on X-ray and ultrasound.

Differential Diagnosis

Tophaceous gout can present with polyarthritis and can mimic other inflammatory polyarthritis such as nodular rheumatoid arthritis and psoriatic arthritis. Pseudogout can also present similarly and concurrently with gout, especially in elderly patient.

Management

This patient can be considered as having "treatment-failure gout" [4]. Gout is considered to be "severe" if the patient has active disease (e.g., recurrent flares, chronic synovitis/arthropathy), tophi or typical erosions on radiograph, and history of uric acid nephrolithiasis or uric acid nephropathy. "Treatment-failure gout" is disabling and is associated with considerable amount of physical, psychological, and socioeconomic burdens to the patient, family, and community. Studies have shown that these patients had significant physical disability, and their SF-36 scores were comparable to population aged 10–20 years older [4, 5].

This patient's treatment options for his acute gout flare are limited by renal insufficiency, precluding the use of NSAIDs or colchicine. Systemic corticosteroids are also not an ideal option given his poorly controlled diabetes. Although intra-articular corticosteroid injections would be preferable, it is impractical in polyarticular flare. Patient was started on IL-1 antagonist, anakinra 100 mg SQ qdaily prn during acute flares.

Table 3.5 Recommended colchicine dosing for treatment of gout in patients with impaired renal function

Creatinine clearance	Colchicine dose
>60 mL/min	0.6 mg po twice daily
40–59 mL/min	0.6 mg po once daily
30–39 mL/min	0.6 mg po every 2 days
11–29 mL/min	0.6 mg po every 2–3 days
<10 mL/min or patients on hemodialysis or patients with severe hepatobiliary dysfunction	Avoid colchicine or limit the dose to 0.6 mg po once or twice per week

Modified from Terkeltaub R. (2012) Gout and other crystal arthropathies, 1st edition. Philadelphia: Elsevier

Patient has several options for the treatment of his chronic gout once his acute flare subsides and opts for pegloticase 8 mg IV every 2 weeks. His serum uric acid level dropped dramatically initially to 1.1 mg/dL (normal serum uric acid <7 mg/dL) but returned to his pretreatment level by his fifth dose. The decision was made to discontinue pegloticase and start febuxostat.

Discussion

Treatment of gout can be divided into treatment of acute and chronic gout. The goal of acute treatment is to rapidly decrease inflammation and pain while the goal of chronic gout is to prevent recurrent gout flares and joint destruction.

Treatment Options for Acute Gout

1. NSAIDs or cox-2 (cyclooxygenase-2-selective) inhibitors: Use with caution among patients with renal insufficiency or CAD.
2. Colchicine: Must be renally dosed (Table 3.5). Based on a study showing equal efficacy but less adverse events, it is now recommended to give colchicine 1.2 mg po × 1 and then 0.6 mg po 1 h later for acute gout flare [6].
3. Systemic or intra-articualr corticosteroids.
4. ACTH is rarely used.

Treatment Options for Chronic Gout

1. Lifestyle modification:
   (a) Aggressive treatment of co-morbidities associated with gout: Obesity, metabolic syndrome, hypertension, diabetes mellitus, hyperlipidemia, coronary artery disease, and congestive heart failure.

(b) Diet: Avoidance of alcohol, high fructose beverages, and purine-rich foods such as red meat, shellfish, and organ meats. Decreased risk of gout has been associated with high intake of vitamin C and low fat/fat-free dairy.

2. Urate-lowering therapy:

   (a) Uricosuric agent: Probenecid.
   (b) Xanthine oxidase inhibitor: (allopurinol/febuxostat)

Allopurinol, a xanthine inhibitor, is approved by the US FDA for treatment of gout with a maximum dose of 800 mg/day. Allopurinol should be initiated at a low dose and slowly titrated to an effective dose in patients with renal impairment to avoid potential allopurinol hypersensitivity syndrome.

Febuxostat is a selective non-purine-based xanthine oxidase inhibitor that was FDA approved in 2009, but unlike allopurinol, it can be used among patients with mild to moderate renal insufficiency.

3. Pegloticase.

Pegloticase was FDA approved in 2010 for refractory chronic gout patients. Humans lack uricase which converts urate into very soluble allantoin that is excreted into urine. Pegloticase is a mammalian recombinant uricase conjugated to ethylene glycol. In two replicate, randomized, double-blind, placebo-controlled trials with a total number of patients of 225, more than one-third of patients treated with pegloticase achieved the target uric acid level of <6 mg/dL at 6 months compared to none in the placebo-treated patients. Patients treated with pegloticase also had significant reduction in tophi and improvement in pain, physical function, and quality of life. Gout flares were the most common adverse events, particularly during the first 3 months of treatment. Infusion reactions occurred in up to 8% of subjects and were the main reason for treatment discontinuation. Even though plasma uric acid levels normalized within the first 24 h in all treated patients, many patients experienced loss of response thought to be due to the development of antibodies against pegloticase. Patients treated with pegloticase also experienced more cardiovascular events and is relatively contraindicated in patients with Class III/IV congestive heart failure [7]. Pegloticase is contraindicated in patients with G-6-PD deficiency due to the risk of hemolysis and methemoglobinemia and should be screened in high-risk population (e.g., African Americans, Mediterranean) prior to treatment initiation [7]. Serum uric levels should be monitored regularly prior to each infusion as rising urate levels may signify development of anti-pegloticase antibodies. Concomitant use of other urate-lowering therapy should be avoided since it may mask the predictable increase in urate levels associated with the development of anti-pegloticase antibodies.

As patients are at an increased risk for acute gout flare during the first 3–6 months after starting urate-lowering therapy, it is recommended that they concomitantly start NSAIDs, cox-2, or Colchicine for prophylaxis.

Recent Developments in the Treatment of Gout

Studies have shown that IL-1 plays a key role in stimulating inflammasome and innate immune response in acute crystal-induced arthritis. This inflammasome, NLRP3, is also implicated in the underlying pathogenesis of other autoinflammatory diseases such as cryopyrin-associated periodic syndrome (CAPS) that respond well to anti IL-1 treatment. Although the FDA has not yet approved these agents for use in gouty arthritis, they have been prescribed off-label and their efficacy has been demonstrated in multiple case reports, retrospective, observational, and open-label cohort studies.

– Anakinra, recombinant IL-1 receptor antagonist (IL-1ra), has been successfully used to treat acute gout flares in patients who have failed or are unable to take or tolerate conventional therapy. It has a rapid onset of action and brief immunosuppressive effect. Anakinra is generally well tolerated, with only mild injection site reactions being reported [8, 9].
– Canakinumab is a fully humanized monoclonal antibody to IL-1β under investigation for the treatment of acute gout. Canakinumab at the dose 150 mg has been shown to have comparable efficacy to intramuscular triamcinolone for the treatment of acute gout flare with no increased incidence of adverse events [10]. It has also been shown to be effective for prophylaxis of acute gout flares during initiation of allopurinol and to be superior to colchicine [10].
– Rilonacept (IL-1 trap), a soluble receptor-Fc fusion protein that blocks both IL-1α and IL-1β, has been studied for the treatment of both acute and chronic gout. Rilonacept improved patient-reported VAS scores for pain and global assessment scores during the 6-week treatment period. It was well tolerated with mild degree of injection site reactions being the most common adverse event [12].

Questions

1. A 17-year-old male is referred for evaluation of intermittent joint pain and swelling. Exam reveals oligoarticular arthritis. Skin exam shows no tophi or skin rash. Initial laboratory studies are only remarkable for uric acid of 11.3 mg/dL. What would be the most appropriate next step in evaluation?
   (a) Urinary uric acid and creatinine
   (b) Enzymatic activity
   (c) Genetic testing
   (d) Kidney biopsy
   (e) Renal ultrasound
2. All of the following are features of uromodulin-associated disorders *except* that
   (a) Hyperuricemia and gout precede clinically evident renal insufficiency.
   (b) It is inherited in an autosomal dominant pattern.
   (c) Fraction excretion of uric acid is increased during the early disease course and will decrease as the CKD progresses.
   (d) Treatment with allopurinol has not been shown to halt the progression of renal insufficiency.
   (e) All patients have a strong family history of gout.

3. What is the mainstay gout therapy in patients with inborn errors in purine metabolism?
   (a) Colchicine
   (b) Enzyme replacement
   (c) Prednisone
   (d) Probenecid
   (e) Allopurinol

4. Hyperuricemia and gout have been associated with various types of GSD, except which type?
   (a) I
   (b) II
   (c) III
   (d) V
   (e) VII

5. Which diagnostic test is most likely to be helpful in establishing the diagnosis of UMOD-associated kidney disease?
   (a) Renal ultrasound
   (b) Fraction excretion of uric acid
   (c) Kidney biopsy
   (d) Genetic analysis
   (e) Enzymatic testing

6. A 35 yo M presents to the clinic with recurrent swollen and painful joints. Past medical history is significant for a recent cardiac transplantation for severe dilated cardiomyopathy. His medications include azathioprine 200 mg/day and prednisone 10 mg/day for immunosuppression. He has been given intermittent short courses of burst steroids with improvement in his joint symptoms. His labs reveal normal CBC, Cr of 2.0, and uric acid of 14.5. What is the most appropriate next step in this patient's long-term management of hyperuricemia?
   (a) Start the patient on allopurinol and decrease azathioprine dose.
   (b) Start the patient on febuxostat.
   (c) Increase prednisone to 30 mg/day for chronic suppression of inflammation.
   (d) Ask nephrology to switch azathioprine to another immunosuppressive agent.
   (e) Initiate pegloticase.

7. A 67 yo M with a history of chronic tophaceous gout, end-stage renal disease on hemodialysis, DM, and HTN presents to the emergency room with a 2-day history of joint pain and swelling in his right wrist, both knees and ankles. He also reports fevers and chills. His vital signs reveal temperature of 102 F, BP of 90/56 mmHg, PR of 115, and RR of 16/min. The patient appears uncomfortable. MSK exam shows active synovitis of the aforementioned joints. His skin is also notable for multiple tophi on his fingers, elbows, knees, and feet. Initial

laboratory studies are pending. Rheumatology service is consulted for management of gout. What is the most appropriate next step of action?

(a) Prescribe systemic corticosteroids.
(b) Perform arthrocentesis.
(c) Prescribe colchicine and send the patient to hemodialysis the following day.
(d) Prescribe anakinra 100 mg SQ daily for 3 days.
(e) Give the patient a single dose of canakinumab.

8. A 71 yo African-American patient with a history of coronary heart disease and CHF, DM, HTN, COPD, and chronic tophaceous gout presents to rheumatology clinic to discuss the new treatment, pegloticase, with you. He has been treated with febuxostat 40 mg/day for the last 4 months. Febuxostat dose was increased to 80 mg/day but he developed pruritic rash. The medication was discontinued and subsequently rechallenged 4 months ago and he has been tolerating it well. His NYHA functional class is II. He is allergic to sulfa drugs and penicillin which cause hives. He also reports a history of G-6-PD deficiency after developing hemolytic anemia requiring hospitalization at the age of 24. Which of the following is the *absolute* contraindication for the use of pegloticase in this patient?

   (a) History of sulfa allergy
   (b) African-American race
   (c) COPD
   (d) Congestive heart failure
   (e) G-6-PD deficiency

9. A 69 yo African-American male with a history of chronic tophaceous gout. The patient has been taking feboxustat 80 mg for the past 6 months. His uric acid levels have ranged from 10.2 to 11.8 mg/dL. His flares remain frequent despite chronic prednisone therapy 10 mg/day. His functional status is severely limited due to frequent gout flares and multiple debilitating tophi. The decision has been made to start him on pegloticase. What test should be ordered before initiating treatment?

   (a) G-6-PD level
   (b) Pulmonary function test
   (c) Chest X-ray
   (d) Renal and bladder ultrasound
   (e) Tuberculosis skin test (PPD)

10. A 58 yo Filipino male patient is scheduled for his third pegloticase infusion tomorrow. His uric acid today increased from 2 weeks ago following the second infusion of 0.2–8.7 mg/dL. His uric acid levels had been below <1 mg/dL after starting pegloticase 6 weeks ago. What is the most appropriate step in management?

    (a) Increase pegloticase dose.
    (b) Change pegloticase to weekly infusion.
    (c) Add febuxostat to pegloticase.

(d) Discontinue pegloticase and check anti-pegloticase antibodies.
(e) Continue pegloticase treatment and check uric acid after the third infusion.

Answer keys: 1(a), 2(c), 3(e), 4(b), 5(d), 6(a), 7(b), 8(e), 9(a), 10(d).

References

1. Lesch M, Nyhan WL. A familial disorder of uric acid metabolism and central nervous system function. Am J Med. 1964;36:561–70.
2. Seegmiller JE, Rosenbloom FM, Kelley WN. Enzyme defect associated with a sex-linked human neurological disorder and excessive purine synthesis. Science. 1967;155(3770):1682–4.
3. Lens XM, Banet JF, Outeda P, et al. A novel pattern of mutation in uromodulin disorders: autosomal dominal medullary cystic kidney disease type 2, familial juvenile hyperuricemic nephropathy, and autosomal dominant glomerulocystic kidney disease. Am J Kidney Dis. 2005;46(1):52–7.
4. Becker MA, Schumacher HR, Benjamin KL, et al. Quality of life and disability in patients with treatment-failure gout. J Rheumatol. 2009;36:1041–8.
5. Lee SJ, Hirsch JD, Terkeltaub R, et al. Perceptions of disease and health-related quality of life among patients with gout. Rheumatology (Oxford). 2009;48(5):582–6.
6. Terkeltaub RA, Furst DE, Bennett K, et al. High versus low dosing of oral colchicine for early acute gout flare. Twenty-four-hour outcome of the first multicenter, randomized, double-blind, placebo-controlled, parallel-group, dose-comparison colchicine study. Arthritis Rheum. 2010;62(4):1060–8.
7. Sundy JS, Baraf HS, Yood RA, et al. Efficacy and tolerability of pegloticase for the treatment of chronic gout in patients refractory to conventional treatment: two randomized controlled trials. JAMA. 2011;306(7):711–20.
8. So A, De Smedt T, Revaz S, et al. A pilot study of IL-1 inhibition by anakinra in acute gout. Arthritis Res Ther. 2007;9(2):R28.
9. Chen K, Fields T, Mancuso CA, et al. Anakinra's efficacy is variable in refractory gout: report of ten cases. Semin Arthritis Rheum. 2010;40(3):210–4.
10. So A, De Meulemeester M, Pikhlak A, et al. Canakinumab for the treatment of acute flares in difficult-to-treat gout arthritis: Results of a multicenter, phase II, dose-ranging study. Arthritis Rheum. 2010;62:2845–9.
11. Schlesinger N, Mysler E, Meulemeester M, et al. Canakinumab reduces the risk of acute gouty arthritis flares during initiation of allopurinol treatment: results of a double-blind, randomized study. Ann Rheum Dis. 2011;70:1264–71.
12. Terkeltaub R, Sundy JS, Schumacher HR, et al. The interleukin 1 inhibitor rilonacept in treatment of chronic gouty arthritis: results of a placebo-controlled, monosequence crossover, non-randomised, single-blind pilot study. Ann Rheum Dis. 2009;68:1613–7.

Chapter 4
Psoriatic Arthritis

Anna Tumyan and Marcy B. Bolster

Abstract Psoriatic arthritis is a chronic inflammatory arthritis associated with psoriasis. Psoriatic arthritis belongs to the group of seronegative spondyloarthropathies and may present with both peripheral joint and axial skeleton involvement. In addition to joint and cutaneous disease, the other common features of psoriatic arthritis include dactylitis and enthesitis, resulting from involvement of surrounding tendons and ligaments as well as nail changes including pitting, ridging, and distal onycholysis. Familial aggregation of cases is common with HLA-B27 positivity reported in 10–25% of patients. There are no validated diagnostic criteria available for psoriatic arthritis and diagnosis should be based on the presence of characteristic clinical manifestations, physical examination, laboratory and imaging findings, and additionally, by the process of elimination of other common inflammatory arthritides. The treatment of patients presenting with more severe joint disease, unresponsive to nonsteroidal anti-inflammatory drugs (NSAIDs), extra-articular manifestations and/or poor prognostic factors require use of systemic disease-modifying anti-rheumatic drugs (DMARDs) and/or biologic agents. Cases related to the presentation of the spectrum of psoriatic arthritis are discussed.

Keywords Psoriatic arthritis • Psoriasis • Inflammatory polyarthritis • Seronegative spondyloarthropathy

A. Tumyan, M.D. (✉)
Department of Internal Medicine,
SIU School of Medicine, Division of Rheumatology,
PO Box 19636, Springfield, IL 62794, USA
e-mail: Atumyan@siumed.edu

M.B. Bolster, M.D.
Division of Rheumatology and Immunology,
Director, Rheumatology Fellowship Training Program,
Medical University of South Carolina, Charleston, SC, USA
e-mail: bolsterm@musc.edu

M. Mahmoudi (ed.), *Challenging Cases in Rheumatology and Diseases of the Immune System*, DOI 10.1007/978-1-4614-5088-7_4,
© Springer Science+Business Media, LLC 2013

Case 1

A 30-year-old male is being evaluated for a 3-year history of worsening lower back pain. The pain is now constant, located in the lower back and left buttock area and is not radiating. The pain is worse at night and in the early morning hours and frequently awakens him at night. He reports significant morning stiffness in the lower back, lasting for several hours and somewhat improved with stretching and taking a hot shower. He also notes difficulty walking due to pain and stiffness in the bottom of his heels.

The heel pain is worse in the mornings upon taking his first steps. He reports that his right second toe has been swollen for the last 2 months. He denies previous back trauma or surgeries. He denies any other joint complaints, fever, muscle weakness, loss of sensation, or problems with bowel or bladder function.

He was previously treated with a course of physical therapy and muscle relaxants, which provided only temporary relief. He currently takes ibuprofen 800 mg three times a day with moderate improvement.

Several months ago he had noted the onset of "scalp irritation" which he initially thought was a reaction to hair products used at that time. He has tried several different brands of shampoo since that time without a change in his symptoms, and he was eventually seen by a dermatologist and diagnosed with psoriasis. He denies other skin rash, nail changes, fever, oral or genital ulcers, dysuria, chest pain, shortness of breath, diarrhea, or hematochezia.

He is a full time ICU nurse and reports difficulty performing his tasks during early morning shifts due to the extent of his back pain and stiffness. He is unmarried and has been in a monogamous relationship for the last 3 years. He denies smoking, alcohol, or illicit drug use. He is otherwise healthy and denies any prior illnesses or surgeries. He denies a history of sexually transmitted disease. His only medication is ibuprofen. He has no known drug allergies. His family history is significant for psoriasis in his mother. Physical examination reveals normal vital signs. He is afebrile. He has tenderness to palpation of the left sacroiliac joint and bilateral heels. Hip examination is unremarkable. He has discomfort in the left buttock upon performing FABER (flexion, abduction, external rotation) maneuver. His spine flexibility is preserved, and a Schober test reveals 5 cm of lumbar distraction. He has diffuse swelling of the right second toe (Fig. 4.1). The scalp examination reveals several erythematous patches with overlying silvery scale. There are no other skin rashes present. His HEENT, cardiovascular, lung, abdominal, and neurologic examinations are unremarkable.

With the Presented History and Physical Examination Findings, What Is Your Working Diagnosis?

The patient is a 30-year-old male with a personal and family history of psoriasis presenting with a several year history of slowly progressive inflammatory lower back pain in association with heel pain and toe swelling. On physical examination he has left sacroiliac joint tenderness and abnormal FABER test (flexion, abduction,

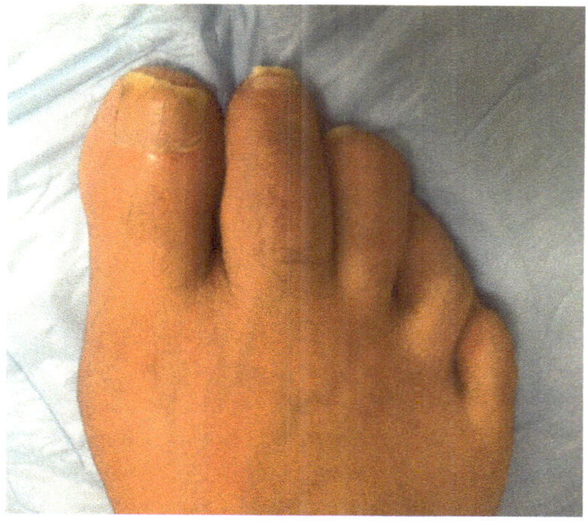

Fig. 4.1 Clinical photograph of the patient demonstrating dactylitis of the right second toe

external rotation also known as Patrick's maneuver), suggestive of left sacroiliitis, bilateral heel tenderness suggestive of plantar fasciitis (enthesopathy) and dactylitis of his second right toe.

Based on the findings of sacroiliitis, dactylitis, and enthesopathy in this patient with a personal and family history of psoriasis the diagnosis of psoriaticarthritis is high on the differential.

Differential Diagnosis

There are several features that help to distinguish inflammatory back pain from mechanical causes of back discomfort including younger age of onset, gradual onset of the symptoms, association with prolonged morning stiffness, worsening of pain and stiffness at night and in early morning hours, and improvement with exercise. Inflammatory back pain may result from involvement of sacroiliac joints leading to sacroiliitis and inflammation of the spine leading to spondylitis.

The differential diagnosis of inflammatory back pain should include seronegative spondyloarthropathies such as psoriatic arthritis, ankylosing spondylitis, inflammatory bowel disease associated arthritis and reactive arthritis (previously known as Reiter's syndrome). Infectious etiologies including pyogenic, mycobacterial and fungal as well as malignant infiltration should be also considered. Sarcoidosis, although uncommonly, may also present with sacroiliitis.

Evaluation and Final Diagnosis

Laboratory testing should include a basic workup with a complete blood count (CBC), complete metabolic panel (CMP) and urinalysis, measurements of inflammatory markers such as erythrocyte sedimentation rate (ESR) and C-reactive protein (CRP), as well as more specific autoimmune serologies including a rheumatoid factor (RF) and anti-cyclic citrullinated peptide (anti-CCP), although they may not be as useful in a patient with spondylitis as opposed to a patient presenting with a peripheral arthritis. HLA-B27 positivity is reported in 10–25% of patients; however, this test is neither sensitive nor specific and is not routinely recommended.

Additional imaging studies should be obtained to evaluate for evidence of joint damage as well as periarticular involvement.

In this case, the CMP, CBC, urinalysis, and inflammatory markers were normal. Testing for RF, anti-CCP antibody, and HLA-B27 was negative. A radiograph of the bilateral sacroiliac joints (taken as a Ferguson view which provides 25–30 degrees of tilt to better visualize the sacroiliac joints) revealed evidence of left sacroiliitis. A radiograph of the lumbar spine was unremarkable with no evidence of shiny corner sign. The latter, also known as a Romanus lesion, represents small erosions at the superior and inferior endplates of the vertebral bodies with surrounding reactive sclerosis and is an early spinal finding in ankylosing spondylitis.

This patient fulfills classification criteria for psoriatic arthritis based on his seronegativity, radiographic findings of left sacroiliitis, dactylitis, enthesopathy, personal and family history of psoriasis.

Case 2

A 42-year-old woman presents to her primary care physician with a 1-year history of painful swelling of her hands, wrists and feet. Her symptoms began with soreness of her hands and feet which initially improved with the use of over the counter NSAIDs. Her arthralgia, however, gradually worsened and over the last several months she also noted swelling of her hands, wrists, and feet. Her symptoms are much worse upon awakening and are associated with 2–3 h of morning stiffness in the affected joints.

Her past medical history is significant for psoriasis diagnosed at age 30 years and managed with topical glucocorticoid ointments. Her skin disease has been stable. She is a substitute preschool teacher who is married and has a 7-year-old child. She denies smoking, alcohol, or illicit drug use.

She denies other skin rashes, fever, alopecia, photosensitivity, oral or genital ulcers, chest pain, shortness of breath, history of serositis, kidney problems, acid reflux, nausea, vomiting, history of inflammatory eye disease, paresthesias, or back pain. She admits to a history of intermittent diarrhea, previously attributed to irritable bowel syndrome. She denies weight loss or hematochezia.

Her family history is not significant. Her medications include ibuprofen and a multivitamin. She has no known drug allergies.

On physical examination she is afebrile and vital signs are normal. Skin examination reveals erythematous plaques with silvery scale involving extensor surfaces of the elbows and knees. Pitting is evident on several of her fingernails. Musculoskeletal examination reveals synovitis of bilateral 2nd–4th metacarpophalangeal (MCP), proximal interphalangeal (PIP) joints and of the left wrist. There is also tenderness of the metatarsophalangeal (MTP) joints to compression. Her grip strength is decreased. There is no spinal or sacroiliac joint tenderness. Her HEENT, cardiovascular, lung, abdominal and neurologic examinations are unremarkable.

With the Presented History and Physical Examination Findings, What Is Your Working Diagnosis?

The patient is a 42-year-old female with a long standing history of psoriasis presenting with symmetrical polyarthritis of small and medium joints. She also has several fingernails with pitting. Although quite different in presentation, this case is also suggestive of psoriatic arthritis as the patient presents with an inflammatory arthritis and nail changes in association with psoriasis.

Differential Diagnosis

The differential diagnosis at this point should include rheumatoid arthritis (RA); systemic lupus erythematous (SLE), other seronegative spondyloarthropathies including reactive arthritis, inflammatory bowel disease associated arthritis and ankylosing spondylitis, Parvovirus B 19-associated arthritis, sarcoid arthropathy, Hepatitis C arthropathy, acute Hepatitis B arthritis and HIVarthropathy.

Evaluation and Final Diagnosis

In this case, the CMP and urinalysis were normal. Her CBC revealed mild normocytic anemia. Her ESR was elevated at 40 mm/h and CRP was normal.

She was noted to have a negative anti-nuclear antibody (ANA), RF, and anti-CCP antibody. Her viral serologies were negative including Parvovirus B19 IgM, HIV, Hepatitis C antibody and Hepatitis B surface antigen.

A radiograph of the chest revealed no evidence of acute cardiopulmonary disease, mediastinal widening or hilar adenopathy. A radiograph of the sacroiliac joints was normal. A radiograph of the hands revealed erosive changes at the MCP and PIP joints with irregular periosteal bony proliferation.

What Is Your Diagnosis and Why?

Psoriatic arthritis is defined as a chronic inflammatory arthritis associated with psoriasis and may present with peripheral joint and/or axial skeleton involvement.

Table 4.1 Classification criteria for psoriatic arthritis (CASPAR) criteria [3]

Inflammatory arthritis (involving peripheral joints and/or spine), or enthesis
Plus 3 or more points from the following categories:
Psoriasis: currently observed *(2 points)*, a personal or family history of psoriasis *(1 point each)*
Typical psoriatic nail changes *(1 point)*: onycholysis, pitting or hyperkeratosis (observed on current physical examination)
Negative RF *(1 point)*
Dactylitis *(1 point)*: either currently observed or previously recorded by a rheumatologist
Radiographic evidence of juxta-articular new bone formation *(1 point)*: on plain radiographs of the hand or foot

Modified from Taylor W, Gladman D, Helliwell P, et al. Classification criteria for psoriatic arthritis: development of new criteria from a large international study. Arthritis Rheum 2006;54:2665–2673

There are no validated diagnostic criteria available for psoriatic arthritis and the diagnosis should be based on the presence of characteristic clinical manifestations, physical examination, laboratory and imaging findings and by a process of elimination of other common inflammatory arthritides.

Historically, the main and most widely used classification criteria (though not validated) for psoriatic arthritis were developed by Moll and Wright in the early 1970s and were based on [1]:

- An inflammatory arthritis (either peripheral arthritis and/or axial involvement with sacroiliitis or spondylitis)
- The presence of psoriasis
- The absence of RF

More recently, classification criteria for psoriatic arthritis (CASPAR criteria), have been developed in an attempt to make the diagnostic criteria for psoriatic arthritis more specific (Table 4.1). The classification criteria incorporate musculoskeletal, dermatologic, and radiographic features and have a high sensitivity and specificity for the diagnosis of both early and late psoriatic arthritis [2].

Several features of psoriatic arthritis are helpful in distinguishing it from other common forms of inflammatory arthritis. Psoriatic arthritis differs from rheumatoid arthritis in terms of its different patterns of presentation including an asymmetric pattern of joint involvement, frequent onset of disease with an oligoarticular (4 or fewer joints) presentation or frequent DIP joint involvement. Rheumatoid arthritis, in contrast, usually presents with symmetrical polyarthritis affecting small and medium joints and sparing of DIP joints. Both diseases may present with cervical spine involvement; however, sacroiliitis or thoracic and/or lumbar spine involvement, which may be seen in psoriatic arthritis, are not typical features of rheumatoid arthritis. Other distinguishing features of psoriatic arthritis include frequent involvement of periarticular structures, such as tendons and ligaments, clinically presenting as dactylitis and enthesitis; rash on the scalp and involvement of nails, causing pitting, ridging, and distal onycholysis.

There are no diagnostic laboratory tests for psoriatic arthritis. Normocytic anemia, elevated inflammatory markers and hypoalbuminemia may be seen in patients with active disease. Hyperuricemia may be present in up to 20% of patients with psoriatic arthritis [4]. Although classified as a seronegative spondyloarthropathy, a small number of patients with psoriatic arthritis (5–10%) may have a positiveRF) and anti-CCP antibodies. Seropositivity (for RF and anti-CCP) is usually associated with female gender and polyarticular disease [5]. A positive HLA-B27 has been reported in 10–25% of patients.

This patient also fulfills classification criteria for psoriatic arthritis based on seronegative symmetrical polyarthritis of small and medium joints, nail dystrophy, and history of psoriasis.

Discussion

Psoriatic arthritis is a chronic inflammatory arthritis associated with psoriasis. Psoriatic arthritis belongs to the group of seronegative spondyloarthropathies and may present with both peripheral joint and axial skeleton involvement. In addition to joint and cutaneous disease, the other common features of psoriatic arthritis include dactylitis and enthesitis, resulting from involvement of surrounding tendons and ligaments as well as various nail changes including pitting, ridging, and distal onycholysis. Familial aggregation of cases is common with a positive HLA-B27 reported in about 10–25% of cases.

Psoriatic arthritis affects men and women equally, with an incidence of 6.6 per 100,000 per year and a prevalence of 1–2 per 1,000. The mean age at onset of psoriatic arthritis is 30–55 years. The estimated prevalence of psoriatic arthritis among patients with psoriasis ranges from 4 to 30%. Although the majority of patients develop psoriasis before the onset of arthritis, the arthritis may precede skin involvement in up to 15% of cases [6].

Patients with psoriatic arthritis present with inflammatory arthritis manifesting by joint pain and swelling, prolonged morning stiffness, as well as joint deformities in more advanced stages of disease. Joint involvement in psoriatic arthritis can vary and may involve peripheral joints and/or the axial spine.

Historically, five patterns of psoriatic arthritis have been recognized; however, these patterns may overlap or change over time in any given patient:

1. Asymmetrical oligoarticular arthritis (4 or fewer joints involved)
2. Symmetrical polyarthritis
3. Distal interphalangealarthropathy
4. Arthritis mutilans
5. Spondylitis with or without sacroiliitis

Monoarticular and oligoarticular arthritis are the most common presenting patterns of psoriatic arthritis and are characterized by male predominance, asymmetric joint distribution and frequent lower limb joint involvement.

Symmetric polyarthritis may be clinically indistinguishable from rheumatoid arthritis and presents with symmetrical involvement of the small and/or medium joints, commonly involving the hand joints. This pattern is characterized by female predominance and the more common development of erosive disease.

Involvement of the DIP joints is a distinctive feature of psoriatic arthritis and has been reported in up to onehalf of patients with psoriatic arthritis. However, the DIP-predominant sub-group of those with psoriatic arthritis represents a much smaller proportion of cases (1–16%). This pattern can occur early in the disease course and commonly be associated with two other significant features of psoriatic arthritis including dactylitis and nail changes.

Arthritis mutilans is a severe form of a destructive erosive arthritis and affects less than 5% of patients. It may manifest with subluxations, "flail" joints and digital telescoping resulting from resorption of bones and the consequent collapse of soft tissues. This phenomenon is also called *doigt en lorgnette* (opera glass finger). It is associated with long-standing disease and more commonly seen in females.

Spondyloarthropathy is uncommon as a predominant feature in psoriatic arthritis; however, axial spine involvement may be seen in 20–40% of cases. Sacroiliac joint involvement in psoriatic arthritis tends to be asymmetric, although patients may also present with bilateral sacroiliitis, and the latter has a stronger association with a positive HLA-B27 [7]. Several features characteristic for spine involvement in psoriatic arthritis, and helpful in distinguishing it from ankylosing spondylitis, include skipped character of lesions and a lower frequency of zygapophyseal joint fusion. The spine disease in psoriatic arthritis tends to be less severe and carries a better prognosis compared to ankylosing spondylitis. The cervical spine is also a common site of involvement and is more likely to become involved with increased disease duration. There are two main types of cervical spine changes described: an ankylosing type, similar to that seen in ankylosing spondylitis, and an erosive/inflammatory type similar to cervical spine involvement seen in rheumatoid arthritis potentially resulting in atlantoaxial or subaxial instability. Because cervical spine involvement can be clinically silent, patients with psoriatic arthritis, particularly those with long-standing disease, should have cervical spineradiographs before undergoing general anesthesia.

The main extra-articular features of psoriatic arthritis are the presence of skin and nail lesions. As noted earlier, although the majority of patients develop skin lesions before the onset of arthritis, in about 15% of cases arthritis precedes the onset of skin disease. The skin lesions may be hidden with common areas including umbilicus, gluteal cleft and scalp, of note. Although earlier reports suggested an association between arthritis disease activity and more severe skin disease, at the present time there is no predictable relationship found between skin and joint manifestations. Nail lesions including pitting, ridging, and distal onycholysis are seen in 80% of patients with psoriatic arthritis and frequently occur in digits with DIP joint involvement.

Dactylitis also so-called a "sausage digit" has been reported in up to 40% of cases of psoriatic arthritis and is one of the important extra-articular features of disease. It presents with complete swelling of a single digit in the hand or foot as a result of both joint inflammation and swelling along the tendon sheath (tenosynovitis). Dactylitis affects more commonly toes than fingers, frequently in association with DIP joint involvement and more destructive radiographic changes.

Enthesis representing an inflammation at the insertion of tendon into bone is another common extra-articular feature and may occur in 20–40% of patients with psoriatic arthritis. It may be the initial manifestation of the disease in a minority of cases. Common sites include Achilles tendon, the plantar fascia insertion into the calcaneus, and ligamentous insertions into pelvic bones.

Other extra-articular manifestations of disease including inflammatory eye disease presenting with conjunctivitis and/or uveitis, urethritis, as well as aortic root dilatation have been also described in patients with psoriatic arthritis, however, with much less frequency.

The etiology and pathophysiology of psoriatic arthritis are not well understood. However, genetic, immunologic and environmental factors are considered important. The role of genetic factors has been demonstrated by clear familial aggregation of both psoriasis and psoriatic arthritis. Environmental factors have also been implicated including infectious agents (streptococcus, HIV) and trauma that may precipitate the onset or a flare of disease activity. Patients presenting with severe skin/joint disease should alert the clinician to test for HIV.

Diagnostic imaging should start with plain radiography. Patients with psoriatic arthritis may demonstrate involvement of peripheral joints as well as axial disease with the presence of both destructive joint and proliferativebone changes; although in early disease the only finding may be of soft tissue swelling.

There are several distinct features differentiating psoriatic arthritis from rheumatoid arthritis including involvement of the DIP joints, an asymmetric distribution of joint involvement, absence of periarticular osteopenia, the presence of bony proliferation near joints (periostitis) and ligament and/or tendon insertion sites (entheses) and bony ankylosis. Erosive disease has been associated with a polyarticular presentation, longer disease duration and dactylitis [8]. In more severe cases osteolysis may occur resulting in the pencil-in-cup deformity or resorption of terminal phalangeal tufts. Along with joint destruction, in periostitis, proliferative new bone formation can occur along the shaft of the bone, often accompanied by soft tissue swelling. Patients with psoriatic arthritis may also develop ankylosis and joint fusion.

Spine involvement in psoriatic arthritis tends to be more asymmetric with a skipped character of lesions, and there may be less extensive involvement of the lumbar spine compared to ankylosing spondylitis [9]. The spine disease in psoriatic arthritis as compared to ankylosing spondylitis tends to have a lesser degree of ankylosis and therefore carries a better prognosis. The cervical spine is also a common site of involvement and may manifest with ankylosing type and an erosive/inflammatory type which can result in atlantoaxial or subaxial instability. Involvement of the sacroiliac joints may be both symmetrical and asymmetrical with the latter being more common (Fig. 4.2). However, joints do not usually fuse, as in ankylosing spondylitis.MRI studies have also demonstrated frequent involvement of extra-articular tissue such as ligaments, periarticular soft tissue, tendon sheaths, and bone [10].

The treatment of psoriatic arthritis is directed at controlling the inflammatory process and depends on several factors including severity of skin and joint disease, presence of extra-articular manifestations as well as poor prognostic fac-

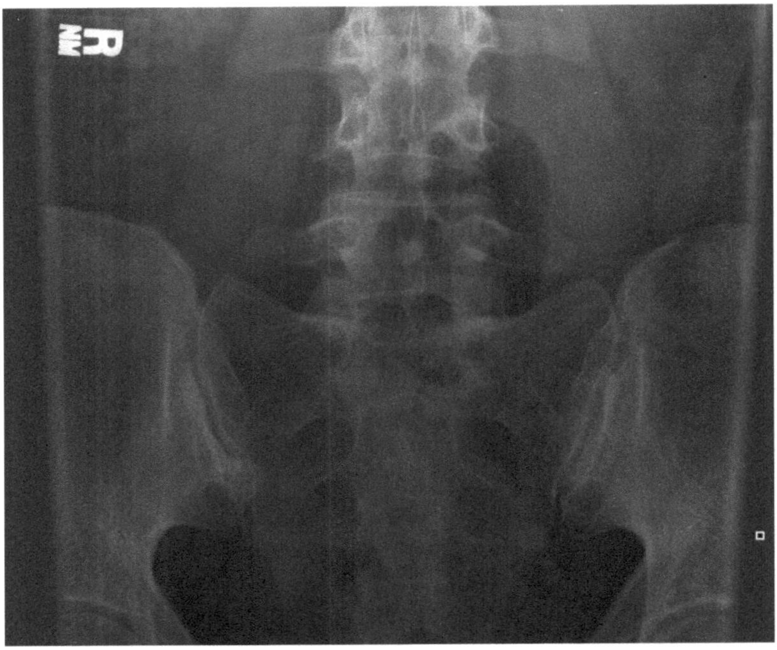

Fig. 4.2 Radiograph of SI joints with Ferguson view in a patient with psoriatic arthritis demonstrating erosive changes or the right sacroiliac joint

tors. Predictive factors for a more severe course of disease include presence of polyarticular disease, elevated levels of acute-phase reactants, evidence of erosive disease, as well as lack of response to initial therapeutic agents. In mild cases of psoriatic arthritis disease control may be achieved with the use of NSAIDs and intermittent intra-articular glucocorticoid injections. Use of oral glucocorticoids in patients with psoriatic arthritis should be avoided as it can be associated with worsening of the skin disease with tapering of the glucocorticoid therapy, possibly causing a generalized erythroderma flare of disease that could require hospitalization.

Patients presenting with more severe joint disease, unresponsive to NSAIDs, extra-articular manifestations and/or poor prognostic factors require use of systemic disease-modifying anti-rheumatic drugs (DMARDs) and/or biologic agents. Drugs such as methotrexate, PUVA (psoralen + ultraviolet A light), retinoic acid derivatives, cyclosporine and leflunomide have been shown to improve both the joint and skin manifestations of psoriatic arthritis. However, none of these medications have been shown to be effective in patients with axial disease or periarticular involvement including enthesitis or dactylitis. Biologic therapy with the Tumor necrosis factor (TNF) antagonists (etanercept, infliximab, adalimumab andgolimumab) has been shown to be effective in the treatment of peripheral arthritis and cutaneous psoriasis in several clinical trials [11]. Anti-TNF therapy has also been shown to be beneficial in patients with axial disease, enthesitis, and dactylitis [12]. Possible adverse effects of TNF therapies include reactivation of latent TB, infection, drug-induced lupus and even the development of psoriasis [13].

Questions

1. All of the following statements are true regarding inflammatory back pain EXCEPT:

   (a) Younger age of onset
   (b) Worsening of pain at night and in the early morning hours
   (c) Improvement of pain with rest
   (d) Prolonged morning stiffness lasting for more than 1 h
   (e) Improvement of pain with activity

2. A 29-year-old homosexual male is evaluated for a 3-month history of progressively worsening skin rash and painful swelling of his hands and feet. He admits also to malaise and about 5 kg of unintentional weight loss since the onset of his symptoms. His past medical history is unremarkable. He is not taking any medications and reports no known allergies. His family history is significant for hypertension and diabetes. He reports occasional alcohol use. He denies smoking or illicit drug use. He had multiple sexual partners in the past and does not use condoms regularly.

   Oh the physical examination he has multiple large erythematous plaques with overlying silvery scale involving his hands, elbows, upper arms, back, abdomen and lower extremities. There is tender swelling of multiple proximal interphalangeal (PIP) and metacarpophalangeal (MCP) joints bilaterally. He has also metatarsalgia (tenderness to squeeze of the metatarsophalangeal joints).

   Which of the following diagnostic studies should be performed next?

   (a) RF
   (b) Anti-CCP
   (c) Anti-nuclear antibody testing (ANA)
   (d) HLA-B27 testing
   (e) Testing for HIV

3. All of the following statements are true regarding radiographic features of psoriatic arthritis EXCEPT:

   (a) Involvement of the DIP joints
   (b) Presence of periarticular osteopenia
   (c) Presence of bony proliferation near joints (periostitis)
   (d) Asymmetric distribution of joint involvement
   (e) Presence of bony ankylosis

4. Which one of the following patterns is the most common presenting feature of psoriatic arthritis?

   (a) Asymmetrical oligoarticular arthritis
   (b) Symmetrical polyarthritis
   (c) Distal interphalangeal arthropathy
   (d) Arthritis mutilans
   (e) Spondylitis with or without sacroiliitis

5. A 42-year-old male is being evaluated for a 6-week history of painful swelling of his left ankle and right knee. Two weeks ago he was evaluated by his primary care physician with an arthrocentesis of the right knee revealing inflammatory fluid, but no evidence for infection and negative crystal analysis. His ESR was elevated at 40 mm/h; CBC, CMP, and urinalysis were unremarkable. His Lyme, Hepatitis, and HIV serologies were negative. He was started on scheduled ibuprofen which provided only minimal relief.

   He admits to a 15-year history of plaque psoriasis previously treated with topical therapy. His skin disease has been worse lately. He is otherwise healthy and reports no major complaints. His medications include ibuprofen and topical steroid ointment for his skin disease. He denies any known allergies. He reports that his mother has psoriasis as well. The family history is otherwise non-contributory. He is married and has 2 children. He denies any alcohol, tobacco, or illicit drug use.

   He is afebrile and vital signs are normal. On his physical examination he is noted to have psoriatic plaques overlying his elbows and knees. There is also swelling, tenderness, and increased warmth of the right knee and left ankle. The rest of the physical examination is unremarkable.

   Which of the following is the most appropriate medical treatment for this patient?

   (a) Prednisone
   (b) Methotrexate
   (c) Sulfasalazine
   (d) Hydroxychloroquine
   (e) Adalimumab

6. Which of the following factors are predictive for a more severe course of disease?

   (a) Presence of polyarticular disease
   (b) Evidence of erosive disease at the time of diagnosis
   (c) Elevated levels of acute-phase reactants
   (d) Lack of response to initial therapeutic agents
   (e) All of the above

7. A 64-year-old male with a 20-year history of psoriatic arthritis and knee osteoarthritis is being seen for a regular follow-up visit. In the past his disease manifested with axial involvement including unilateral sacroiliitis and asymmetric spondylitis. He has also a previous history of enthesitis. His disease has been

stable for years on his current therapy with an anti-TNF inhibitor. He continues to have some limitations in the range of motion in his neck and lower back; however, he denies any significant pain or morning stiffness. His major complaint remains chronic bilateral knee pain, which is worse with activity and improves with rest. His left knee is especially painful and prevents him from ambulation. His recent knee X-Rays revealed severe osteoarthritic changes in the left knee and moderate changes in the right. He is scheduled for a left total knee arthroplasty in a month.

He is otherwise doing well and reports no major complaints. He denies any chest pain, leg swelling, and shortness of breath, cough, or urinary complaints.

His past medical history is significant for a nonobstructive coronary artery disease and mild emphysema. He is a former smoker and denies alcohol or illicit drug use. His family history is unremarkable.

On physical examination he has limited extension and flexion in the cervical and lumbar spine. The extension of the neck is also painful. His Schober test reveals 3 cm of distraction, which is unchanged from his previous visit. There is crepitus in both knees; however, no effusion is present. Cardiovascular, pulmonary, and neurologic examinations are unremarkable.

His EKG is normal and lab work reveals normal CBC and CMP.

Which of the following perioperative diagnostic tests should be performed in this patient?

(a) Spirometry
(b) Echocardiogram
(c) Cervical spine radiograph with flexion and extension views
(d) Urinalysis
(e) All of the above

8. All of the following statements are true regarding extra-articular manifestations of psoriatic arthritis EXCEPT:

(a) Enthesitis
(b) Dactylitis
(c) Nail dystrophy: onycholysis, pitting or hyperkeratosis
(d) Erythema nodosum
(e) Uveitis

9. A 35-year-old male with a long standing history of psoriasis is being evaluated for a 6-month history of inflammatory back pain. He denies any other joint complaints. He took naproxen in the past, which helped with the back pain; however, it caused nausea and abdominal pain and therefore was discontinued by the patient. He had also tried Tylenol which provided no relief. Review of systems is otherwise unremarkable.

His past medical history is significant for psoriasis diagnosed in his early twenties. He reports no significant family history. He denies any known allergies. He does not take any prescription medications. He denies use of tobacco, alcohol, or illicit drug use.

His physical examination is significant for left sacroiliac joint tenderness. He has no evidence of peripheral arthritis. His left sacroiliac joint X-Ray is unremarkable; however, a subsequent MRI is done and is consistent with early erosive changes of the left sacroiliac joint.
Which of the following is the most appropriate medical treatment for this patient?

(a) Prednisone
(b) Methotrexate
(c) Sulfasalazine
(d) Etanercept
(e) Meloxicam

10. Which of the following statements are true regarding psoriatic arthritis?

(a) May present with both peripheral joint and axial skeleton involvement
(b) Frequently involves periarticular structures, such as tendons and ligaments and nails
(c) Familial aggregation of cases is common
(d) HLA-B27 positivity reported in 10–25% of patients
(e) Classified as a seronegative spondyloarthropathy
(f) All of the above

Answers: 1. (c), 2 (e), 3 (b), 4 (a), 5 (b), 6 (e), 7 (c), 8 (d), 9 (d), 10 (f).

References

1. Moll JM, Wright V. Psoriatic arthritis. Semin Arthritis Rheum. 1973;3:55–78.
2. Chandran V, Schentag CT, Gladman DD. Sensitivity and specificity of the CASPAR criteria for psoriatic arthritis in a family medicine clinic setting. J Rheumatol. 2008;35:2069–70.
3. Taylor W, Gladman D, Helliwell P, et al. Classification criteria for psoriatic arthritis: development of new criteria from a large international study. Arthritis Rheum. 2006;54:2665–73.
4. Bruce IN, Schentag CT, Gladman DD. Hyperuricemia in psoriatic arthritis: prevalence and associated features. J Clin Rheumatol. 2000;6:6–9.
5. Candia L, Marquez J, Gonzalez C, et al. Low frequency of anti-cyclic citrullinated peptide antibodies in psoriatic arthritis but not in cutaneous psoriasis. J Clin Heumatol. 2006;12:226–9.
6. Scarpa R, Oriente P, Pucino A, et al. Psoriaticarthritisinpsoriaticpatients. Br J Rheumatol. 1984;23:246–50.
7. Torre Alonso JC, Rodriguez Perez A, Arribas Castrillo JM, et al. Psoriatic arthritis (PA): a clinical, immunological and radiological study of 180 patients. Br J Rheumatol. 1991;30:245–50.
8. Marsal S, Armadans-Gil L, Martinez M, et al. Clinical, radiographic and HLA associations as markers for different patterns of psoriatic arthritis. Br J Rheumatol. 1999;38:332–7.
9. Helliwell P, Hickling P, Wright V. Do the radiological changes of classic ankylosing spondylitis differ from the changes found in the spondylitis associated with inflammatory bowel disease, psoriasis, and reactive arthritis? Ann Rheum Dis. 1998;57:135–40.
10. Olivieri I, Barozzi L, Favaro L, et al. Dactylitis in patients with seronegative spondylarthropathy: assessment by ultrasonography and magnetic resonance imaging. Arthritis Rheum. 1996;39:1524–9.

11. Heiberg MS, Kaufmann C, Rødevand E, et al. The comparative effectiveness of anti-TNF therapy and methotrexate in patients with psoriatic arthritis: 6 month results from a longitudinal, observational multicenter study. Ann Rheum Dis. 2007;66(8):1038.
12. Antoni CE, Kavanaugh A, Kirkham B, et al. Sustained benefits of infliximab therapy for dermatologic and articular manifestations of psoriatic arthritis: results from the infliximab multinational psoriatic arthritis controlled trial (IMPACT). J Arthritis Rheum. 2005;52(4):1227.
13. Cullen G, Kroshinsky D, et al. Psoriasis associated with anti-tumour necrosis factor therapy in inflammatory bowel disease: a new series and a review of 120 cases from the literature. Aliment Pharmacol Ther. 2011;34(11–12):1318–27. doi:10.1111/j.1365-2036.2011.04866.x. Epub 2011 Sep 29.

Part II
Arthritis and Systemic Diseases

Chapter 5
Immunoglobulin G4 (IgG4) Related Disease

Krati Chauhan, Phil A. Hart, and Vaidehi R. Chowdhary

Abstract IgG4-related disease (IgG4-RD) is a recently recognized syndrome characterized by frequent elevation of serum Ig4 levels and typical pathology of the affected organs. Biopsy shows lymphoplasmacytic inflammation, frequent eosinophils, storiform fibrosis, obliterative phlebitis and abundant IgG4-positive staining plasma cells. Disease manifestations often respond dramatically to steroid therapy.

Keywords IgG4 • Aortitis • Autoimmune pancreatitis • Orbital pseudolymphoma

Case 1

A 59-year-old male presented with elevated creatinine of 6 months duration, discovered at the time of a routine physical. He complained of recent onset of fatigue and severe muscle pains in thighs. The thigh pain that had been present for many years was worse in the last 6 months. He would occasionally get "sinus headaches" and had experienced multiple attacks of sinusitis in the past. He denied a history of fever, weight loss, skin rashes, joint pains and visual complaints. Review of systems was otherwise negative.

He was extensively evaluated elsewhere and a presumptive diagnosis of vasculitis was made. Cyclophosphamide and prednisone therapy was advised and he sought a second opinion at our hospital.

K. Chauhan, M.D. (✉) • V.R. Chowdhary, M.D.
Division of Rheumatology, Department of Medicine, Mayo Clinic College of Medicine,
200 First Street SW, Rochester, MN 55905, USA
e-mail: chauhan.krati@mayo.edu; chowdhary.vaidehi@mayo.edu

P.A. Hart, M.D.
Division of Gastroenterology, Department of Medicine, Mayo Clinic College of Medicine,
Rochester, MN, USA

M. Mahmoudi (ed.), *Challenging Cases in Rheumatology and Diseases of the Immune System*, DOI 10.1007/978-1-4614-5088-7_5,
© Springer Science+Business Media, LLC 2013

Past Medical History

Past medical history was complex and significant for the following: (1) Pituitary insufficiency: This was diagnosed 14 years prior to presentation. Evaluation revealed a peri-pituitary mass and thickened pituitary stalk. Biopsy of the stalk showed dense fibrous tissue with lymphocytic infiltrate. (2) Sinusitis status post two sinus surgeries. Maxillary sinus biopsy at surgery had shown polypoid respiratory mucosa with chronic inflammation, numerous eosinophils, and non-necrotizing granulomatous inflammation. Definitive vasculitis and areas of necrosis were not seen. (3) Coronary artery disease. (4) Asthma. (5) Chronic peripheral eosinophilia ranging from 8.7 to 17.6% (normal 0–7%).

Physical Exam

Vitals: Height: 184.0 cm. Weight: 95.40 kg. BMI: 28.178 kg/m^2. Temperature: 36.6 °C. Pulse Rate: 77/min, regular, Blood Pressure: 121/60 mmHg, (Right arm) standing. General: Well developed, well nourished, in no acute distress. Eyes showed mild ptosis of left lid (present since birth) with normal fundus and visual field examination. A small shotty node was palpated in the inguinal region with no other lymphadenopathy. ENT, thyroid, skin, lung, heart, abdomen, joint, neurologic, and spine examinations were normal.

Laboratory values: Hemoglobin, white blood cell count and platelet count were normal. Differential count showed eosinophilia (eosinophils 1.36×10^9/L, normal $0.05–0.50 \times 10^9$/L) and a peripheral blood smear showed rouleaux formation. ESR and CRP were elevated at 104 mm/at 1 h (normal 0–22 mm/1 h) and 3.7 mg/dL (normal < 0.8 mg/dL) respectively. Serum creatinine was 2.6 mg/dL (normal 0.8–1.3 mg/dL, patient's baseline 1.2 mg/dL) and BUN 41 mg/dL (normal 8–24 mg/dL). Urinalysis showed protein/osmolality ratio of 0.54 (normal < 0.12), but was otherwise normal. 24-h urinary protein was 964 mg (normal 0–150 mg in 24 h). Other blood chemistries namely liver biochemistries, uric acid, serum electrolytes and serum glucose were unremarkable. Hepatitis serologies were negative for HBsAg and HCV. Serum protein electrophoresis showed polyclonal hypergammaglobulinemia, immunofixation and urine protein electrophoresis were normal. Autoantibodies, namely rheumatoid factor, antinuclear antibodies, dsDNA and anti-neutrophil cytoplasmic antibodies (ANCA) were negative.

Renal ultrasound showed bilateral cortical thinning and possible focal scarring lower pole right kidney. The right kidney measured 10.9 cm, and left kidney 12.4 cm. Unenhanced CT chest and abdomen showed paraspinal masses along the thoracic spine at about the level of T7 through T10. The appearance of masses was felt to be suspicious for lymphoma. Soft tissue thickening adjacent to the left lateral border of the descending thoracic aorta, abdominal aorta level of the mesenteric and renal artery origins, and above the aortic bifurcation was noted. Diffuse pancreatic atrophy and uniform wall thickening of the distal stomach and gastric antrum were seen. Although the findings were nonspecific, a possibility of gastric lymphoma was suggested.

Differential Diagnosis

The patient presented with renal failure of recent onset, paraspinal soft tissue masses, aortic thickening and a past medical history of pituitary insufficiency, sinusitis, lung disease (asthma), suggestive of a multisystem disease process.

1. *Vasculitides*: Vasculitic processes like granulomatosis with polyangiitis (GPA, formerly Wegener's) can present with pituitary involvement, sinusitis, and renal insufficiency. Kidney involvement typically presents with glomerulonephritis, red blood cells and casts are usually seen in urine that were absent in this case. Histopathology of kidney shows pauci-immune, segmental necrotizing crescentic glomerulonephritis and biopsy from other organs shows necrotizing granulomatous inflammation. Tumor like masses have been reported in GPA and are seen most commonly in breast or kidney. A positive PR3 and c-ANCA is seen in most patients with multisystem GPA whereas this patient had negative tests.

   Polyarteritis nodosa (PAN) can cause renal insufficiency with normal urinary sediment and negative ANCA serology. PAN is typically associated with hepatitis B infection which was absent in this patient and would not explain other organ involvement (pituitary, sinusitis and paraspinal masses).

   Peripheral eosinophilia, sinusitis and history of asthma can be seen in Churg–Strauss vasculitis. Lung abnormalities include non-cavitatory nodules, pleural effusion or infiltrates. Mononeuritis multiplex is the most common neurologic involvement and pituitary disease is rare. Biopsy shows necrotizing vasculitis with eosinophilia.

   Aortic thickening can be seen in large vessel vasculitis like temporal arteritis or Takayasu's disease; however, patient's clinical scenario was not consistent with large vessel disease.
2. *Granulomatous Disorders*: Sarcoidosis can present with granulomatous hypophysitis. Lung involvement manifest as bilateral hilar adenopathy and/or interstitial lung disease which were not seen in his case. Kidney involvement may include nephrocalcinosis or rarely granulomatous lesions. Aortic thickening is exceedingly rare and there were no articular or cutaneous manifestations of sarcoid.
3. *Hematologic diseases*: Lymphoma as suggested in multiple imaging studies needs to be considered in the differential. Infiltration from lymphomatous processes can present with renal insufficiency, paraspinal masses, and peripheral eosinophilia. However, the patient's distant pituitary disease would remain unexplained by lymphoma. Histiocytic disorders can involve the pituitary; however, other characteristics were not noted. Hypereosinophilic syndromes can present with multiorgan manifestations; however, the organs involved were not typical for this condition.

4. *Miscellaneous*: Retroperitoneal fibrosis (RPF) can present with aortic thickening and renal insufficiency secondary to ureteral obstruction. Although aortic thickening was noted the fibrotic changes of RPF were not seen. RPF can be associated with other fibroinflammatory processes like sclerosing mesenteritis and IgG4 related disease (IgG4RD). The pancreatic atrophy noted in abdomen raises the possibility of autoimmune pancreatitis (AIP), the pancreatic manifestation of IgG4-RD; however, this is a nonspecific finding and can be seen in those with a history of pancreatic disease or advanced age. In addition to pancreatic disease, IgG4-RD can involve pituitary, lungs, kidney, aorta, salivary glands, biliary tree and eye. The diagnosis is made on the basis of typical organ involvement supported by serologic, radiographic and histopathologic findings.

Lastly the present episode of renal insufficiency may be completely independent of previous medical problems and other renal diseases like chronic tubulointerstitial nephritis would need to be excluded. Renal biopsy would be a helpful investigation.

Working diagnosis: Atypical GPA or a low grade lymphoma.

Workup: The following additional tests were obtained. Angiotensin converting enzyme (A.C.E) 31 U/L (Normal, 7–46 U/L), total immunoglobulin 1,390 mg/dL (Normal 600–1,500 mg/dL), IgG1 473 mg/dL (Normal 490–1,140 mg/dL), IgG2 599 mg/dL (Normal 150–640 mg/dL), IgG3 49.0 mg/dL (Normal 20–110 mg/dL), and IgG4 833 mg/dL (Normal 8.0–140.0 mg/dL).

Imaging

1. MRI chest and abdomen: In addition to findings noted on CT scan MRI showed diffuse pancreatic atrophy with slight dilatation and irregularity of the main pancreatic duct. There was abnormal perfusion to both kidneys with bilateral cortical infarcts.
2. MRA thoracic and abdominal aorta: There was asymmetric wall thickening in the aortic arch, more prominent along the left side. Circumferential wall thickening of the descending thoracic aorta extending from the level of the pulmonary arteries to the level of the diaphragm, abdominal aorta at the level of the celiac artery origin and extending to the level of the bifurcation with involvement of the origin and proximal left renal artery (see Fig 5.1a) was noted.

Biopsy: Biopsy of the paraspinal mass was obtained and previously obtained biopsies were reviewed.

1. Renal Biopsy: Glomeruli were obsolescent with features of hypertensive nephrosclerosis. There were no features to suggest vasculitis. Immunofluorescent and electron microscopy showed no evidence of immune complex deposits.
2. Fine needle aspiration and biopsy of paraspinal mass: Chronic lymphoplasmacytic infiltrate and storiform fibrosis (see Fig. 5.1b). Immunoperoxidase studies showed a mixed population of T cells (CD3 positive) and B cells (CD20 positive).

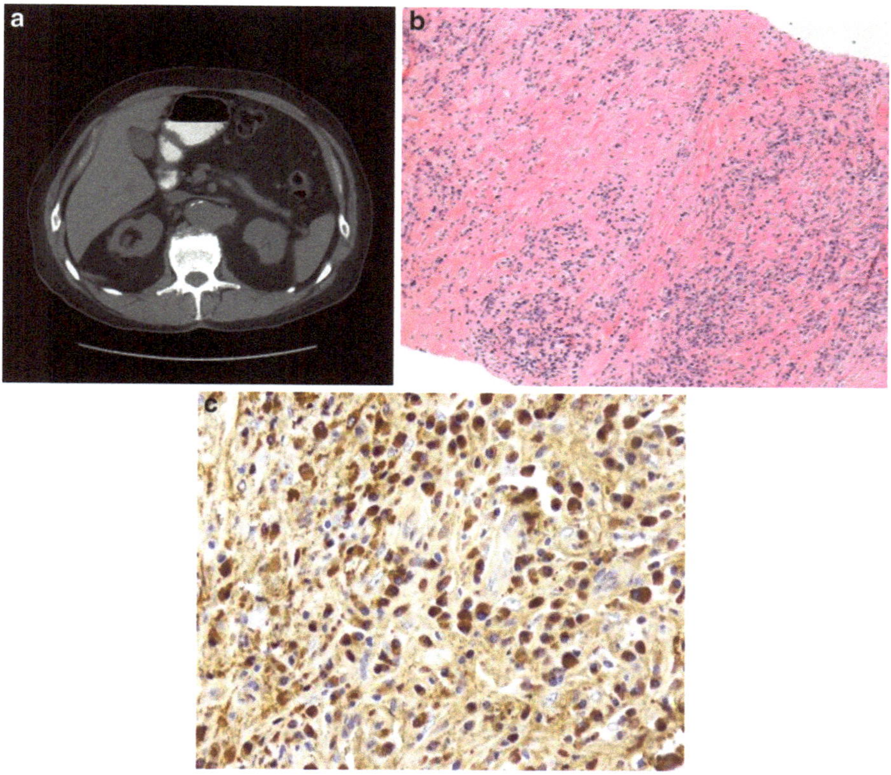

Fig. 5.1 (**a**) CT chest (non-contrast) showing thickening of aorta. (**b**) Biopsy of right paraspinal soft tissue mass showing lymphoplasmacytic infiltrate and classic storiform fibrosis. (**c**) Abundant IgG4+ staining plasma cells on immunohistochemical stain (power ×40)

The plasma cells were polyclonal for kappa and lambda immunoglobulin light chains. Immunohistochemical stain for IgG4, showed abundant IgG4-positive staining plasma cells (see Fig. 5.1c).

What Is Your Diagnosis and Why?

A unifying diagnosis for this patient's clinical scenario, including peripheral eosinophilia, aortitis, paraspinal pseudotumors, and pancreatic atrophy, could be explained by IgG4-RD. Although membranous nephropathy and tubulointerstitial nephritis can be seen in IgG4-RD, the renal biopsy did not suggest either of these etiologies. Rather, the renal insufficiency was felt to be secondary to extension of the periaortic process along the renal blood vessels causing segments of ischemia and/or infarction. In the setting of serum IgG4 elevation greater than two times the upper limit and supportive histopathology and immunohistochemistry, the diagnosis of IgG4-RD is confirmed. The patient was treated with steroids and had reduction in serum creatinine levels, IgG4 levels that subsequently normalized and size of the paraspinal masses. He relapsed following discontinuation of steroids, but responded to re-induction with steroids and addition of mycophenolate mofetil. He has remained in clinical is serologic remission without disease relapse or new organ involvement for last 7 years.

Final Diagnosis

IgG4 related disease.

Case 2

A 65-year-old woman presented for evaluation of progressive lacrimal gland enlargement and diplopia of 3 months duration.

Past Medical History

1. Irritable bowel syndrome.
2. Generalized lymphadenopathy that was stable in size for more than 5 years.
3. Recurrent urinary tract infections.

Physical Exam

General: no distress; HEENT: bilateral proptosis, no oral lesions; Lymph: palpable, small left inguinal node, otherwise no cervical, supraclavicular, axillary, or right inguinal lymphadenopathy
Laboratory analysis: The following basic studies were within normal limits: hemoglobin, white blood cell count, platelet count, blood chemistries, and TSH level. Additional studies included: ESR 17 mm/h, CRP 3.99 mg/L (normal <3.0 mg/L), rheumatoid factor 63 IU/mL (normal <15 IU/mL), and negative ANA antibodies. Urinalysis with microscopy was normal.

Imaging

Chest X-ray: Normal. CT head and neck: showed bilateral enlargement of the lacrimal glands and extraocular muscles concerning for lymphoma. PET scan: Increased uptake in the pancreatic head and tail and less intense activity in the enlarged lymph nodes.

With the Presented Data What Is Your Working Diagnosis?

This patient presented with bilateral lacrimal gland enlargement and generalized lymphadenopathy. The term orbital pseudotumor (OP) is used to describe inflammation of orbital structures or adnexa simulating a tumor. Clinical features are pain, proptosis, diplopia, decreased visual acuity, and swelling around the eyes and orbit. Several conditions can cause OP.

Abscesses or cellulitis of the eye can present as orbital pseudotumor. Noninfectious causes include sarcoidosis, GPA, thyroid ophthalmopathy, lymphoma, and other metastatic malignancies. Often a biopsy is required to make the diagnosis and exclude malignancy. In this patient the lack of hilar lymphadenopathy or interstitial lung disease makes sarcoidosis unlikely, and, normal urinary sediment, lack of ear, lung or kidney involvement makes GPA unlikely. Thyroid ophthalmopathy can precede, coincide, or follow the diagnosis of hypo- or hyperthyroidism. Most patients with thyroid ophthalmopathy will provide a history of Grave's; however, some may have Hashimoto's disease, or even be in a euthyroid state. In these euthyroid patients the presence of anti-thyroid receptor antibodies supports the diagnosis. Lid lag and lid retraction are characteristic findings of this condition. Orbital lymphoma is the most common malignant tumor of the orbit and is typically non-Hodgkin's lymphoma. Biopsy is necessary to demonstrate this diagnosis. It can be associated with systemic lymphoma in 1/3 of cases, so evaluation is required to exclude distant disease. Orbital involvement can be seen in IgG4-RD and biopsy is needed to make the diagnosis.
Working diagnosis: Orbital pseudotumor, worrisome for lymphoma.
Workup: MRI abdomen/MRCP showed a distal common bile duct stricture, and a hypointense mass-like area in the head of the pancreas, delayed enhancement, and multifocal strictures of the main pancreatic duct. These radiographic findings were consistent with diagnosis of autoimmune pancreatitis. Serum IgG4 level was elevated at 153 mg/dL (normal 8.0–140.0 mg/dL). Previous lymph node biopsies were reviewed and showed reactive hyperplasia without evidence of malignancy. The right lacrimal gland and inferior rectus muscle were biopsied and showed dense lymphocytic infiltrates with abundant (>10/hpf) IgG4-positive plasma cells.

What Is Your Diagnosis and Why?

The mildly elevated serum IgG4, radiographic findings of autoimmune pancreatitis and abundant IgG4 positive cells on biopsy confirm the diagnosis of IgG4-related orbital pseudotumor.

Final Diagnosis: IgG4-Related Orbital Pseudotumor

Treatment with prednisone resulted in improvement in lymphadenopathy, proptosis, resolution of the biliary stricture, and improvement in the radiographic appearance of the pancreas abnormalities. She relapsed during steroid taper and was treated with rituximab. Clinical and serologic response was noted following the fourth infusion. The orbital pseudolymphoma and submandibular gland enlargement resolved, and she has been without disease relapse with more than 2 years of follow-up.

Discussion

History, Definition, and Prevalence

The history of IgG4-RD is intimately linked to that of autoimmune pancreatitis (AIP). In 1995, Yoshida et al. described a case of pancreatitis with hypergammaglobulinemia, autoantibodies, dramatic response to steroids and coined the term "autoimmune pancreatitis." In 2001 the association of elevated serum IgG4 with sclerosing pancreatitis was noted. Kamisawa and colleagues, in 2003 described the systemic nature of this disease and introduced the term IgG4 related autoimmune disease. Since then many names have been used to describe this entity including IgG4-associated disease, IgG4 syndrome, hyper IgG4 disease, IgG4 positive multiorgan lymphoproliferative syndrome (MOLPS), IgG4-related systemic sclerosing disease, IgG4 related systemic disease, IgG4-related autoimmune disease and systemic IgG4-related plasmacytic syndrome (SIPS). In an effort to simplify the nomenclature the term IgG4-related disease has been accepted to describe the syndrome [1]. The disease is only currently being recognized and exact incidence and prevalence is not known. Much literature on this entity comes from Asia especially Japan and the incidence is estimated to be 0.28–1.08/100,000 population [1].

Signs and Symptoms

IgG4-RD commonly develops in organs with ductal/glandular complexes like pancreas, salivary glands (exceptions aorta, retroperitoneum, etc.), results in their tumorous swelling, is associated with elevated serum IgG4 levels (>135 mg/dL) and has a characteristic pathology on biopsy of involved organs [2]. The pathologic features described include diffuse lymphoplasmacytic infiltrates, obliterative phlebitis, a characteristic pattern of fibrosis called storiform referring to radial arrangement of fibroblasts, reminiscent of blades of a pinwheel, and abundant, IgG4 positive staining plasma cells.

The disease commonly affects middle aged males; the mean age at diagnosis for AIP is 59–68 years and the male to female ratio is 4–8:1. It can involve various organs such as pancreas (AIP), bile ducts (IgG4 related sclerosing cholangitis), salivary glands (chronic sclerosing sialadenitis and Mikulicz disease), lacrimal gland (chronic sclerosing dacryoadenitis, orbital pseudotumor), aorta (inflammatory aneurysm, noninfectious aortitis), lung (nodular or diffuse inflammation), kidney (tubulointerstitial nephritis) and fibroinflammatory syndromes like retroperitoneal fibrosis, sclerosing mediastinitis, etc. The following discussion will focus on the rheumatic manifestations of this disease.

Salivary and Lacrimal Gland Disease

1. *Mikulicz disease* (*MD*): In 1888 Johann von Mikulicz-Radecki described the case of a man with bilateral parotid and submandibular gland enlargement which was later referred to as MD. In 1933 Sjogren described keratoconjunctivitis sicca (KCS) and enlarged salivary glands. Later in 1950 Morgan and Castleman examined cases of MD and concluded that this was one manifestation of Sjogren syndrome (SS) and MD came to be synonymous with SS. However, MD is a distinct entity from SS and the following differences between the two have been described [3]. MD is more common in men whereas SS is female predominant. Swelling of salivary glands is persistent in MD, whereas patients with SS have recurrent but not persistent enlargement. Symptoms of KCS are prominent in SS but not in MD. Allergic manifestations are more common in MD compared to SS (40% vs. 7% respectively). Antinuclear antibodies, anti-Ro, anti-La antibodies are more frequent in SS. Serum levels of IgG4 are frequently elevated in MD but normal in SS. Histopathology of salivary gland in MD shows lymphocytes with numerous plasma cells, abundant IgG4+ positive staining plasma cells with an increased ratio of IgG4+/IgG cells. In contrast tissue infiltration in SS is predominantly lymphocytic with minimal IgG4 tissue infiltration. Response to steroid is dramatic in MD with reduction in salivary gland swelling and improved function in contrast to SS patients who are frequently unresponsive. Recently, the term MD has been replaced with by IgG4-related sialadenitis to fit the common nomenclature for IgG4-RD.

Kuttner's tumor or chronic sclerosing sialadenitis is another manifestation of IgG4-RD. The term Küttner's tumor refers to enlargement of the submandibular gland, irrespective of the etiology, and is most commonly due to sialoliths. It is important to recognize IgG4 associated sialadenitis as the disease is steroid responsive thus potentially avoiding unnecessary surgery. Organ histology shows interlobular fibrosis, follicular hyperplasia, obliterative phlebitis and abundant IgG4+ plasma cells.

Eye Disease

IgG4-RD is increasingly recognized as a cause of previously idiopathic orbital disease, and can often accompany salivary gland disease. The pathologic changes in the lacrimal glands (i.e., IgG4-related dacryoadenitis) are similar to those seen in IgG4-RD sialadenitis. An IgG4-related orbital pseudotumor, as presented in Case 2, is an inflammatory mass consisting of lymphoplasmacytic infiltrate, fibrosis, and

IgG4 infiltration that can affect a combination of the lacrimal gland, extraocular muscles (IgG4-related orbital myositis), and other portions of the orbit. These abnormalities are collectively referred to as IgG4-related ophthalmic disease. Similar IgG4-related pseudotumors have been described in other organs including the lung, liver, and breast.

Aorta

Aortic involvement can be seen in several patients and is considered under following subheadings.

1. *IgG4 associated aortitis*: Noninfectious aortitis can be seen in a variety of rheumatic diseases like giant cell arteritis, Takayasu's arteritis, systemic lupus erythematosus, rheumatoid arthritis, etc. Pathology shows either giant cell or lymphoplasmacytic inflammation. IgG4 related aortitis is described in the subset with lymphoplasmacytic inflammation and frequently involves thoracic aorta. It is a very rare manifestation and is seen in 0.5–1.6% of all thoracic aortic resections and 9% of all thoracic noninfectious aortitis. Involvement of the aortic arch and saccular form are more commonly seen in IgG4-thoracic aortic aneurysm (TAA), in contrast to non-IgG4-TAA [4].
2. *Inflammatory abdominal aortic aneurysm* (*IAAA*): The term inflammatory aortic aneurysm is applied to abdominal aortic aneurysm characterized by a thick aneurysmal wall, perianeurysmal or retroperitoneal fibrosis, and adhesions to surrounding organs. The triad of back or abdominal pain, weight loss and elevated acute phase reactants is highly suggestive of IAAA. As with thoracic aortitis this is an extremely rare manifestation and seen in 0.3% of abdominal aortic aneurysms and is commonly asymptomatic. Allergic disorders and autoimmune diseases are higher in IgG4 AAA and other risk factors for atherosclerosis lower. Typically IAAA and periaortitis have more inflammation in adventitia. IgG4 related IAAA show frequent eosinophilic infiltration, lymph follicle formation, obliterative phlebitis and higher numbers of IgG4 positive cells compared to non-IgG4 related AAA. The presence of eosinophils and focal granulomatous inflammation in some suggests that in some cases the IgG4 plasma cells may be occurring in the setting of a localized allergic/hypersensitivity reaction. A media-predominant form of IgG4-related aortitis as seen in thoracic aorta has not yet been reported in the abdominal aorta. Surgery is difficult; steroids may help reduce the inflammation but paradoxically can increase risk of rupture due to wall thinning.

Retroperitoneal Fibrosis

IgG4 related RPF is a subset of "idiopathic" RPF. Imaging findings show that the disease presents more commonly with inflammatory masses rather than diffuse involvement, often involving the abdominal aorta, the kidneys or the ureters. Patients frequently develop renal failure as a consequence of ureteral obstruction, and unfortunately in patients with dense fibrosis this can occasionally be irreversible despite steroid treatment. Patients may also have involvement of other organs and response to steroid therapy is good. It should be noted that obliterative phlebitis may not be seen in needle biopsy specimen due to small size.

Pathophysiology: Much of the literature on pathogenesis and treatment comes from AIP. The hallmark serologic abnormality of this disease is elevated IgG4 levels.

Biology of IgG4

There are four subclasses of immunoglobulin G (IgG) numbered 1 through 4 in order of their discovery and serum concentrations. IgG1 is most abundant constituting 43–75% of total IgG and IgG4 responsible for <5%. Over time the cut-off values have changed based on variations in assays utilized, but the current normal range for IgG4 levels in adults >18 years of age is 2.4–121 mg/dL (Mayo Medical Laboratories). In the normal state, levels of IgG4 do not fluctuate much and are tightly regulated. IgG4 antibodies are unusual in that they cannot form large immune complexes or bind C1q to activate classical complement pathway [5]. The effector function is also reduced compared to other immunoglobulin subtypes due to reduced binding to Fcγ receptors.

IgG4 arises after prolonged antigenic stimulation. Elevated levels are found in atopic dermatitis, allergies and parasitic diseases and are also associated with elevated IgE. IgG4 levels also increase during allergen desensitization which suggests a protective or an anti-inflammatory role for IgG4. However, in pemphigus vulgaris and pemphigus foliaceus a direct pathogenic role has been demonstrated, with an IgG4 antibody directed against desmoglein mediating direct disruption of the epithelial layer. It is unclear if the elevated IgG4 levels in IgG4-RD are pathogenic or represent a compensatory protective response.

Genetic susceptibility plays a role and several HLA and non-HLA genes have been described. Autoantibodies to lactoferrin and carbonic anhydrase have been described in patients with AIP and molecular mimicry with H pylori could potentially explain this association. Majority of studies show that Th2 immune response is activated in these patients and peripheral blood mononuclear cells isolated from patients produce high levels of Th2 cytokines IL-4, IL-5, IL-10 and IL-13. Of specific interest, IL-10 enhances IgG4 production from B cells. The Th2 shift in immune response also increases IgE levels and eosinophil organ infiltration that is commonly seen in these patients. TGF-β is a powerful pro-fibrotic cytokine that is elevated in patients and may mediate the fibrosis seen in various organs.

Table 5.1 Clinical diagnostic criteria for IgG4-RD (adapted from [6])

1. Clinical examination showing characteristic diffuse/localized swelling or masses in single or multiple organs
2. Hematological examination shows elevated serum IgG4 concentrations(135 ≥ mg/dl)
3. Histopathologic examination showing:
   (a) Marked lymphocyte and plasma cell infiltration and fibrosis
   (b) Infiltration of IgG4+ plasma cells: ratio of IgG4+/IgG + cells > 40% and >10 IgG4+ plasma cells/HPF

Definite diagnosis: criteria (1) + (2) + (3)
Probable diagnosis: criteria (1) + (3)
Possible diagnosis: criteria (1) + (2)

Diagnostic Evaluation

Characteristic organ involvement, elevated serum IgG4 levels, typical histopathology and immunohistochemistry are supportive of a diagnosis of IgG4-RD. Diagnostic criteria for AIP are the best-described; however, a recent international consensus on these criteria was not reached until recently. Criteria for diagnosis of IgG4-RD and lesions in various organs like kidney, Mikulicz disease have been proposed and summarized in Table 5.1 [6].

There are numerous nonspecific serum abnormalities seen in patients with AIP and IgG4-RD, including peripheral eosinophilia, elevated IgE, gamma globulin, and total IgG levels, and autoantibodies (ANA and rheumatoid factor). When considering a diagnosis of IgG4-RD without pancreatic involvement, histologic evaluation of available tissue is incredibly helpful. All features of the described pathology above may not be present in tissues depending on the sample organ (e.g., obliterative phlebitis is not seen in lymph nodes). Immunohistochemistry staining for IgG4 plasma cells is often helpful, with evaluation including the number of positive staining plasma cells per hpf as well as the ratio of IgG4+/IgG plasma cells per hpf. Abnormal cutoffs of >10 IgG4-positive staining plasma cells and a ratio of >40% have been used historically; however, there are now different cutoff values in the absolute number of IgG4-positve cells based on the type and method of tissue sampled [7].

Treatment

There are no approved treatments for IgG4-RD and all agents described here are off-label. Corticosteroids are the mainstay of therapy and diagnosis should be reconsidered in patients with no objective response to steroids. Organ involvement can be investigated by imaging and PET may be helpful in fully defining disease extent and activity. Although steroids are accepted by most as first line treatment for IgG4-RD, there are no prospective data to support this practice. Moreover, there is not a global consensus regarding the starting dose, tapering regimen, or duration of steroid treatment. Adding to the confusion is the fact that spontaneous remissions in AIP have been described. A large Japanese study involving 563 patients showed spontaneous remission in 74% of patients [8].

Treatment Strategy

The two main philosophies for steroid treatment include providing a lower dose for a longer duration of time vs. high dose prednisone with a more rapid taper. The Japanese approach consists of treatment with prednisolone (0.5 mg/kg) for 2–4 weeks, tapered over 3–6 months to 5 mg daily [9]. In contrast, our approach has been to treat with 40 mg prednisone for 4 weeks then following demonstration of clinical response to taper by 5 mg per week without providing maintenance treatment (duration of 11 weeks) [10]. Remission rates are >95% with both of these strategies.

The Japanese strategy involves maintenance therapy with 2.5–5 mg steroids for 6 months to 3 years. The relapse rate appeared to be lower in their patients who did receive maintenance steroids compared to those treated with a shorter duration of steroids. However, since almost a quarter of these patients relapsed despite long-term steroid therapy, we have not typically offered our patients maintenance therapy.

Treatment of Relapses: Most relapses occur in the first 3 years following diagnosis and are steroid responsive. Relapses can involve organs different organs than those at the initial presentation, with pancreas and biliary disease seen most frequently. Our approach has been to start patients on an immunomodulator (typically Azathioprine 2–2.5 mg/kg/day for 12–18 months) following their first or second relapse. Other immunosuppressants that have been used with success, but in which supportive data are limited include mycophenolate mofetil (750 mg twice daily), methotrexate, cyclophosphamide, imatinib, tocilizumab and bortezomib. Recently, rituximab, an anti-CD 20 monoclonal antibody has shown promising results in patients with IgG4-RD with and without AIP.

Disease Monitoring

Serum IgG4 levels are not reliable for monitoring therapy response or predicting disease relapse. Despite clinical and radiographic remission, levels can remain elevated in over half of patients following treatment. Additional studies to identify a more reliable marker of disease activity are needed.

Conclusion

IgG4-RD is a newly emerging and fascinating disease characterized by multiorgan involvement, typical histology and frequently elevated serum IgG4 levels. More studies are needed regarding natural history and treatment of rheumatic manifestations. The role of IgG4 in disease pathogenesis needs to be explored further.

Questions

1. All of the following can be seen in patients with IgG4-RD except-
   (a) Autoimmune pancreatitis
   (b) Orbital pseudotumor
   (c) Salivary gland enlargement
   (d) Glomerulonephritis with necrotizing granulomatous vasculitis
2. Tissue biopsy in patients with IgG4-RD may show the following histopathologic features except-
   (a) Lymphoplasmacytic infiltrates
   (b) Non-caseating granulomas
   (c) Storiform fibrosis
   (d) Obliterative phlebitis
3. Levels of serum IgG4 can be elevated in all except-
   (a) Parasitic infections
   (b) Sarcoidosis
   (c) Atopic dermatitis
   (d) Allergic disorders
4. Choose the best correct response, Sjogren syndrome patients –
   a) Are predominantly male
   (b) Have persistent parotid swelling
   (c) Have positive ANA, anti-Ro and anti-La
   (d) Respond dramatically to steroids
5. All of the following are supportive of a diagnosis of IgG4-RD with the exception of –
   (a) Serum IgG4 level of 200 mg/dL
   (b) Radiographic evidence of diffuse pancreatic enlargement
   (c) Steroid-responsive lymphadenopathy and submandibular enlargement
   (d) 5 IgG4-positive plasma cells/hpf, 20% ratio of IgG4+/IgG cells/hpf from a lymph node biopsy

6. Orbital pseudotumor can be seen in all except-
   (a) Sarcoidosis
   (b) Non-Hodgkin's lymphoma
   (c) Granulomatosis with polyangiitis
   (d) Myasthenia gravis
7. Corticosteroid therapy is associated with the following adverse effects except-
   (a) Hyperglycemia
   (b) Hypothyroidism
   (c) Cushing's syndrome
   (d) Hypercholesterolemia
8. Choose the best response, IgG4-RD is-
   (a) More common in women
   (b) Typically unresponsive to steroids
   (c) Always presents with pancreatitis
   (d) Associated with allergic disorders
9. IgG4 antibodies are directly pathogenic in-
   (a) Pemphigus foliaceus
   (b) IgG4-RD
   (c) Atopic dermatitis
   (d) Contact allergy
10. Thoracic aortitis can be seen in all except-
    (a) Horton disease
    (b) IgG4-RD
    (c) Cogan's syndrome
    (d) Marfan syndrome

Answers: Q.1. (d), Q2. (b), Q.3. (b), Q.4. (c), Q.5. (d), Q.6. (d), Q.7. (b), Q.8. (d), Q.9. (a), Q.10. (d).

Acknowledgments We gratefully acknowledge assistance from Dr. James E. Huprich, Dr. Thomas C. Smyrk and Dr. Suresh T. Chari. VRC is funded by National Institute of Arthritis and Musculoskeletal Diseases—K23 AR057815-01A1, Ronald F. Kinney Executive Dean for Research Career Development Award, Mayo Foundation.

References

1. Umehara H, Okazaki K, Masaki Y, et al. A novel clinical entity, IgG4-related disease (IgG4RD): general concept and details. Mod Rheumatol. 2012;22(1):1–14.
2. Masaki Y, Kurose N, Umehara H. IgG4-related disease: a novel lymphoproliferative disorder discovered and established in Japan in the 21st century. J Clin Exp Hematop. 2011;51(1):13–20.

3. Masaki Y, Dong L, Kurose N, et al. Proposal for a new clinical entity, IgG4-positive multiorgan lymphoproliferative syndrome: analysis of 64 cases of IgG4-related disorders. Ann Rheum Dis. 2009;68(8):1310–5.
4. Stone JH, Khosroshahi A, Deshpande V, Stone JR. IgG4-related systemic disease accounts for a significant proportion of thoracic lymphoplasmacytic aortitis cases. Arthritis Care Res (Hoboken). 2010;62(3):316–22.
5. Aalberse RC, Stapel SO, Schuurman J, Rispens T. Immunoglobulin G4: an odd antibody. Clin Exp Allergy. 2009;39(4):469–77.
6. Umehara H, Okazaki K, Masaki Y, et al. Comprehensive diagnostic criteria for IgG4-related disease (IgG4-RD), 2011. Mod Rheumatol. 2012;22(1):21–30.
7. Deshpande V, Zen Y, Chan JK, et al. Consensus statement on the pathology of IgG4-related disease. Mod Pathol. 2012;25(9):1181–92. doi: 10.1038/modpathol.2012.72.
8. Kamisawa T, Shimosegawa T, Okazaki K, et al. Standard steroid treatment for autoimmune pancreatitis. Gut. 2009;58(11):1504–7.
9. Kamisawa T, Okazaki K, Kawa S, et al. Japanese consensus guidelines for management of autoimmune pancreatitis: III. Treatment and prognosis of AIP. J Gastroenterol. 2010;45(5):471–7.
10. Pannala R, Chari ST. Corticosteroid treatment for autoimmune pancreatitis. Gut. 2009;58(11):1438–9.

Chapter 6
Sarcoidosis

Christian M. Sebat and Richart W. Harper

Abstract Sarcoidosis is a systemic granulomatous disease of unknown causes that can afflict virtually every organ system in the body. The infiltrating granulomas and chronic persistent inflammation in tissues and organs are presumed to be the consequence of an abnormal systemic and/or local immune response to either one or multiple unknown antigens in genetically susceptible adolescents and adults. The precise etiology of sarcoidosis has eluded the best minds in Medicine for over a century but that does not preclude our ability to diagnose sarcoidosis in a timely manner. The following two cases are representative of the difficult challenges frequently encountered in the diagnosis and management of this disease with protean and seemingly unrelated clinical manifestations.

Case 1

A 40-year-old Caucasian female was referred to UC Davis Pulmonary Clinic for an abnormal chest X-ray. Several months prior to her clinic visit, she noticed increasing fatigue, which progressively worsened to the point that she could "sleep all day." She had associated drenching night sweats on a regular basis. She unintentionally lost 15

C.M. Sebat, D.O. (✉)
University of California, Davis, CA, USA

Division of Pulmonary, Department of Internal Medicine Critical Care and Sleep Medicine, UC Davis Medical Center, 4150 V Street, Suite 3400 Sacramento, CA 95817, USA

Mather VA Medical Center, Northern California Health Care System (NCHCS), Mather, CA, USA
e-mail: csebat@ucdavis.edu

R.W. Harper, M.D.
University of California, Davis, CA, USA

Division of Pulmonary, Department of Internal Medicine Critical Care and Sleep Medicine, UC Davis Medical Center, 4150 V Street, Suite 3400, Sacramento CA 95817, USA

M. Mahmoudi (ed.), *Challenging Cases in Rheumatology and Diseases of the Immune System*, DOI 10.1007/978-1-4614-5088-7_6,
© Springer Science+Business Media, LLC 2013

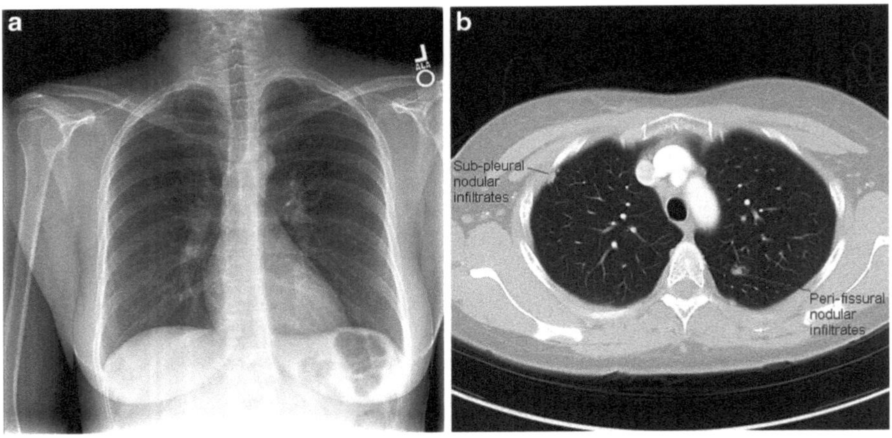

Fig. 6.1 (**a**) Chest X-ray depicting mild mediastinal lymphadenopathy. (**b**) Computed tomography of the chest depicting nodular infiltrates

pounds during this period. Several weeks prior to her clinic visit, she experienced temporary disorientation earlier in the afternoon that culminated in a syncopal episode at dinner that evening. A chest X-ray was obtained by her primary care provider for evaluation of her syncope, which prompted the referral for consultation (Fig. 6.1a). The patient has a history of irritable bowel syndrome, allergic rhinitis, and gastroesophagel reflux disease (GERD). She never smoked cigarettes or used illicit drugs, works as an administrative assistant at a local hospital, and denied any out of state travel in last couple years. She does not own any pets and lives alone in a newly constructed apartment in Sacramento, CA. Her current medications includes fexofenadine 180 mg tablet daily, fluticasone 50 mcg nasal spray daily, loratadine 10 mg daily, and omeprazole 20 mg daily. She has not taken diet drugs. Review of symptoms was negative for shortness of breath, poor appetite, palpitations, chest pain/pressure, peripheral edema, orthopnea, paroxysmal nocturnal dyspnea, cough, wheeze, or pleurisy.

Physical examination revealed a healthy appearing woman sitting comfortably and able to answer all questions. She had a temperature of 36.9, blood pressure of 130/73 mmHg, heart rate of 85 beats/min, a respiratory rate of 16 breaths/min, and an oxygen saturation of 100% on room air. Lungs were clear to auscultation without wheezes or crackles bilaterally. No heart murmurs or gallops were heard. Abdomen was normal without hepatomegaly or splenomegaly. Her extremities were without clubbing, cyanosis, or edema. No skin rash was found and neurologic assessment was normal. The patient's complete blood count and comprehensive metabolic panel were normal.

With the Presented Data What Is Your Working Diagnosis?

The patient's complaints of chronic fatigue, night sweats, and abnormal chest X-ray strongly suggest an illness with systemic manifestations. Infection and cancer come immediately to mind. Lymphoma or lung cancer can explain the hilar fullness and

"B" symptoms. Alternatively, a connective tissue disease or vasculitis such as granulomatosis with polyangitis (Wegener's granulomatosis) can present with similar very nonspecific symptoms and parenchymal lung involvement. Her history of irritable bowel syndrome may actually be undiagnosed inflammatory bowel disease, which can manifest with associated interstitial lung disease. Since the patient lives in the Northern California Central Valley, a diagnosis of cocidioidomycosis must be entertained along with pulmonary tuberculosis. Pulmonary arterial hypertension, primary or secondary, should be considered and can give rise to bilateral hilar fullness and her symptoms of syncope. Sarcoidosis can also present with nonspecific systemic symptoms such as fatigue, fever and weight loss as predominant features. Her chest X-ray findings in this case are consistent with this diagnosis as well. Finally, either primary HIV infection, immunodeficiency related chronic indolent infections, or lymphoproliferative disorders should be included in the working diagnosis.

Differential Diagnoses

1. Lymphoma or lung cancer
2. Sarcoidosis
3. Coccidioidomycosis or other fungal infections
4. Tuberculosis
5. Granulomatosis with polyangitis
6. HIV, lymphocytic interstitial pneumonia, or primary pulmonary lymphoma
7. Pulmonary arterial hypertension, primary or secondary

Workup

After review of the medical record, history and physical examination, initial investigation focused on her cardiac system. Electrocardiogram revealed a normal sinus rhythm and normal axes. Echocardiogram revealed normal biventricular function with normal cardiac chamber sizes and normal estimated right ventricular systolic pressure. A computed tomographic (CT) scan of her chest (Fig. 6.1b) revealed upper and mid-lung zone clusters of nodular infiltrates with bilateral hilar and mediastinal lymphadenopathy. Pulmonary arteries were normal in size and no bronchiectasis was found. Pulmonary function tests demonstrated an isolated mild decrease in her DLCO (16.6 mL/mmHg/min which is 66% predicted). Serum ANCA, serine proteinase-3 (PR-3) and myeloperoxidase (MPO) antibody levels were not elevated. Angiotensin converting enzyme (ACE) level was normal at 46 U/L (Normal: 9–67 U/L). HIV ELISA antibody test was nonreactive.

After 8 weeks, fiber-optic bronchoscopy revealed normal proximal airways and a bronchoalveolar lavage (BAL) demonstrated 365 WBC/mL (No well established normal's due to wide variation in techniques) with 15% lymphocytes and 74% macrophages (Normal alveolar WBC differential is >90–95% macrophages).

The alveolar lymphocyte CD4:CD8 cell ratio was 2.8. Bacterial, fungal, and mycobacterial stains and cultures did not demonstrate organisms. The bronchial mucosa was normal on visual inspection. Endobronchial and transbronchial biopsies of the right middle and lower lobes, respectively, demonstrated normal bronchial mucosa and lung parenchyma. A endobronchial ultrasound-guided needle aspiration of the right hilar and subcarinal lymph nodes demonstrated noncaseating aggregates of epithelioid cells suggesting granulomas without evidence of malignancy. Stains for bacteria, fungal, and acid-fast bacilli were negative, and flow cytometry from the lymph node aspiration did not support a diagnosis of lymphoproliferative disease.

What Is Your Diagnosis and Why?

Sarcoidosis is the most likely diagnosis but must be a diagnosis of exclusion. The noncaseating granulomas found on mediastinal lymph node aspiration, radiographic findings, and the patient's age support a presumptive diagnosis of sarcoidosis. What is distinctive in this case is the absence of common presenting symptoms of pulmonary sarcoidosis despite her radiographic studies. There was no history of cough or chest pain but dyspnea was probably present and caused the patient to feel fatigued with activities of daily living.

The bronchoscopic evaluation was non-diagnostic for infection, decreasing the likelihood of mycobacterial or fungal etiologies. Serologies and normal renal function did not support granulomatosis with polyangiitis (Wegener's granulomatosis), the most likely vasculitis given her clinical presentation, chest X-ray findings, and pathology results. Cytologic and flow-cytometric analysis of the needle aspiration from the enlarged mediastinal lymph nodes did not support a diagnosis of malignancy or lymphoproliferative disorder.

Discussion

Sarcoidosis is believed to be an abnormal systemic or local granulomatous immune response to either one or multiple unknown antigens in a genetically susceptible individual. The key effector cell in sarcoidosis is the CD4+ T cell, which communicate with activated alveolar macrophages to initiate formation of granulomas and sustain chronic inflammation. In affected organs that can include the lungs (most often), liver, bone, heart, central nervous system, gastrointestinal tract, and eyes. Classically, the granulomatous inflammation occurs via differentiation of the CD4+ T cells into type 1 helper T cells to produce interleukin-2 and interferon-gamma. This augments macrophage-derived TNF-alpha. However, other cell types may be as important or more important in the pathogenesis of this disease.

Presentation and Diagnosis

Evidence strongly suggests that interactions between specific environmental exposures and genetic factors are important. There is a higher incidence of sarcoidosis in African-Americans, and Northern Europeans than in other ethnic populations. Monozygotic twins of patients with sarcoidosis are at higher risk of developing sarcoidosis. Also, specific human leukocyte antigen (HLA) class II molecules place patients at higher risk of developing the disease, portend a poorer prognosis, or both. However, reports of occupational, environmental, or temporal-related case clustering of sarcoidosis suggest important environmental factors are critical as well [1].

Sarcoidosis is often suspected after incidental findings of bilateral hilar lymph node enlargement and/or parenchymal reticulo-nodular infiltrates are noted on chest radiography. However, it is rare that a diagnosis of sarcoidosis can be made based on clinical presentation alone [2, 3]. It is strongly recommended that a more definitive diagnosis be made in appropriate cases with a biopsy of an affected organ to demonstrate noncaseating epithelioid cell granulomas. It is critical that other granulomatous diseases are excluded as the finding of granulomas can occur in other diseases (Table 6.1). A careful history including occupational and environmental exposures will help to narrow the differential.

Special mention should be made of Löfgren's syndrome. This combination of fever, erythema nodosum, polyarthritis, and chest radiograph showing bilateral hilar lymphadenopathy with or without parenchymal infiltrates is a unique presentation of sarcoidosis that does not require tissue biopsy for confirmation of diagnosis. Some authors suggest that Heerfordt's syndrome (uveitis, parotiditis, and fever), or a gallium-67 scintigraphy that demonstrates the combined "lambda-panda" sign (gallium uptake in the bilateral hilar lymph nodes in combination with parotid and lacrimal gland uptake) are specific to sarcoidosis alone, but this is not universally accepted. For our patient, the radiographic findings along with fatigue and drenching night sweats mandated that we exclude malignancy, infection, and other inflammatory etiologies.

In the absence of other sites for biopsy, bronchoscopy with transbronchial lung biopsies has become essential to confirm the presence of noncaseating granulomas and to exclude other possible etiologies. Chest computed tomography will often reveal bilateral mediastinal lymph node enlargement and/or upper lobe predominant fibro-nodular infiltrates in a peri-lymphatic distribution and can guide bronchoscopic or other invasive testing, especially lymph node sampling. Endobronchial ultrasound-guided transbronchial needle aspiration of mediastinal lymph nodes appears to increase the diagnostic yield of lymph node sampling in patients with suspected sarcoidosis when compared to blind bronchoscopic needle aspiration [4]. Bronchoalveolar lavage (BAL) is useful when cell counts suggest an alternative diagnosis such as eosinophilic processes when eosinophils are found, or infection when actual pathogens are found, e.g., Coccidioides immitis spherules, and highly suggested when neutrophils are plentiful. The normal BAL cell count is 98–99% alveolar macrophages with only 1% neutrophils. Flow cytometry from the BAL showing a CD4/CD8 ratio >3.5 is highly specific for sarcoidosis, but less useful if the ratio is lower.

Table 6.1 Differential diagnosis for granulomas based on organ involvement (adapted from [1])

Lung	Lymph node	Skin	Liver	Bone marrow
Mycobacteria	Mycobacteria	Mycobacteria	Mycobacteria	Mycobacteria
Endemic fungi	Brucellosis	Endemic fungi	Brucellosis	Endemic fungi
P. jerovicii	Toxoplasmosis	Berylliosis	Schistosomiasis	Mononucleosis
Hypersensitivity pneumonitis	Hodgkin's	Heavy metal exposure	Crohn's disease	CMV
Berylliosis	Non-Hodgkins	Foreign body reaction	Primary biliary cirrhosis	Hodgkin's
Heavy metal exposure	Cat-scratch disease	Rheumatoid nodules	Hodgkin's	Non-Hodgkins
Drug reactions			Non-Hodgkins	Drug reactions
Foreign body aspiration				
Chronic ILD				
Rheumatoid nodules				

Because any organ system can be variably involved in sarcoidosis, there are a myriad of possible clinical presentations. Patients can be asymptomatic or present with protean and nonspecific manifestations as seen in this case. Constitutional symptoms such as fever, fatigue, malaise and weight loss can occur in up to 30% of patients with sarcoidosis and is more common in African-Americans or Asian Indians. More than 90% of patients will have pulmonary involvement, but may not present with respiratory symptoms. One-third to one-half of all sarcoidosis patients will present with typical respiratory symptoms including wheeze, dry cough, dyspnea on exertion, or chest pain. Liver involvement is almost as common as pulmonary involvement, up to 80% of all liver biopsy specimens, but rarely causes any symptoms or morbidity. Clinical evidence of cardiac involvement is rare and can range from benign arrhythmias to sudden death as a consequence of heart block. Other common presentations include ocular (uveitis), neurologic (Bell's palsy, lymphocytic meningitis), or dermatologic involvement (lupus pernio, "livid papillary psoriasis" of Mortimer's Malady, erythema nodosum), nondestructive arthritis, and even endocrine manifestations (hypercalcemia, deregulated calcitriol production or simply nephrocalcinosis +/− kidney stones due to excessive urinary calcium excretion in the absence of overt hypercalcemia).

A broad screen for the burden of organ involvement should be done once a diagnosis of sarcoidosis is made (Table 6.2). A complete blood count to include white cell, red blood cell, and platelet counts will suggest bone marrow involvement. A comprehensive metabolic panel can suggest other organ involvement such as hepatobiliary inflammation, renal dysfunction causing electrolyte derangement or acid-base disturbances, and hypercalcemia due to a high burden of granulomatous disease. Pulmonary function tests can be normal. The most common abnormal findings in sarcoidosis patients are reduced DL_{CO} (<80% of predicted) and low slow vital capacity (<80% predicted). Approximately 30% of patients will have evidence of primary or concurrent obstruction (airway involvement or extrinsic compression) leading to mixed obstructive and restrictive lung physiology [5], the former due to granulomatous infiltration of the bronchial airways and 20% may have clinically significant airway hyperactivity that may fool the clinician into thinking of asthma. Chest X-ray can be normal (Scadding stage 0), show hilar adenopathy (stage I), hilar adenopathy and parenchymal infiltrates (stage II), parenchymal infiltrates alone (stage III), or pulmonary fibrosis (stage IV). This staging system is a radiographic description and should not be considered analogous to staging in cancer. Therefore, the physician is not compelled to treat a patient with sarcoidosis to prevent a progression from, for example, stage II to stage III. However, the initial radiographic stage at diagnosis does correlate with the likelihood of PFT abnormalities and correlates inversely with the likelihood for the resolution of radiographic pulmonary abnormalities over time [1].

Specific clinical presentations will warrant additional tests that will not be done routinely on all sarcoidosis patients. In this patient, the initial presentation of syncope suggested possible cardiac involvement. Although only approximately 5% of patients

Table 6.2 Recommended initial clinical evaluation.

History with particular focus on occupational and environmental exposures
Posteroanterior and lateral chest radiographs
Pulmonary function tests (spirometry, lung volumes, DLco)
Complete blood count
Serum chemistries (alkaline phosphatase, alanine and aspartate aminotranferase, creatinine, BUN, calcium)
Urine analysis
ECG
Complete ophthalmologic exam
Serum angiotensin-converting enzyme
PPD or Quantiferon-gold
Other tests based on history or physical exam (echocardiogram, MRI brain, 24-h urine for calcium)

with sarcoidosis have clinical evidence of cardiac disease, up to 40% will have evidence of cardiac sarcoidosis on advanced imaging [6]. Conduction system abnormalities, ventricular arrhythmias, and congestive heart failure are among the most common clinical manifestations [6]. Cardiac sarcoidosis is confirmed when endomyocardial biopsy demonstrates non-caseating epithelioid cell granulomas with a histologic or clinical diagnosis of extracardiac sarcoidosis. However, endomyocardial biopsy is insensitive due to the patchy nature of the disease with biopsy revealing non-caseating granulomas in a minority of patients with cardiac sarcoidosis [6]. Cardiac sarcoidosis should be considered in a young patient with advanced second or third degree heart block, monomorphic ventricular tachycardia, or dilated cardiomyopathy in the absence of early onset coronary artery disease. In patients with extra-cardiac sarcoidosis and no cardiac symptoms, an electrocardiogram and echocardiogram are reasonable choices to screen for disease with regular or annual monitoring if they remain asymptomatic. If cardiac sarcoidosis is suspected by symptoms then advance imaging should be pursued. Fluoro-deoxyglucose positron emission tomography (FDG PET) is sensitive for identifying active inflammation but Cardiac magnetic resonance imaging (MRI) has the advantage of identifying characteristic cardiac lesions of varying age and has superior specificity [6]. Gallium-67 Scintigraphy is used when cardiac involvement is strongly suspected as its specificity is good and it has the advantage of being used to assess response to therapy but its sensitivity is low [6]. For our patient, the ECG and echocardiogram were unremarkable and the patient's symptoms were most consistent with vasovagal syncope. Based on the history and initial cardiac findings, no further cardiac evaluation was performed.

Our patient carried a diagnosis of irritable bowel syndrome. The liver is commonly involved in sarcoidosis, causing intra-hepatic cholestasis from the granulomatous disease burden. This can manifest as vague abdominal pain, pruritis, and/or jaundice which can lead to cirrhosis and/or portal hypertension. However, sarcoidosis involves the intestines less than 1% of the time. A comprehensive metabolic panel is a reasonable screen for hepatic involvement.

Management

Most patients diagnosed with sarcoidosis will require no therapy or require therapy for a relatively short period of time. Though, up to one-third of patients will require long-term or lifelong treatment with immunosuppressive agents, most often oral corticosteroids. Once a diagnosis of sarcoidosis is made, the decision to treat pharmacologically is determined by the persistence of symptoms, the specific organs involved, or deterioration of organ function upon subsequent monitoring. The specific indications for starting therapy are controversial, but it is generally accepted that cardiac disease, neurologic disease, or eye disease not responding to topical therapy should be treated with systemic immunosuppression. For organs affected by sarcoidosis, frequent monitoring of symptoms and disease activity should be performed to ensure disease activity is controlled or to identify clinical deterioration from inadequately controlled sarcoidosis early. Serum angiotensin-converting enzyme (ACE) levels can be used to follow sarcoidosis disease activity in a patient if their ACE level was elevated during their initial presentation. However, it is not sensitive or specific enough to serve as a diagnostic marker of disease [1]. ACE can be elevated in diabetes mellitus, coccidioidomycosis and other conditions.

Our patient's primary disease manifestation was in the pulmonary parenchyma and mediastinal lymph nodes based on laboratory evaluation. The absolute absence of pulmonary symptoms, and overt involvement of other organs can reasonably justify observing this patient with serial pulmonary function testing. Typically, 3–6 month serial pulmonary function tests are sufficient for the first year. If the patient remains stable during this time, the frequency of monitoring can be extended. For Stage I disease, 6 month follow-up is recommended, whereas every 3 month follow-up is recommended for Stage II and Stage III disease. If pulmonary function deteriorates during this time (decreasing DLco, more lung volume restriction), and/or the patient has an increase in symptoms causing significant impairment of daily activities, or both, then treatment with corticosteroids to induce a clinical remission is indicated.

Extra pulmonary signs and symptoms should be monitored particularly if the eyes and central nervous system are involved. Chronic fatigue and night sweats are difficult to treat and are usually transient. The isolated reduced DL_{CO} on pulmonary function testing we detected in our patient definitely raises the specter of pulmonary vascular disease with pulmonary hypertension, and would prompt echocardiography to further evaluate. Since the estimated right ventricular systolic pressure on our patient's echocardiogram was normal and the patient did not complain of exertional dyspnea, a right heart catheterization to evaluate for sarcoidosis-associated pulmonary hypertension was not performed. However, if fatigue persists and the patient develops new dyspnea on exertion out of proportion to PFT and echocardiographic abnormalities, then right heart catheterization would be a reasonable diagnostic test for pulmonary arterial hypertension that can be related to pulmonary sarcoidosis.

Most patients will respond rapidly to corticosteroids with resolution of their symptoms in 3–6 months. The optimal dose and duration has not been established, but prednisone at 40 mg (0.5–1.0 mg/kg) by mouth daily is a typical starting dose

[1]. The general principle is to taper prednisone every 2–4 weeks to a minimum effective dose. A return of symptoms during the taper should prompt the physician to increase the prednisone to the last effective dose. For patients that require more than 15 mg per day for greater than 3 months, prophylaxis against Pneumocystis jerovicii should be initiated (co-trimoxazole one tablet three times a week). Treatment for 1 year is recommended with close monitoring for 2 years after the cessation of prednisone. If the patient's disease is persistent for more than 1 year, or frequently exacerbates during the observation period, consideration should be made to initiate a steroid-sparing agent. No comparative trials have established a superior alternative agent, but azathioprine, hydroxychloroquine, methotrexate, mycophenolate mofetil, and leflunomide have all been used with success. Despite the sound biological evidence in favor of anti-TNF-alpha therapy, clinical studies have been underwhelming regarding the role of these agents for the treatment of sarcoidosis.

Follow-Up

With regards to our patient, based on her minimal symptoms and subtle objective abnormalities we elected to observe her with regular clinic follow-up and repeat pulmonary function tests. At 6 months, her pulmonary function remains unchanged and clinically her weight is stable with her fatigue and night sweats diminishing without pharmacologic therapy.

Case 2

A previously healthy 49-year-old Caucasian woman presented with a painless rash on her face, neck and shoulders in conjunction with numbness around her right eye and forehead for 1 month. There had been no change in her personal hygiene habits (e.g., soap or cosmetics), no new medications or antibiotics, no history of tanning or recent excessive sun exposure. She denied fevers, chills, weight loss, poor appetite, or other constitutional symptoms. She had no visual acuity loss, diplopia, changes in sense of smell, hearing or taste. The rest of her review of systems was unremarkable. There was no recent travel, hiking trips or pets in the household. On physical examination she was afebrile with normal vital signs. Head and neck exam revealed pink small papular lesions 2–3 mm in diameter on her face including the eyelids, nares and neck. There was numbness over the V1 branch of the right trigeminal nerve but no other cranial nerve deficits were noted and there was no tenderness over the scalp. Pupils were 2 mm bilaterally, reactive to light with normal extra-ocular muscle movements. There was no conjunctival injection, edema or exophthalmoses identified. Funduscopic exam was normal, no visual field deficits or problems with visual acuity were found. Oropharyngeal exam was normal. No lymphadenopathy was palpated. Lung, cardiac, and abdominal exams were normal. Her skin exam revealed a warm, non-tender, blanching, 2–3 mm, pink, papular, erythematous rash on the shoulder and upper trunk. The extremities were without clubbing, dystrophic nails, cyanosis, or edema.

What Is Your Working Diagnosis? What Is the Differential Diagnosis?

The combination of a papular dermatologic eruption and focal neurologic deficit is concerning for a disseminated infection such has histoplasmosis, coccidioidomycosis, cryptococcosis, or syphilis. Additionally, the skin findings may be suggestive of molluscum contagiosum or a paraneoplastic syndrome such as leukemia cutis with spread to the meninges and focal cranial nerve compression. Systemic inflammatory diseases such as Dermatomyositis, Behcet's syndrome, Sjogren's syndrome, and sarcoidosis should also be considered.

Work-Up

To paraphrase Willy Sutton, go to where the money is—the skin rash. A biopsy of her skin rash revealed non-caseating epithelioid granulomatous inflammation with bacterial, fungal, and acid-fast stains negative for organisms (Fig. 6.2a). MRI of her brain revealed an orbital mass approximately 5 × 8 mm on the right, medially and posterior to the globe that was ill defined and partially eroding into the ethmoid sinus (Fig. 6.2b). Due to the finding of granulomatous inflammation in the skin a computed tomography (CT) scan of her chest revealed bilateral nodular parenchymal lung infiltrates without mediastinal or hilar lymphadenopathy (Fig 6.2c). Complete blood count was unremarkable and a comprehensive metabolic panel was within normal limits without renal, liver or electrolyte abnormalities. An anti-nuclear antibody titer was <1:20. Pulmonary function tests demonstrated a mildly decreased DLCO (20.1 mL/mmHg/min which is 74% predicted) otherwise normal spirometry and lung volumes.

What Is Your Diagnosis? Why?

The granulomatous inflammation in the skin on histological evaluation without evidence of vasculitis or infection based on bacterial, fungal, or acid-fast staining in the setting of pulmonary parenchymal changes and an orbital mass suggests the diagnosis of cutaneous sarcoidosis with orbital manifestations of V1 nerve compression and asymptomatic pulmonary involvement.

Discussion

In this discussion we will cover aspects of cutaneous, ocular and neurosarcoidosis. Please see the previous case discussion for information regarding more common aspects and discussion of sarcoidosis.

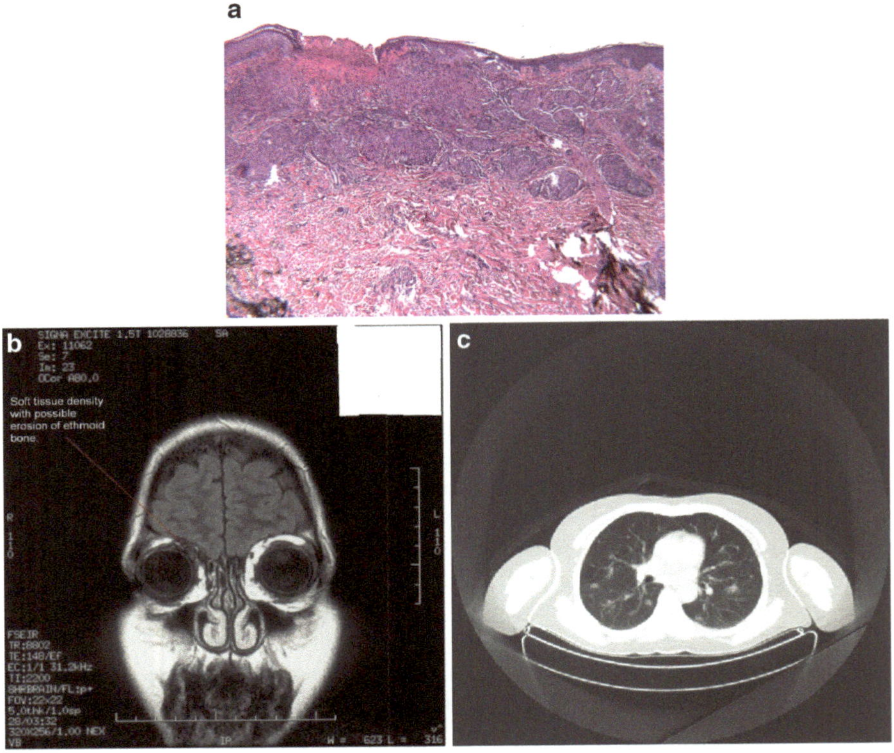

Fig. 6.2 (**a**) Dermatopathology of the skin rash. (**b**) MRI with T1 weighted image showing soft tissue density on the medial side of the right orbit. (**c**) CT chest demonstrating bilateral nodular infiltrates

Presentation

The neurologic and cutaneous manifestations in this patient posed a diagnostic challenge and illustrates the variety of extra-pulmonary organ systems that sarcoidosis can affect. A myriad of skin findings can occur in sarcoidosis but it remains a diagnosis of exclusion. Cutaneous manifestations can occur in up to 20% of patients with sarcoidosis [7] and are divided into "specific" and "nonspecific" lesions. Specific skin rashes demonstrate non-caseating epithelioid granulomas on skin biopsy without an apparent alternative diagnosis. Nonspecific lesions include erythema nodosum, which is estimated to occur in up to 25% of patients with sarcoidosis and generally associated with a very good prognosis [7] particularly if Lofgren's syndrome is present. In contrast, lupus pernio, another nonspecific skin lesion consisting of violaceous, indurated papules, nodules, and plaques most commonly on the face over the nose and into the nostrils, is associated with severe pulmonary and/or upper airway involvement [7]. Other nonspecific findings are rarer and include erythema multiforme, prurigo, or Sweet's syndrome.

Ocular manifestations are often overlooked in sarcoidosis, and can affect any part of the eye. The globe, orbit, and adnexal structures can also be involved. Sarcoidosis affects the eye in approximately 10 to as high as 50% of patients depending on the case series [8]. In patients with ocular sarcoidosis, anterior uveitis is the most common manifestation, followed by vitreitis, fundus and choroidal lesions. Orbital and adnexal lesions are relatively rare in patients with ocular sarcoidosis [8]. There are no pathognomonic findings of ocular sarcoidosis but there are numerous observations when taken together in the context of systemic disease consistent with sarcoidosis that can be strongly suggestive. These findings are beyond the scope of this chapter, but with regard to our patient, a recent case series of 30 patients with specifically orbital or adnexal disease found that sarcoidosis most commonly affected the lacrimal gland and 85% of lesions were well circumscribed on computed tomography [8].

Asymptomatic central nervous system involvement in patients with sarcoidosis is not uncommon. Evidence of neurosarcoidosis has been found in up to 14% of patients with systemic sarcoidosis in post-mortem analysis [9]. Sarcoidosis can affect any part of the central and peripheral nervous system. When symptomatic, the cranial nerves are most commonly involved in 50–75% of patient with neurosarcoidosis [9]. Facial nerve palsy is the most common cranial nerve manifestation. Sarcoidosis can also cause parenchymal brain lesions with a variety of manifestations such as cognitive and behavioral disturbances, seizures, signs of basal ganglia dysfunction, hypothalamic/pituitary deregulation, and focal neurological deficits. Meningeal disease can occur leading to aseptic meningitis or hydrocephalus and the spinal cord, peripheral nerves, and muscles can also be involved.

Work-Up

Skin lesions are evaluated clinically and either punch or excisional wedge biopsies are sufficient to identify noncaseating granulomas. A search for additional evidence to support a diagnosis of sarcoidosis should be done, e.g., bilateral hilar adenopathy on chest X-ray. If adenopathy is present, additional investigations should be made to exclude malignancy. Finally, alternative diagnoses should be excluded including bacterial, fungal, AFB staining and culture of biopsies and perhaps vasculitis or connective tissue disease serology's performed if clinically indicated.

Suggestive ocular signs in sarcoidosis include yellow waxy retinal spots, nodular iritis with mutton fat keratic precipitates, nodular trabecular infiltrates, vitreous snow ball and string of pearl opacities, retinal periphlebitis, perivascular "candle wax drippings" [10]. Certainly, consultation with an opthamologist is strongly recommended.

A diagnosis of neurosarcoidosis is "probable" when there is pathologic confirmation of systemic sarcoidosis, the clinical syndrome and diagnostic evaluation suggest neurosarcoidosis, and alternative diagnoses have been excluded. This diagnosis becomes "definite" when a patient has had a beneficial response to immunotherapy over a 1 year observation period [9]. A brain, meningeal, or spinal cord biopsy is not usually readily obtainable and can carry significant morbidity. Therefore, we rely greatly on biopsies from alternative organ sites, clinical picture, and imaging modalities. Magnetic resonance imaging (MRI) without and with gadolinium is the imaging modality of choice most often showing linear and nodular leptomeningeal and perivascular enhancement with a predilection for the basal meninges, midline structures (hypothalamus, optic chiasm, pituitary), and penetrating vascular paths (Virchow-Robin spaces) [9]. This finding is almost imperceptible on unenhanced images. Contrast enhanced computed tomography can be used if there is a contraindication to MRI or gadolinium but visualization of the base of the brain, posterior fossa, cranial nerves is impeded by bone artifact. These leptomeningeal findings can also be seen in meningeal carcinomatosis, lymphoma, leukemia, tuberculosis, and fungal meningitis. Therefore, a high index of suspicion for these diagnoses should be held while in the work-up and treatment phase, as these diagnoses can certainly also develop in an immunosuppressed patient. Additional MRI imaging findings include parenchymal enhancing lesions, Dural enhancing lesions, abnormal T2 signal in white matter without enhancement, and hydrocephalus [9]. Some of these findings can also occur in the spinal cord mostly commonly the cervical cord. Positron emission tomography (PET) is not typically used in the work-up of neurosarcoidosis but can be helpful in identifying alternative sites for biopsy. Cerebral spinal fluid studies (CSF) are nonspecific but often show lymphocytic pleocytosis, elevated opening pressures and protein levels, and classically low glucose concentrations (<2/3 of the plasma glucose). The differential diagnosis should include TB and Cryptococcosis. CSF angiotensin converting enzyme levels are not sensitive enough to be used in the diagnosis of sarcoidosis [9].

Management

Oral corticosteroids for disfiguring skin manifestations remain the treatment of choice with use of steroid-sparing agents such as methotrexate for recalcitrant cases. Anti-TNF-alpha agents may have a promising future as steroid-sparing agents as well. However, for limited cutaneous disease topical steroids or intra-lesional steroid injections are effective therapies along with tetracycline-based antibiotics (minocycline) and antimalarials (chloroquine or oxychloroquine) [7].

Asymptomatic patients incidentally found to have neurosarcoidosis should be monitored closely with repeat imaging and clinical exams with a decision to treat based on the lesions location and/or changes in character or size over-time that predispose to significant morbidity. All symptomatic patients with neurosarcoidosis should be treated immediately, keeping in mind that infections and neoplasia can mimic sarcoidosis and may transiently get better with corticosteroid therapy only to subsequently worsen with potentially devastating consequences. Delaying therapy in a symptomatic patient can result in significant deterioration in neurologic function leading to a permanent neurological changes and disabilities, including coma. Corticosteroids remain the drug of choice for acute symptoms of neurosarcoidosis [9]. They have a rapid onset and there is a plethora of case series and anecdotal evidence supporting their efficacy. In severe acute neurosarcoidosis we typically give intravenous methylprednisolone at a dose of 1 g or 20 mg/kg daily for 3–5 days followed by 0.5–1 mg/kg daily tapered down based on symptom improvement over 4–6 weeks to a maintenance dose of approximately 15 mg of oral prednisone equivalent daily with regular follow-up office visits prior to further taper [9]. If the patient fails to respond or re-exacerbates after steroid taper, the majority of patients, we will typically add a steroid-sparing agent such as cyclophosphamide, methotrexate, azathioprine, or mycophenolate mofetil. Antimalarials such as chloroquine and hydroxychloroquine have been shown to have some efficacy in steroid-refractory neurosarcoidosis. The tumor necrosis factor-alpha inhibitors, namely, infliximab, have an evolving body of evidence for use in neurosarcoidosis and pulmonary sarcoidosis either primarily or in corticosteroid-resistant cases [9]. Monitoring the patient's response to therapy with gadolinium enhanced MRI may be helpful to determine duration of therapy or titration of dosing when patients clinical symptoms are unreliable.

Follow-Up

Our patient's skin manifestations were treated with topical corticosteroid creams with excellent results. Her pulmonary parenchymal abnormalities have been managed conservatively with serial pulmonary function tests, which thus far have demonstrated stability of lung function over 3 months. She is currently being evaluated by ophthalmology and neurosurgery for biopsy and/or resection of the orbital mass.

Questions

1. Which of the following choices is an appropriate annual screening test to help prevent sarcoidosis-associated morbidity?

   (a) ACE level
   (b) 24-h urine calcium excretion
   (c) CT chest with IV contrast
   (d) Thallium nuclear myocardial perfusion study

2. Which of the following choices is the most common pulmonary function test abnormality seen in patients with pulmonary sarcoidosis?

   (a) Normal pulmonary function
   (b) Obstructive airway deficit alone
   (c) Obstructive deficit with decreased DLCO
   (d) Restrictive deficit with decreased DLCO

3. Regarding the incidence or prevalence of sarcoidosis; all of the following answers are true, except?
   (a) Populations of African-American and Northern European descent have a higher prevalence of sarcoidosis then other populations.
   (b) Incidence of developing sarcoidosis is higher amongst monozygotic twins of patient's with sarcoidosis when compared to the general population.
   (c) There is a higher incidence of sarcoidosis amongst HIV positive patients when compared to the general population.
   (d) Incidence cases of Sarcoidosis have been found to cluster around occupational, environmental, and temporally related events.
4. Scadding staging of chest X-rays in patients with sarcoidosis is useful when predicting?
   (a) Risk of cardiovascular mortality
   (b) Risk of progression to central nervous system involvement
   (c) Pulmonary function test abnormality
   (d) Chances of spontaneous resolution of radiographic findings
5. When using an echocardiogram to evaluate patients with sarcoidosis which of the following statements is most accurate?
   (a) Myocardial wall thinning is the most common finding in cardiac sarcoidosis
   (b) Tricuspid valve regurgitant jet velocities tend to underestimate peak right ventricular systolic pressures
   (c) Pulmonary involvement of sarcoidosis tends to obscure echocardiographic windows
   (d) Echocardiographic screening for sarcoidosis associated pulmonary hypertension should be done annually
6. Which of the following is not a pathologic finding in "specific" cutaneous manifestations of cutaneous sarcoidosis?
   (a) Epithelioid histiocytes
   (b) Non-caseating necrosis
   (c) Giant cells
   (d) Spherules on fungal stain
7. All of the following syndromes/findings are specific enough for sarcoidosis to obviate biopsy, except.
   (a) "Lambda Panda" sign on Gallium-67 Scintigraphy
   (b) Leptomeningeal thickening and beading on MRI brain
   (c) Heerfordt's syndrome
   (d) Lofgren's syndrome

8. A diagnosis of probable neurosarcoidosis is made when all of the following criteria are met, except.
   (a) Clinical syndrome, objective exam, and radiology suggest neurosarcoidosis
   (b) Extra-neurologic tissue biopsy findings are consistent with neurosarcoidosis
   (c) Patient has experienced a beneficial response to immunotherapy over 1 years time
   (d) Alternative diagnoses have been excluded
9. Which of the following is the most common clinical finding in patients with symptomatic neurosarcoidosis?
   (a) Cranial nerve involvement
   (b) Hydrocephalus
   (c) Aseptic meningitis
   (d) Seizures
   (e) Parkinsonian features
10. All of the following are accepted therapies for cutaneous sarcoidosis except.
   (a) Topical clobetasol
   (b) Minocycline
   (c) Plaquenil
   (d) Fluoroquinolones
   (e) Anti-TNF-alpha therapy

Answers to questions: 1(b), 2(d), 3(c), 4(d), 5(b), 6(d), 7(b), 8(c), 9(a), 10(d).

References

1. Baughman RP, Culver DA, Judson MA. A concise review pulmonary sarcoidosis. Am J Respir Crit Care Med. 2011;183:573–5812.
2. Statement on sarcoidosis. Joint Statement of the American Thoracic Society (ATS), the European Respiratory Society (ERS) and the World Association of Sarcoidosis and Other Granulomatous Disorders (WASOG) adopted by the ATS Board of Directors and by the ERS executive committee, February 1999. Am J Respir Crit Care Med. 1999;160(2):736–55.
3. Iannuzzi MC, Rybicki BA, Teirstein AS. Sarcoidosis. N Engl J Med. 2007;357(21):2153–65.
4. Tremblay A, Stather DR, MacEachern P, Khalil M, Field SK. A randomized controlled trial of standard vs endobronchial ultrasound-guided transbronchial needle aspiration in patient with suspected sarcoidosis. Chest. 2009;136:340–6.
5. Morgenthau AS, Iannuzzi MC. Recent advances in sarcoidosis. Chest. 2011;139(1):174–82.
6. Youssef G, Beanlands RSB, Birnie DH, Nery PB. Cardiac sarcoidosis: applications of imaging in diagnosis and directing treatment. Heart. 2011;97:2078–87.
7. Lodha S, Sanchez M, Prystowsky S. Sarcoidosis of the skin: a review for the pulmonologist. Chest. 2009;136:583–96.
8. Demirci H, Christianson MD. Orbital and adnexal involvement in sarcoidosis: analysis of clinical features and systemic disease in 30 cases. Am J Ophthalmol. 2011;151:1074–80.
9. Terushkin V, Stern BJ, Judson MA, Hagiwara M, Pramanik B, Sanchez M, Prystowsky S. Neurosarcoidosis: presentations and management. Neurologist. 2010;16:2–15.
10. Cowan CL. Review for disease of the year: differential diagnosis of ocular sarcoidosis. Ocul Immunol Inflamm. 2010;18(6):442–51.

Chapter 7
Systemic Lupus Erythematosus

Roshan Dhawale

Abstract Systemic lupus erythematosus (SLE) is the prototypic autoimmune disease characterized by the production of autoantibodies to components of the cell nucleus in association with diverse clinical manifestations encompassing almost all organ systems. SLE is a complex disease with variable presentations, course, and prognosis characterized by remissions and flares. The extreme heterogeneity of the disease has led some investigators to propose that SLE represents a syndrome rather than a single disease. Here we present two cases describing the complexity and heterogeneity of the disease.

Keywords SLE • Lupus • Pregnancy • Lupus nephritis • Alveolar hemorrhage • Systemic lupus erythematosus

Case 1

The patient is a 21-year-old African-American woman who presented initially at an outpatient rheumatology practice. She was noted to be 14 weeks pregnant. She was diagnosed with Systemic Lupus Erythematosus (SLE) based on symptoms of polyarticular symmetrical inflammatory joint pains, discoid rashes, alopecia and generalized myalgias. Her serological profile and diagnostic testing was significant for a high titer positive antinuclear antibody (ANA) of 1:640 speckled and homogenous (normal <1:80 titer), a negative anti-smith (anti-Sm), a positive anti-Ro antibody 4.8 (normal <2 U/mL), negative anti-La antibody, positive anti-double-stranded DNA antibodies (dsDNA)

R. Dhawale, M.D., M.P.H. (✉)
Division of Rheumatology and Clinical Immunology, University of Pittsburgh Medical Center, 3500 Terrace Street, South BST 7th Floor, Pittsburgh, PA 15261, USA
e-mail: dhawaler@upmc.edu

M. Mahmoudi (ed.), *Challenging Cases in Rheumatology and Diseases of the Immune System*, DOI 10.1007/978-1-4614-5088-7_7,
© Springer Science+Business Media, LLC 2013

600 (normal <30 IU/mL), negative rheumatoid factor (RF) and low complements (C3 and C4) of 57 and 3 (normal C3 90–180 mg/dL and C4 16–47 mg/dL), respectively. She was begun on prednisone 20 mg twice daily and clinical improvement closely followed. A month later, she developed a urinary tract infection (UTI) and pyelonephritis when her urinalysis tested positive for protein, blood, red blood cells and leucocyte esterase (LE). She was hospitalized at an outside facility, treated with antibiotics and discharged. On routine follow-up, she was found to have persistently elevated blood pressures (BP) up to 160–170 s systolic and 90–100 s diastolic, for which she was referred to our tertiary care facility for diagnostic work up and management.

Past medical history, Social and Family history: She had no other significant past medical history and no allergies. Medications included Prednisone 20 mg twice daily and Nitrofurantoin (Macrobid) for UTI. This was her first pregnancy. She did not smoke, consume alcohol or use recreational drugs. She was unemployed with no significant past environmental exposure. She had a remote family history of SLE.

Review of systems (ROS): Positive for fevers prior to diagnosed UTI, occasional myalgias, hair loss, improvement in rashes, fatigue, occasional chills, shortness of breath, and cloudy urine. Rest of the complete ROS was negative.

Physical findings: Afebrile, BP: 156/92 mmHg, Heart rate: 96, Oxygen saturation: 97%. General appearance revealed an anxious appearing young African American woman in no acute distress. She had patchy alopecia, no currently observed rashes, and joint examination revealed no synovitis, tenderness or deformity. She had a gravid abdomen, appropriate for gestational age, non-tender, lungs significant for a few basilar crackles, tachycardia on cardiac examination, but no murmurs or gallops. No jugular venous distension, 1+ edema noted on lower extremities, all peripheral pulses were palpable. Rest of examination, including neurological system was normal.

Diagnostic testing: She had a normal white cell count, hemoglobin of 8.0 (normal 11.8–14 g/dL), normal platelets, normal electrolytes, creatinine of 0.8 (normal <1.2 mg/dL), BUN of 10 (normal 8-24 mg/dL), urinalysis was significant for 6–10 red blood cells (RBC), 2+ protein and 3+ blood, negative for leucocyte esterase or nitrite, 0–5 white blood cells (WBC). 24 h quantification of protein revealed nephrotic range proteinuria >8 g protein. She also had a positive anti-dsDNA 300 (normal <30 IU/mL), low complements C3 and C4 of 50 and 3, respectively (normal C3 90–180 mg/dL and C4 16–47 mg/dL), elevated sedimentation rate (ESR) of 74 (normal <20 mm/h) and C-reactive protein (CRP) 1.2 (normal <0.2 mg/dL). Protein electrophoresis was unremarkable, as was acute hepatitis panel testing. Human immunodeficiency virus (HIV) and syphilis testing was negative. Blood and urine cultures negative.

Impression: Likely developed Lupus Nephritis (LN) or Preeclampsia from pregnancy.

Plan: The patient was scheduled for an immediate kidney biopsy. The biopsy results revealed class IV LN with a full-house immune-fluorescence staining pattern, mostly consistent with active disease and no chronic changes identified. Majority of the glomeruli were found to have endocapillary and/or crescentic changes. Decision was made to give 1 g of intravenous methylprednisolone for three days followed by an IV equivalent of prednisone at 1 mg/kg/day and start patient on Azathioprine (Imuran) for the active nephritis. Due to anti-Ro positivity, fetal heart monitoring was done which revealed no evidence of heart block. Anti-hypertensive drugs were initiated and the patient was discharged.

On outpatient follow-up, the patient was found to be intolerant of Imuran, and through multiple discussions between specialists and field experts, the patient was switched to Tacrolimus (Prograf) which was increased gradually to 4 mg twice daily with toxicity monitoring lab tests being performed regularly. Proteinuria decreased to <3 g. Other active SLE symptoms resolved. For 7 weeks, the patient had stabilized at home but then re-presented to the hospital with shortness of breath, anxiety, and chest pain. At this point, she was on 60 mg of prednisone daily.

Laboratory data: Noted to have an increase in 24 h proteinuria, now at >7 g and had also developed thrombocytopenia with platelets of 60,000 (normal 156,000–369,000/μL) and anemia with hemoglobin of 7.3 g/dL. Chest X ray was normal. Creatinine remained stable. Prograf levels were therapeutic 5.2 (normal 4–16 ng/mL).

With Presented Data, What Is Your Working Diagnosis?

This is a 21-year-old pregnant woman with SLE and LN on treatment, who now presents with shortness of breath, new onset thrombocytopenia, persistently elevated blood pressure, and increased proteinuria.

Differential Diagnosis

This includes worsening active and worsening LN, thrombotic thrombocytopenia purpura, microangiopathic hemolytic anemia, or preeclampsia.

Work Up

Hemolysis parameters were normal, including fibrinogen, fibrin split products and haptoglobin. Peripheral smear revealed few schistocytes. Antibodies to check for heparin-induced thrombocytopenia were negative. Chest pain work up was negative. No significant serological changes were found. ADAMTS 13 enzyme activity was 29 (normal <30%), auto-antibody levels of 22.7 (normal <12 U/mL) found slightly elevated, repeat testing normal and TSH was normal. Echocardiogam and CT angiography were negative. Prednisone, supportive measures and BP management were continued.

What Is Your Diagnosis and Why?

Microangiopathic hemolytic anemia: This could be related to the use of Prograf or worsening SLE activity and remain on the differential diagnosis. Prograf was discontinued.

Preeclampsia: Pregnancy related preeclampsia could certainly be the cause for the patient's clinical deterioration.

Worsening LN: Patient been treated with Prograf and prednisone but may have failed initial therapy. Prograf use has not been well established as therapy for inducing remission as yet. Pregnancy had limited the use of other immunosuppressive regimes.

TTP: Few schistocytes, no significant reduction in ADAMTS activity making it less likely.

Follow-Up

Despite supportive measures, the platelets continued to decrease, blood pressures remained elevated and eventually the decision was made to deliver the baby by cesarean section at around 28 weeks with patient's consent. Once the baby was delivered, detailed discussions were carried out with the patient wherein she was offered Cyclophosphamide (Cytoxan) intravenous infusions at 0.5–1 g/m^2 monthly dosing or Mycophenolate mofetil (Cellcept) goal dose of 3 g. She elected for the latter, and hydroxychloroquine was added. Within few days post-delivery, patient dramatically improved in terms of proteinuria, her BP stabilized and platelets increased. She was discharged with outpatient rheumatology and nephrology follow-up. Over time, the patient did well with slow but sustained renal recovery.

Our final diagnosis is a case of worsening active LN and preeclampsia of pregnancy. Delivery of the fetus and change in therapy for LN were likely what lead to improvement in her case.

Discussion

Pregnancy in lupus patients continues to be a diagnostic and treatment conundrum for practicing rheumatologists, in particular LN. Most of our discussion is focused on LN with a few words on lupus and pregnancy.

(a) Lupus and pregnancy: Available data seems to suggest that there is an increase in flares during pregnancy (particularly in the first half of pregnancy), as well as immediate postpartum for a period of 2 months [1]. A number of studies find that the rate of flares in pregnant women appears to be significantly more than in nonpregnant women. Fertility in these women is normal, except during periods of severe disease activity. Risk factors for SLE activity during pregnancy appear to be status of disease in six months preceding conception, and preexisting renal disease [2]. A greater prevalence of preeclampsia and pregnancy induced hypertension has been found in SLE women based on a number of studies.

(b)Lupus nephritis in pregnancy: This presents a difficult and challenging problem for clinicians given the limitations on use of immune agents for induction and maintaining remission in patients. LN can be classified into six groups as below based on severity of lesions found [3].

Classification

Table 7.1 reviews the classification of LN. Class I LN shows normal findings at light microscopy, but abnormal mesangial deposits by immunofluorescence. Class II LN may be associated with necrosis of cells in the capillary walls, of fibrinoid nature, with hyaline thrombi due to an excess of subendothelial immune complexes, with or without proliferative changes. Class III LN is characterized by segmental or global endo/extracapillary proliferation with active sclerosing lesions. Class IV is >50% diffuse with segmental or global lesions. Subendothelial deposits are very frequent, with infiltration of inflammatory cells and proliferation. Proliferation and necrosis can be segmental (class IV-S) or global (class IV-G). Differentiation of IV-S from IV-G is important from a prognostic point of view. The majority of class IV cases (65%) are IV-G. Class IV-S cases are characterized by higher hematuria, less proteinuria, fewer deposits, but more necrosis. In the presence of monocyte infiltration, outcomes are worse. Class VI is associated with >90% glomerulosclerosis. Characteristic features at immuno-fluorescence include deposits of IgG, IgM, and IgA; complement factors C3 and C1q; and immunoglobulin light chains [4].

Activity and chronicity indexes are provided to the clinician, as they represent predictors, although weak, of long-term prognosis. A value of 1+ corresponds to an involvement of <25%, 2+ to 25–50%, and 3+ to >50%. Negative prognostic indices include crescents in more than 30% of the glomeruli, a chronicity index >5, male sex, and a higher lesion activity in the glomeruli.

Pathophysiology

Immune complex formation and deposition in the kidney results in intra-glomerular inflammation with recruitment of leukocytes and activation and proliferation of resident renal cells [5]. A plethora of humoral and cellular elements contributes to glomerular injury. Intense inflammation may destroy resident renal cells by necrosis or apoptosis, resulting in fibrinoid necrosis. In a few patients, intense capillary inflammation results in rupture of the capillary wall and the capsule itself with epithelial cells, mononuclear cells, fibrin basement membrane material, and collagen accumulating in the urinary space of the glomerulus causing crescentic glomerulonephritis (GN). When injury is less intense, endocapillary cells respond by proliferating and producing extracellular matrix (proliferative lesions). Extreme injury or protracted inflammation activates a final common pathway of all types of glomerular injury, resulting in atrophy and scarring [6].

The location of immune complex deposition and formation is closely linked to histopathology and the intensity of the inflammatory response. Deposition of immune complexes in the mesangium is characteristic of mesangial LN. Immune complex deposition in the sub-endothelial area of the capillary loops results in proliferative LN (focal or diffuse) with exuberant glomerular hypercellularity. This hypercellularity is due to proliferation of mesangial and endothelial cells and leukocytic infiltrates, resulting in compromised capillary flow and renal function. Subepithelial deposits along peripheral glomerular capillary loops that are diffusely thickened and the lack of inflammatory infiltrate are characteristic of membranous nephropathy [6].

Work Up

Proteinuria of various levels is the dominant feature of LN and is usually accompanied by glomerular hematuria [7]. Nephritic syndrome accounts for an additional 30–40% of patients; rapidly progressive GN is rare and accounts for <10% of presentations. Generally, untreated patients with mesangial nephritis have small amounts of proteinuria (<1 g/day) with hematuria, but typically no cellular casts. Patients with membranous glomerulopathy have proteinuria often at nephrotic range, but otherwise unremarkable urine sediments. C3 tends to be normal, and anti-dsDNA antibodies when present are usually found in low titers. In contrast, patients with proliferative nephritis have hypertension, nephritic urine sediment with various degrees of proteinuria, often nephrotic, low C3, and typically high titers of anti-dsDNA antibodies. In patients who have been previously treated with steroids, the findings in the urinalysis may be more subtle than previously and require a high index of suspicion for diagnosis.

Urinalysis is the most important and effective method to detect and monitor disease activity in LN [7]. Hematuria (usually microscopic) indicates inflammatory glomerular or tubulointerstitial disease. Dysmorphic erythrocytes may be seen. Granular and fatty casts reflect proteinuric states, whereas RBC, WBC, and mixed cellular casts reflect nephritic states. Broad and waxy casts reflect chronic renal failure. In severe proliferative disease, urine sediment containing the full range of cells and casts can be found (telescopic urine sediment) as a result of severe glomerular and tubular ongoing disease superimposed on chronic renal damage.

Table 7.1 Revised World Health Organization (WHO) classification of LN according to International Society of Nephrology/Renal Pathology Society 2003

WHO class	Description
Class I	Minimal mesangial LN
Class II	Mesangial proliferative LN
Class III	Focal proliferative LN
Class IV	Diffuse proliferative LN
Class V	Membranous LN
Class VI	Advanced sclerosing LN

Table 7.2 Indications for Renal biopsy

Nephritic urine sediment (glomerular hematuria and cellular casts)
Glomerular hematuria with proteinuria greater than 0.5–1 g/day
Glomerular hematuria with proteinuria less than 0.3–0.5 g/day, and low C3 or positive anti-double-stranded DNA (dsDNA)
Proteinuria greater than 1 to 2 g/day (especially if C3 is low or anti-dsDNA antibodies are present or both)

Renal Biopsy

The Table 7.2 refers to common indications for biopsy in LN patients [6].

Treatment

In order to be clinically relevant to our case, we chose to focus on treatment of LN in pregnant patients only. Pregnant patients with active SLE and mild disease generally are managed with corticosteroids. In moderate-to-severe disease, such as active LN or other serious manifestations, corticosteroids, azathioprine, cyclosporine (rarely), and intravenous gamma globulin may be acceptable for the fetus. Generally speaking, Cyclophosphamide and Methotrexate are contraindicated (US Food and Drug Administration or FDA category D-positive evidence for risk), whereas Mycophenolate mofetil is also category D with known fetal risk. Hydroxychloroquine (Plaquenil) is a Category C (risk cannot be ruled out), but has been found to be useful in SLE patients to prevent flares during pregnancy and no increase in teratogenic effects were noted. Tacrolimus is FDA category C; its use for LN has not been well established, particularly in United States, to be used only when benefits outweigh risks.

The American Academy of Pediatrics (AAP) recommends that nursing is permissible for women receiving corticosteroids, but the interval between dose and nursing should be at least 4 h if the prednisone dose is more than 20 mg/day. Because azathioprine may be excreted in breast milk, this is not recommended with breastfeeding. Infant risk cannot be ruled out with Mycophenolate. Hydroxychloroquine is thought compatible with breastfeeding per AAP. While low concentrations are found in breast milk, it should be undertaken with caution due to slow elimination and potential for cumulative toxicity [6].

Summary and Conclusion

LN in pregnancy is a serious disease and options for treatment are limited due to the teratogenecity associated with several drugs which are prototypically used for induction or maintenance of disease remission. Early diagnosis, good conception planning (best when disease has been inactive for 6 months or more), close monitoring for worsening disease activity and preeclampsia, and careful drug selection are cases which may have the best outcomes.

Case 2

A young 19-year-old Caucasian male presented with 3 week history of progressively worsening hemoptysis, fever, chills, fatigue, and joint pains. The joint pains primarily involved both his hands, wrists, elbows, feet and ankles, associated with swelling and warmth for the past 5–6 weeks. He began coughing up blood in small quantities about 3 weeks prior to presentation, and accompanying fever, malaise and fatigue. He was given a short 7 day course of prednisone by his primary care physician for a presumed post-infectious syndrome/viral arthritis and a course of amoxicillin for bronchitis. There was minimal production of greenish expectoration admixed with bright red blood. The symptoms had got worse over the prior week and the patient presented to the emergency room of our tertiary care hospital.

Past medical, Family and Social history: Significant for anxiety and chronic migraines. No medications on presentation, no allergies. Family history was relevant for a maternal uncle with rheumatoid arthritis per mother's report. Mother had two unexplained miscarriages. Social history significant for a 4 pack years of smoking, moderate alcohol consumption twice a month and no recreational drug use.

Review of systems (ROS): A complete review revealed fatigue, fever up to 100.8F, occasional chills at bedtime, rashes over face and chest, photosensitivity, oral ulcers, and mild early hair loss. He had also noticed recent onset of color changes to his fingers and toes (consistent with raynaud's phenomenon), shortness of breath, mostly on exertion and rarely at rest, but denied skin thickening, heartburn, difficulty with swallowing, sick or tuberculosis exposure, recent incarceration or cyanosis. No cardiac symptoms. Rest of the complete ROS was negative.

Physical examination: Temperature: 100.2F, BP: 146/82 mmHg, HR: 108, Oxygen saturations: 90% on 6 L oxygen nasal cannula. General appearance was remarkable for a fatigued young Caucasian male in mild respiratory distress. Chest exam revealed coarse crackles bilaterally, post-expiratory wheezing, tachycardia on cardiac exam without murmurs. Abdominal and extremity exam was normal. Spine examination was normal. Skin relevant for erythematous maculopapular raised rash over the anterior chest, arms, forearms, cheeks and forehead in a photosensitive distribution. Small areas of patchy hair loss were identified. A small oral ulcer was identified on the right side of the tongue. Small 1 cm tender and mobile lymph nodes were appreciated in cervical chain bilaterally. Joint examination revealed tenderness, warmth and synovitis over the proximal interphalangeal (PIP) and metacarpophalangeal joints (MCP) over both hands and the wrists. Grip strength noted to be 4/5. Tenderness over shoulders, ankles and knees were noted with small effusions at knee joints bilaterally. No muscle weakness or neurological findings.

Diagnostic testing: Blood work revealed a low white cell count of 3,200 (normal 4,200–10,400/μL) with a lymphocytic depletion of 10% (normal 20–45%). He had anemia with Hgb of 9.0 (normal 12–14.5) and a low platelet count 120,000 (normal 156,000–369,000/μL). On chest X-ray, he had patchy airspace consolidation bilaterally. On chest computed tomography (CT) scanning, he had patchy fluffy-appearing alveolar infiltrates on both sides, more on the right than the left side. Impression was consistent with bilateral pneumonia, hemorrhage, vasculitis or heart failure. Echocardiogram was normal. ECG showed sinus tachycardia without other changes. No pulmonary embolism identified.

Impression: Bilateral severe pneumonia or diffuse alveolar hemorrhage.

Plan: The patient developed acute respiratory decompensation and with oxygenation dropping to high 70s, needed urgent intubation in emergency department and required an intensive care unit (ICU) admission. He was begun on broad spectrum empiric antibiotics and continued on aggressive intravenous hydration since heart failure was thought unlikely. Bronchoscopy revealed bright red blood and minimal yellowish expectoration. Samples were sent for gram stain, culture and other microbiology, including acid fast staining. Blood and urine cultures were sent. All attempts were focused on stabilizing his medical condition. No vasopressor drugs were found necessary. On the ventilator, he required 80% FiO_2 levels to maintain saturation.

Laboratory data: Cultures were negative, including acid fast staining for bacilli (AFB). ANA testing was positive at 1:1,280 homogenous pattern (normal titer <1:80), anti-Sm positive at 65 (normal <20 U/mL), anti-dsDNA negative, complements C3 and C4 were 60 and 12 respectively (normal C3 90–180 mg/dL and C4 16–47 mg/dL), urinalysis was unremarkable. RF was low positive at 24 (normal <20 U/mL) with negative anti-Ro and La antibodies. Serum was negative for anti-topoisomerase (Scl-70), centromere, histone, Jo-1 (synthetase) antibodies, and RNA polymerase III antibodies. Anti-U1-ribonucleoprotein (Sm/RNP) antibodies were positive at 38 (normal <20 U/mL). Thyroid antibodies negative. Acute hepatitis panel and HIV negative. Blood and urine cultures negative. Given above presentation and serologies, a panel for antiphospholipid antibodies was sent. Urine toxicology was negative.

With Presented Data, What Is Your Working Diagnosis?

This is a young 19-year-old Caucasian male presenting with features suggestive of a connective tissue disease, and evidence of respiratory failure with CT scan findings consistent with bilateral alveolar infiltrates accompanied by fever and malaise. Infection or inflammation is the chief consideration in this case.

Differential Diagnosis

The differential diagnosis of this patient includes bilateral multi-lobar pneumonia, diffuse alveolar hemorrhage from SLE, antiphospholipid antibody syndrome, or pulmonary vasculitis/capillaritis from a pulmonary-renal syndrome or ANCA vasculitides. Opportunistic or fungal infections seemed less likely in absence of an immune deficiency syndrome, chronic use of corticosteroids or environmental exposure.

Work Up

Anticardiolipin antibodies (aCL) tested positive aCL IgG at 32 (normal <15 GPL U/mL), IgM 45 (normal <15 MPL U/mL), IgA 12 (normal <15 APL U/mL), beta-2 glycoprotein I (B-2 GPI) IgM of 58 (normal <17 SMU), B-2 GPI IgA of 22 (normal <20 SAU) and B-2 GPI IgG 64 (normal <16 SGU), whereas a complete lupus anticoagulant (LAC) panel was negative. ESR was 82 (normal <20 mm/h) and CRP was 2.8 (normal <0.2 mg/dL). Anti-neutrophilic cytoplasmic antibodies (ANCA) were negative, as were the anti-glomerular basement membrane antibodies (anti-GBM). Cardiac enzymes negative. The negative sputum cultures, including AFB staining and fungal cultures, negative systemic cultures bright red blood noted on bronchoschopy and decreasing hemoglobin suggested hemorrhage.

What Is Your Diagnosis and Why?

1. Infection: Pneumonia, while appeared promising initially with a few antecedent infectious symptoms, now seems less likely given negative cultures, lack of improvement with antibiotics, presence of active bleeding on bronchoscopy and no risk factors suggesting an immune-compromised state.
2. Diffuse alveolar hemorrhage (DAH) from SLE: This could be a possibility given the patient's clinical presentation suggesting a connective tissue disease (arthritis, rashes, raynaud's, photosensitivity, serologies, fatigue) and association with DAH.

3. Pulmonary/Renal syndrome or ANCA vasculitides: This also remains a possibility, but less likely given negative ANCA antibodies and no evidence of renal involvement. However, limited disease may sometimes present with only lung involvement. Notably, there were no lung nodules.
4. Antiphospholipid antibody syndrome (APS): This can be associated with dramatic pulmonary presentation as above and on occasion, is labeled as a catastrophic APS when multi-organ system or life threatening involvement is present with a high mortality.
5. Heart failure: Least likely given young age, normal two-dimensional echo and cardiac enzymes.

Follow-Up

The presentation was found most consistent with diffuse alveolar hemorrhage from SLE. However, a manifestation of APS could not be ruled out. Patient was started on high doses of intravenous (IV) Methylprednisolone 1 g for three days, followed by an IV equivalent of 1 mg/kg/day of prednisone. He was also begun on plasma exchange daily to start with, followed by every other day exchanges after initial period. A decision was made to begin the patient on intravenous monthly Cyclophosphamide using National Institute of Health (NIH) protocol at 0.75 g/m^2 given the life threatening nature of DAH with informed consent from the family. Intravenous hydration and bladder protection using Mesna (Uromitexan) were used. Supportive measures and antibiotics were continued until the infection was ruled out. Patient had slow but significant improvement over three weeks. After rehabilitation, the patient was discharged on an intended plan of 4–6 months of IV Cyclophosphamide, hydroxychloroquine 400 mg daily and prednisone 30 mg twice daily with slow taper. APS antibodies were confirmed and anticoagulation was initiated later. Several months afterwards, he was doing well, on low dose Prednisone and had been switched to Azathioprine (Imuran) for maintenance.

Our final diagnosis is diffuse alveolar hemorrhage from SLE and/or possibly APS.

Discussion

Diffuse alveolar hemorrhage (DAH) is a rare but potentially catastrophic complication of SLE. Mortality has been reported to be 50–90% in various series. Clinical features are nonspecific, but diffuse alveolar infiltrates on imaging, hypoxemia, dyspnea, and anemia are characteristic. Alveolar hemorrhage usually occurs in patients with a known history of SLE, high titers of anti-dsDNA antibodies, and active extrapulmonary disease. Fiberoptic bronchoscopy with bronchoalveolar lavage (BAL) and/or transbronchial lung biopsy is usually adequate to substantiate the diagnosis in patients with suspected alveolar hemorrhage. Lung biopsy specimens show extensive hemorrhage within alveolar spaces and capillaritis. Deposits of IgG, C3, or immune complexes have been found in 50% of patients with alveolar hemorrhage complicating SLE [6]. Although more commonly seen in previously diagnosed lupus patients, it can also serve as the initial presenting manifestation in up to 10–20% of patients based on published case series.

DAH may also be associated with APS characterized by alveolar infiltrates and diagnosed by serial BALs indicative of increasing hemorrhagic appearance and confirmation with hemosiderin-laden macrophages and serial increase in RBC counts. Biopsy may not be required, but can show alveolar hemorrhage, microvascular thrombosis and occasionally pulmonary capillaritis. Exact incidence is unknown in primary and secondary APS [8].

Pathophysiology

Pulmonary capillaritis appears to be the histological hallmark of DAH in the setting of antiphospholipid (aPL) antibodies. It is characterized by infiltration of neutrophils into the lung interstitium, causing structural necrosis and loss of capillary integrity. This, in turn, leads to extravasation of red blood cells into the alveolus. It is speculated that aPL induces an up-regulation of vascular endothelial cell adhesion molecules and thus incites neutrophil migration to the interstitium, leading to the changes described earlier and subsequent hemorrhage [9]. Complement C5 activation, leading to neutrophil activation and mobilization to the alveolar septum, may also contribute to DAH in the setting of APS, a hypothesis extrapolated from studies on the role of complement in aPL-mediated pregnancy loss.

Work-Up

Initial presentation prompts the clinician to begin with imaging such as radiograph of the chest, followed by a CT scan or magnetic resonance imaging of the chest. BAL is generally useful to exclude infections. Persistently bloody fluid and hemosiderin laden macrophages help to confirm DAH. Additionally, serological studies for SLE and APS are necessary if the diagnosis has not been established previously. The lung biopsy can be either consistent with either pulmonary capillaritis in 14% of cases or bland hemorrhage in 72% of cases [10]. It is also important to look for other causes such as ANCA-associated vasculitis, coagulopathies and TTP as part of the evaluation.

Treatment

High dose corticosteroids traditionally used alone have been associated with high mortality outcomes. Concomitant cyclophosphamide has improved the prognosis significantly [11]. Other alternatives have been use of mycophenolate and cyclosporine (not very commonly used). DAH is also one of the few indicators to use phasmapharesis in SLE which has been shown to improve survival. Intravenous immunoglobulin has been used with improvement in regression of DAH.

Summary and Conclusion

DAH is a rare but sometimes life-threatening manifestation of SLE and/or APS. A high index of suspicion should be used when diagnosing this condition in previously diagnosed patients or likely candidates. Once infection is ruled out, the patient should be started promptly on immunosuppressive treatment in order to give them the best chance of survival and long term outcome. Medical stabilization and supportive respiratory care are often critically necessary. Use of CD-20 B-cell antagonist Rituximab appears to be promising for the treatment of DAH based on recent case reports [12].

Questions

1. When is it most likely for renal disease to present after diagnosis?
   (A) First 2 years
   (B) 2–5 years
   (C) 5–8 years
   (D) >10 years
   (E) No particular pattern observed
2. Which of the following statements is correct?
   (A) Preeclampsia appears to be more common in pregnant SLE women
   (B) Renal disease prior to pregnancy is a good prognostic marker
   (C) Cyclophosphamide is safe during pregnancy and lactation
   (D) Flare status is not dependent on preconception disease activity
   (E) Breast feeding is contraindicated in women with SLE
3. Which of these are useful to diagnose renal disease in SLE? Choose all that apply.
   (A) Urinalysis
   (B) Kidney biopsy
   (C) Quantification of protein
   (D) Complements and dsDNA
   (E) All of the above

4. Which of the following are true about oral contraceptives and hormone replacement therapy (HRT) in SLE women? Choose all that apply.

   (A) OC pills can be used in mild or inactive SLE women
   (B) OC pills can be used when patient also has anti-phospholipid antibodies
   (C) OC pills can be associated with flares in SLE with low disease activity
   (D) There is a possibility that HRT may induce lupus flares
   (E) Progestin only supplements likely may be used safely by SLE women

5. Which patients are more likely to have worse renal disease?

   (A) African American race
   (B) Associated anti-phospholipid antibodies
   (C) Higher levels of dsDNA
   (D) Poor initial response initial response to immunosuppressive therapy
   (E) All of the above

6. Which of the following is the most common pulmonary manifestation in SLE?

   (A) Pulmonary fibrosis
   (B) Shrinking lung syndrome
   (C) Diffuse alveolar hemorrhage
   (D) Pleurisy
   (E) Pulmonary embolism

7. What is generally considered the incidence of DAH in SLE?

   (A) 2–5%
   (B) 10–20%
   (C) 20–40%
   (D) 40–50%
   (E) >50%

8. What is the preferred treatment for APS in the presence of well established clinical thrombotic events?

   (A) Aspirin alone
   (B) Clopidogrel (Plavix) alone
   (C) Long term anticoagulation with Warfarin (Coumadin)
   (D) Aspirin plus Clopidogrel
   (E) Corticosteroids

9. Poor prognostic indicators for DAH in SLE include: Choose all that apply.

   (A) Renal failure
   (B) Need for mechanical ventilation
   (C) Thrombocytopenia
   (D) Neuropsychiatric lupus
   (E) All of the above

10. DAH is more commonly seen in SLE with: Choose all that apply.
    (A) Elevation in dsDNA titers
    (B) Hypocomplementemia
    (C) Hypercomplementemia
    (D) Rheumatoid factor
    (E) Antinuclear antibody levels

Answer Key: 1 (A), 2 (A), 3 (E), 4 (A), (D) and (E), 5 (E), 6 (D), 7 (A), 8 (C), 9 (E), 10 (A) and (B).

References

1. Gargenstein M, Pollak VE, Kark RM. SLE and pregnancy. NEJM. 1962;267:165–9.
2. Clowse ME, Magder LS, Witter F, Petri MA, et al. The impact of increased lupus activity on obstetric outcomes. Arth Rheum. 2005;52(2):514–21.
3. Weening JJ, D'Agati VD, Schwartz MM, et al. For the International Society of Nephrology Working Group on the Classification of Lupus Nephritis; Renal Pathology Society Working Group on the Classification of Lupus Nephritis. The classification of glomerulonephritis in systemic lupus erythematosus revisited. Kidney Int. 2004;65:521–30.
4. Seshan SV. Classification of lupus glomerulonephritis and predictors of prognosis—an update. Program and abstracts of the 7th international congress on SLE and related conditions; 2004; New York, NY
5. Grande JP, Balow JE. Renal biopsy in lupus nephritis. Lupus. 1998;7:611–7.
6. Firestein GS, Kelley WN, Budd RC, Harris ED. Pathogenesis of SLE; clinical features and treatment of SLE. Chapter 74/5 Kelley's textbook of rheumatology, 8th ed. W.B. Saunders Company; 2008. pp 1233–1300.
7. Austin HA. Clinical evaluation and monitoring of lupus kidney disease. Lupus. 1998;7:618–21.
8. Ford HJ, Roubey RA. Pulmonary manifestations of APS. Clin Chest Med. 2010;31(3):537–45.
9. Deane KD, West SG. Antiphospholipid antibodies as a cause of pulmonary capillaritis and diffuse alveolar hemorrhage: a case series and literature review. Semin Arthritis Rheum. 2005;35(3):154–65.
10. Kamen DL, Strange C. Pulmonary manifestations of SLE. Clin Chest Med. 2010;31(3):479–88.
11. Schwab EP, Schumacher Jr HR, Freundlich B, et al. Pulmonary alveolar hemorrhage in systemic lupus erythematosus. Semin Arthritis Rheum. 1993;23:8–15.
12. Pottier V, Pierrot M, Subra JF, Mercat A, Kouatchet A, Parrot A, Augusto JF. Successful Rituximab in a lupus patient with diffuse alveolar hemorrhage. Lupus. 2011;20(6):656–9.

Chapter 8
Systemic Sclerosis

Corey M. Hatfield and Marcy B. Bolster

Abstract Systemic sclerosis (SSc) can be divided into two main phenotypes: diffuse and limited variants. The terms diffuse and limited refer to the extent of skin involvement. Limited SSc is what was formerly known as the CREST (Calcinosis, Raynaud phenomenon, Esophageal dysmotility, Sclerodactyly, Telangiectasias) syndrome. There are several illnesses that might mimic SSc like morphea, nephrogenic systemic fibrosis, and eosinophilic fasciitis. This is a case based review of SSc, diffuse and limited phenotypes.

Keywords Diffuse and limited systemic sclerosis • CREST • Scleroderma

Case 1

A 67-year-old female is evaluated by her primary care provider for changes of her skin which began with her hands and arms. At first she thought it felt like her fingers, hands, and arms were swollen but then the skin began to feel thick and hard. The skin of her feet, legs, and chest soon underwent similar changes. Her fingers started to tingle and change color with exposure to the cold. At times the fingertips appear blue, white, and/or red depending on how cold she is. Her husband, also present, mentions that her face looks younger and that her double chin has disappeared. She can no longer straighten the fingers of either hand completely. She has occasional pain in her ankles but is otherwise pain-free. She denies chest pain, shortness of breath, gastroesophageal reflux, or constipation. She denies a history of kidney problems. Her family physician found her to be anemic with a hemoglobin of 9.0 g/dl

C.M. Hatfield, D.O. (✉) • M. B. Bolster, M.D.
Division of Rheumatology, Medical University of South Carolina,
96 Jonathan Lucas St., Ste 912, MSC637, Charleston, SC 29425, USA
e-mail: hatfiel@musc.edu; bolsterm@musc.edu

M. Mahmoudi (ed.), *Challenging Cases in Rheumatology and Diseases of the Immune System*, DOI 10.1007/978-1-4614-5088-7_8,
© Springer Science+Business Media, LLC 2013

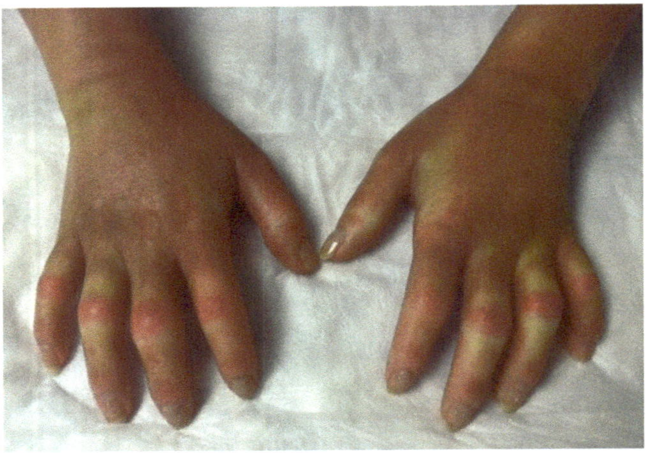

Fig. 8.1 Patient with systemic sclerosis (SSc) with skin thickening apparent on the dorsum of the hands and forearms

(11–16 g/dl). A colonoscopy and EGD were performed and the EGD revealed an area of vascular ectasia in the stomach that was oozing and required cauterization. She was started on omeprazole 20 mg once daily.

Her past medical history is significant for breast cancer. She underwent a bilateral mastectomy 3 years ago and completed chemotherapy 2 years ago. She is now thought to be cancer free. She also has diabetes and hypertension. Her mother died at age sixty-one due to breast cancer. Her father was known to have rheumatoid arthritis. He died at the age of seventy-six from heart problems. She is a retired nurse who is married. She does not use tobacco products or drink alcohol. She has two sons and one daughter who are healthy. She has no known allergies. In addition to the omeprazole, she takes metformin, valsartan, and hydrochlorothiazide.

On physical examination, she is afebrile, blood pressure is 115/56 mmHg, pulse 80 beats per minute, and respiratory rate 18 breaths/min. Examination of the skin reveals telangiectasias on her face. She has hyper and hypo-pigmentation on her anterior chest and on the posterior aspects of her lower legs ("salt & pepper" changes). Abdominal striae are noted. The skin of her fingers is thick, extending from the fingers proximally up the arm to just above each elbow (Figs. 8.1 and 8.2).

The skin of the toes is similar and the tightness extends proximal to each knee. The skin of her anterior chest and face are also tight. She does not have digital pitting or ulcerations. The HEENT, cardiac, lung, abdominal and neurological examinations are normal. The musculoskeletal examination reveals flexion contractures at the proximal interphalangeal joints of both hands (Fig. 8.2). Her wrist and ankle range of motion is reduced. She is able to fully extend and flex both elbows and knees. There is no joint swelling or tenderness. She does not have tendon friction rubs.

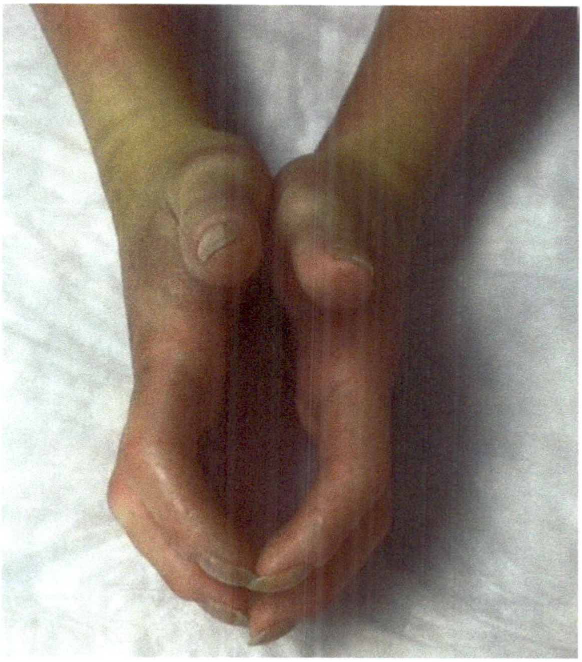

Fig. 8.2 Sclerodactyly with flexion contractures of the PIP joints

With the History and Examination Presented, What Is Your Working Diagnosis?

This is a 67-year-old female with Raynaud phenomenon, skin thickening, and anemia secondary to a GI bleed. The skin examination reveals skin thickening proximal to the elbows and knees and telangiectasias. Given the history and physical exam findings, we feel certain that this patient has a fibrosing skin disorder. She has a family history of rheumatoid arthritis. She has digital vasospasm in response to cold (Raynaud phenomenon). With Raynaud phenomenon and a family history of autoimmunity we are concerned that she may have an autoimmune disease.

Differential Diagnosis

Scleroderma and diseases that can cause scleroderma-like skin changes would be at the top of our differential diagnosis. Could she have diffuse or limited cutaneous systemic sclerosis (SSc)? Other fibrosing skin conditions included in the differential diagnosis would include: eosinophilic fasciitis, generalized morphea, scleromyxedema, scleredema, and nephrogenic systemic fibrosis (Table 8.1).

Table 8.1 Systemic sclerosis

	Morphea	Scleredema	Scleromyxedema	Nephrogenic systemic fibrosis	Eosinophilic fasciitis
Skin	Pigmented, thickened	Indurated, doughy, woody	Popular, waxy	Woody	Indurated, woody, groove sign
Distribution	Patchy, trunk, linear, en coup de sabre	Neck, back, face	Face, neck, arms, fingers	Extremities, trunk; face spared	Extremities, trunk; hands/feet spared
Abnormal lab findings	Anti-topoisomerase II antibodies	Monoclonal gammopathy	Monoclonal gammopathy	Renal insufficiency	Eosinophilia, elevated aldolase
Complications	N/a	Loss of motion of shoulders	Severe contractures	Severe contractures	N/a
Neurologic findings	Present only in coup de sabre form on the face	N/a	Seizures, delirium, coma	Peripheral neuropathy	Carpal tunnel syndrome
Associated diseases	N/a	Infection, diabetes	Multiple myeloma	Renal failure, gadolinium exposure	Cytopenias, aplastic anemia

Evaluation

Laboratory testing should start with basic labs including complete blood count (CBC) with differential, comprehensive metabolic profile (CMP), and urinalysis. These tests may be helpful in identifying the presence of and extent of visceral involvement.

Additional serologic testing should include an antinuclear antibody (ANA), as well as an extractable nuclear antigen panel (ENA). The ENA panel contains the following:

- Anti-Smith antibody
- Anti-Scl-70 antibody (anti-topoisomerase I)
- Anti-Sjogren Syndrome A (SSA) antibody, also known as anti-Ro antibody
- Anti-Sjogren Syndrome B (SSB) antibody, also known as anti-La antibody
- Anti-Ribonucleoprotein antibody

We were considering that this patient may have a form of scleroderma or a disease that might mimic scleroderma so there are a few other studies to pay particular attention to and additional testing that needs to be obtained. The anti-Scl-70 antibody is associated with the diffuse cutaneous variant of SSc and the development of interstitial lung disease (ILD). Anti-RNA polymerase III is also associated with diffuse cutaneous SSc as well as scleroderma renal crisis. Patients with limited cutaneous SSc are more likely to have an anti-centromere antibody [1].

Patients with scleroderma are at risk for developing pulmonary arterial hypertension and interstitial lung disease so all patients should undergo pulmonary function testing including lung volumes and diffusion capacity, a 6 min walk test and an echocardiogram. A high resolution CT scan of the chest may be warranted depending on the results of the aforementioned studies.

In the case of our patient, the complete metabolic panel, and urinalysis were normal. Her complete blood count revealed anemia. She was anti-nuclear antibody (ANA) positive, 1:640 with a speckled pattern on immunofluorescence. Her anti Scl-70 antibody was negative. Anti-RNA polymerase III antibody was positive. Pulmonary function testing (PFT) was performed and her forced vital capacity (FVC) was 83 % predicted and diffusion capacity was 85 % predicted. Her diffusion capacity, forced expiratory volume in 1 second (FEV1) and FEV1/FVC ratio were normal. An echocardiogram revealed a normal left ventricular ejection fraction, normal right ventricular pressures and volumes, normal valvular function, and no evidence of a pericardial effusion.

What Is Your Final Diagnosis and Why?

SSc is the most likely diagnosis at this time given her signs and symptoms. Important considerations would include whether she has diffuse or limited cutaneous disease, and in this case, given that she has truncal involvement and skin thickening proximal

Table 8.2

1980 ACR Criteria for systemic sclerosis (scleroderma, SSc) (i)
Major criterion
Proximal skin thickening (proximal to the metacarpophalangeal joints)
Minor criteria
Sclerodactyly
Digital pitting scars
Bibasilar pulmonary fibrosis
SSc diagnosis is confirmed with the presence of one major criterion or two minor criteria

to the knees and elbows, she meets the classification criteria for diffuse cutaneous SSc. Diffuse cutaneous SSc is distinguished from limited cutaneous SSc by the distribution of skin thickening. Patients with diffuse disease will have skin changes proximal to the elbows and knees. They may also have truncal involvement. Patients with limited cutaneous SSc, formerly referred to as CREST (Calcinosis, Raynaud phenomenon, Esophageal dysmotility, Sclerodactyly, Telangiectasia) syndrome, will have similar skin thickening but without truncal involvement and not occurring proximal to the elbows or knees. Our patient meets American College of Rheumatology (ACR) criteria for the diagnosis of SSc since she fulfills one major criterion [2] Table 8.2.

Our patient has Raynaud phenomenon which may occur as a primary or secondary condition. In this case, the patient has secondary Raynaud phenomenon in association with diffuse cutaneous SSc, and approximately 95 % of patients with SSc have Raynaud phenomenon. However in any patient presenting with Raynaud phenomenon who has a paucity of other symptoms or signs, objective testing to include ANA and wide-field nailfold capillaroscopy can have prognostic value. A positive ANA and/or nailfold capillary changes using wide-field microscopy are predictive of the development of a connective tissue disease in a patient with Raynaud phenomenon [3, 4].

Patients with either limited or diffuse cutaneous SSc may develop interstitial lung disease. ILD occurs more commonly in patients with diffuse skin changes. Having an RNA polymerase III antibody is thought to be perhaps protective against ILD. Patients are at highest risk for the development of ILD within the first 4 years following disease onset [5]. This patient denies shortness of breath, she was RNA polymerase III antibody positive, and her pulmonary function testing is normal, but given the fact that she has diffuse skin changes and recent onset of disease she is still considered to be at risk for developing ILD.

The patient did have a positive anti-RNA polymerase III antibody. The presence of this autoantibody and her diffuse skin disease both portend an increased risk for the development of scleroderma renal crisis [2]. The creatinine and urinalysis are normal. Scleroderma renal crisis typically occurs early in the disease course of a patient with diffuse cutaneous disease. Symptoms of renal crisis might include shortness of breath, pulmonary edema, lower extremity edema, headaches, seizures, and visual disturbances with funduscopic changes similar to what is seen in malignant hypertension. The heralding sign of scleroderma renal crisis however is an elevated blood pressure. Even a mild elevation of blood pressure in someone who is usually normotensive or traditionally has a "low blood pressure" should raise clinical suspicion. A variant known as normotensive scleroderma renal crisis is thought to occur more often in patients who have been treated with 15 mg/day or more of prednisone, or its equivalent [6].

Case 2

A 43-year-old African-American male is referred to rheumatology clinic because his fingers began to feel puffy and tight. He has noted loss of grip strength and dexterity over the last several months. Now he cannot completely straighten his fingers. For the past 10 years he has experienced Raynaud phenomenon. He has never had digital pits or ulcers. He has learned to manage this cold induced vasospasm by avoiding cold exposure and keeping his core temperature warm. He has had gastroesophageal reflux since he was in college. He takes esomeprazole 40 mg once/day which controls his heartburn. He has lost approximately 10 pounds unintentionally over the last 6 months. He denies chest pain, but he has noted more shortness of breath with exertion over the last 6–8 weeks.

His past medical history is significant for GERD and Raynaud phenomenon as stated above. He had his appendix removed at the age of 15. No other surgeries. He has no known family history of autoimmune disease. His mother had diabetes and hypertension. His father had glaucoma and elevated triglycerides. This patient is a nonsmoker who drinks 1–2 alcoholic beverages each week. He has seasonal allergies but no known drug allergies. The only medication he takes regularly is the omeprazole 40 mg once each day. Occasionally he takes loratidine 10 mg as needed for seasonal allergies.

On physical examination he is afebrile. Blood pressure is 138/76 mmHg with a pulse of 88 beats per minute. He is breathing 18 times/min. In general he is in no acute distress and appears his stated age. There are vesicular breath sounds throughout all lung fields. His heart rate is normal with a regular rhythm. There is a II/VI systolic ejection murmur heard best at the left lower sternal border, and it is nonradiating. The murmur does not radiate to the carotids. Bowel sounds are normal in all four quadrants. No abdominal masses or organomegaly is appreciated. On skin examination he has multiple telangiectasias on his face, anterior chest, and on the dorsal and palmar surfaces of both hands. The skin of the fingers is tight symmetrically. This tightness extends proximally from the fingers to just past the wrists. His feet have similar findings with skin thickening of the toes extending proximally to just above the ankles. No digital pitting or ulceration. The skin on the face is tight as well and his oral aperture appears reduced. Just distal to the left olecranon process he has a subcutaneous lesion that is firm to palpation and nontender. There is no joint swelling but he does have reduced range of motion of both his wrists and ankles. There are flexion contractures of the PIP joints bilaterally.

With the History and Examination Presented, What Is Your Working Diagnosis?

This is a 43-year-old gentleman with a documented history of Raynaud phenomenon and GERD. Over the last several months he has noted changes in his fingers that have resulted in a loss of dexterity and grip strength. His skin examination is significant for tightening of the skin of the fingers and toes. He also has flexion contractures of the fingers. He is dyspenic with exertion and on exam he has a II/VI systolic ejection murmur. This condition involves multiple systems including his skin, musculoskeletal, GI, pulmonary, and cardiovascular systems. We suspect he may have an autoimmune disease.

Differential Diagnosis

The differential diagnosis list for this case would be similar to that described in Case 1. Both diffuse and limited cutaneous SSc require consideration as well as the diseases that may mimic SSc (Table 8.1).

Evaluation

The evaluation of this patient would be similar to that described in Case 1 (see above). His complete blood count, complete metabolic panel, and urinalysis were unremarkable. The ANA test was positive with a titer of 1:1,280 in a centromere pattern. In this case the RNA polymerase III antibody and the ENA panel were negative. His pulmonary function testing was normal except that his diffusion capacity was low, only 40 % of predicted. A transthoracic echocardiogram was obtained revealing tricuspid regurgitation and his peak right ventricular systolic pressure (PRVSP) was estimated to be 52 mmHg. The right atrium and right ventricle appeared to be enlarged. He did not have a pericardial effusion. Right heart catheterization was performed and confirmed that this patient has pulmonary arterial hypertension. The pulmonary capillary wedge pressure was normal. The mean pulmonary arterial pressure was 45 mmHg (9–18 mmHg). A plain radiograph of the left elbow/forearm confirmed that the palpable lesion found on his exam just distal to the left olecranon process was an area of calcinosis.

What Is Your Final Diagnosis and Why?

In this case we have all of the classic findings of a patient with limited cutaneous SSc (formerly known as CREST). He has an area of calcinosis, Raynaud phenomenon, esophageal reflux, sclerodactyly, and telangiectasias. The positive ANA with the centromere pattern is another common feature in patients with the limited variant. This patient's dyspnea is attributable to pulmonary hypertension. This was suspected based on his PFTs which showed a reduced diffusion capacity with otherwise normal lung function tests. The echocardiogram was also suggestive of pulmonary hypertension with elevated right sided pressures (PRVSP). The right heart catheterization confirms that this patient has pulmonary arterial hypertension.

Discussion

SSc is a disease characterized by the presence of thickened, hardened skin.

There are two subsets of SSc: diffuse cutaneous SSc (dcSSc) and limited cutaneous SSc (lcSSc) determined on the basis of the extent and distribution of skin involvement.

The systemic manifestations of SSc are diverse. Most prominent are abnormalities of the circulation (i.e., Raynaud phenomenon) and involvement of the musculoskeletal, renal, pulmonary, cardiac, and gastrointestinal systems, with fibrotic and/or microvascular complications. The etiology of the disease is unknown. The peak age of onset is 30–50 years with a female predominance. Patients with scleroderma will typically have a positive ANA. The most specific ANA immunofluorescence patterns in SSc are nucleolar and centromere. An anti-centromere antibody is most commonly seen in those patients with the limited variant [2]. Anti-Scl-70 antibody and anti-RNA polymerase III antibody are seen most often in patients with diffuse cutaneous disease. Anti-Scl-70 is associated with an increased risk for developing interstitial lung disease. A positive RNA polymerase III antibody is considered to be a risk factor for scleroderma renal crisis and is associated with a reduced likelihood for development of ILD.

Skin manifestations of SSc include skin thickening, digital pitting/ulceration, telangiectasias, and calcinosis. Skin thickening typically begins in the fingers and toes and gradually progresses more proximally. If the skin thickening extends proximally beyond the elbows or knees then this would be consistent with having diffuse cutaneous SSc. Truncal involvement would also indicate that a patient has diffuse cutaneous SSc. Thickening of the skin on the face can be seen in either diffuse or limited cutaneous SSc. Patients with limited cutaneous SSc will have neither skin thickening proximal to the elbows or knees nor truncal involvement. Skin changes in SSc may progress over the first 2 years following onset of the disease. Patients may appear to have limited skin involvement in the beginning but go on to progress to having diffuse skin changes over the course of the first 2 years of disease. The presence of tendon friction rubs can suggest that further skin changes are likely and that the patient will go on to develop diffuse cutaneous SSc. Telangiectasias may be observed on the fingers, palms, chest, face, and oral mucosa in patients with either limited or diffuse cutaneous disease (Fig. 8.3).

Calcinosis is another skin complication seen in some patients with SSc. The etiology of calcinosis in connective tissue diseases is not known. Deposits of calcium

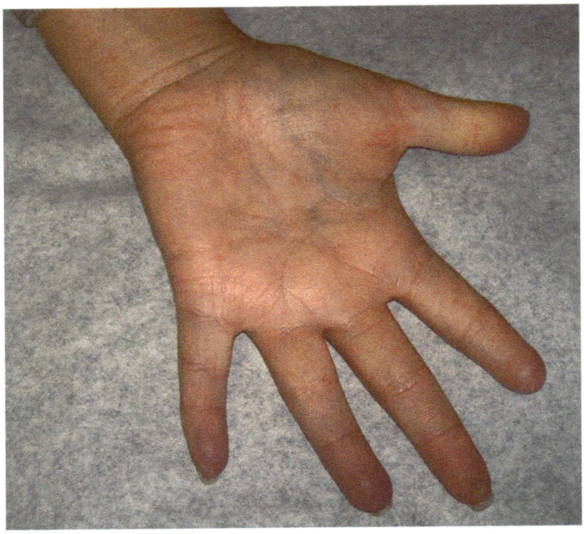

Fig. 8.3 Palmar telangiectasias

hydroxyapatite crystals can occur in the digital pads (calcinosis cutis), periarticular tissues, sites of repeated pressure or trauma (e.g., olecranon bursa), extensor surfaces of the forearms, prepatellar and infrapatellar bursal areas, and the buttocks. The size of these calcium deposits varies from tiny punctuate lesions to large masses (tumoral calcinosis). Calcinosis may cause the overlying skin to ulcerate and white/milky drainage may exude from these lesions. If secondary bacterial infections occur, treatment with antibiotics and in some cases surgical debridement may be required.

Almost every patient with SSc will have cold induced vasospasm of the digital arteries; this is known as Raynaud phenomenon. The arterial vasospasm may lead to well-demarcated tri-phasic color changes (white, blue, red) of the fingers starting distally and progressing proximally. Larger vessels like the ulnar arteries may also be involved, and can contribute to the presence of ischemic digital ulcers [7]. The ischemic injury is the result of both arterial vasospasm and anatomic narrowing due to vascular intimal proliferation, medial hypertrophy, and adventitial fibrosis. Patients with digital pits and/or ulcers may benefit from vasodilator therapy, aspirin, digital sympathectomy and/or arterial bypass surgery. Digital ulcers may become infected and require antibiotic treatment. Digital pitting is one of the diagnostic criteria for SSc and relates to the ischemic tissue injury resulting from Raynaud phenomenon (Table 8.2).

Pulmonary disease is now the leading cause of mortality in patients with SSc. Interstitial lung disease (ILD), characterized by basilar pulmonary fibrosis, occurs in both the limited (lSSc) and diffuse (dSSc) cutaneous phenotypes. ILD is thought to occur more frequently in patients with anti-topoisomerase I antibody and in those with diffuse skin disease [2]. Patients usually develop ILD within 4 years of the onset of disease. African American males in the fifth and sixth decades of life have the highest risk of developing severe lung disease [5]. Pulmonary function testing in all patients with scleroderma is recommended. A reduction in the diffusion capacity for carbon monoxide (DL_{co}) is the earliest and most sensitive abnormality, but is not specific for ILD in these patients [8]. An isolated reduction of DL_{CO} may also suggest pulmonary hypertension. Reduction in the total lung capacity (TLC) with reduced FVC and a normal FEV1/FVC ratio is indicative of the restrictive pattern one expects to see in ILD, including patients with scleroderma. PFT abnormalities may occur prior to the onset of respiratory symptoms. If the pulmonary function tests are abnormal, High Resolution CT (HRCT) scan of the chest is recommended. HRCT of the chest may reveal ground glass opacification indicative of an inflammatory alveolitis and/or fine fibrosis. Other possible HRCT findings in patients with SSc associated ILD includes subpleural cysts, reticular fibrosis, traction bronchiectasis, and honeycombing.

Scleroderma patients are at increased risk for the development of pulmonary arterial hypertension (PAH), most often in the setting of limited cutaneous disease (lSSc) with little or no ILD. Although PAH is more common in patients with the limited cutaneous phenotype of scleroderma (lSSc) it may occur in anyone with SSc. Secondary causes of pulmonary hypertension would include interstitial lung disease, valvular heart disease, and left ventricular diastolic dysfunction. Symptoms of PAH include: dyspnea, fatigue, syncope, light-headed sensation, atypical chest pain and/or lower extremity swelling. Pulmonary function testing may demonstrate a reduction in the diffusion capacity. An echocardiogram is recommended for screening patients for pulmonary hypertension. The echocardiogram may however either under- or over-estimate the peak right ventricular systolic pressure. Sometimes the interpreting cardiologist cannot comment on the right-sided pressures because of a lack of tricuspid regurgitation. When suspected, right heart catheterization must be done to confirm pulmonary arterial hypertension. The diagnosis of PAH requires a mean pulmonary artery pressure greater than or equal to 25 mmHg at rest with a pulmonary capillary wedge pressure less than or equal to 15 mmHg [9]. The right heart catheterization is considered the diagnostic gold standard for diagnosing PAH. A right heart catheterization will also be helpful in ruling out other causes of PAH including left ventricular diastolic dysfunction, which occurs not infrequently in scleroderma patients. Other cardiac manifestations of scleroderma include heart failure, conduction block and arrhythmias, all resulting from fibrosis and myocardial ischemia believed to be due to non-epicardial coronary artery disease. Arterial vasospasm of different vascular beds, such as coronary, renal and intestinal arteries may also be observed.

Gastrointestinal motility is delayed in nearly all patients with scleroderma, and the entire GI tract may be affected. An estimated 30–40 % of patients will have subclinical esophageal dysmotility [10]. The lower esophageal sphincter (LES) pressure is also reduced. An incompetent LES combined with the esophageal dysmotility leads to gastroesophageal reflux and subsequently increases the risk of aspiration and the development of pneumonitis and/or pneumonia. Intestinal dysmotility may lead to constipation and can also result in a pseudo-obstruction. Pseudo-obstruction is a very serious condition in which patients develop nausea, vomiting, bloating, obstipation and abdominal pain. Pseudo-obstruction may be difficult to distinguish from a true anatomical obstruction, particularly in patients who have undergone previous abdominal or pelvic surgery, but the former is due to a functional ileus and conservative management is imperative.

Occult or overt GI bleeding may occur. Blood loss may be the result of erosive esophagitis, gastritis, mucosal telangiectasias, Mallory-Weiss tear, or gastric antral vascular ectasia (GAVE), also known as the "watermelon stomach." Be cautious when considering anticoagulation/DVT prophylaxis in patients with SSc given these multiple sources for possible gastrointestinal blood loss. GAVE can lead to profound blood loss requiring multiple blood transfusions.

Patients with scleroderma may experience early satiety, bloating and delayed gastric emptying, each of which may diminish caloric intake. Gastroparesis and delayed intestinal motility can reduce the absorption of medications and nutrients. The oral aperture may be reduced due to the skin tightening, contributing to inadequate oral intake.

Prior to the introduction of angiotensin converting enzyme (ACE) inhibitors, renal crisis was the leading cause of mortality in patients with scleroderma. Scleroderma renal crisis still occurs but is being recognized sooner and treated aggressively with ACE inhibitors and, thus, outcomes have improved. Approximately 10 % of patients with SSc will develop renal crisis, usually within 3 years of disease onset [11]. A patient with scleroderma renal crisis typically presents with new onset hypertension. Laboratory abnormalities of renal crisis may include [12]:

- Microangiopathic anemia (schistocytes on peripheral blood smear)
- Thrombocytopenia
- Elevated serum creatinine
- Proteinuria (usually mild)
- Active urinary sediment with RBCs and RBC casts (or bland microhematuria)

The take home point here is to closely follow the blood pressure of all patients with scleroderma. Evaluate even small increases in blood pressure thoroughly. Start ACE inhibitors early and increase the dosage as necessary if renal crisis is suspected. Remember scleroderma renal crisis is more likely to be seen in patients with diffuse SSc.

Musculoskeletal involvement is common in patients with SSc. Manifestations include arthralgia, inflammatory arthritis, flexion contractures, and tendon friction rubs. The progressive skin thickening/fibrosis can lead to joint flexion contractures. The proximal interphalangeal (PIP), elbow, and knee joints are commonly affected. Tendon friction rubs occur most commonly in patients with diffuse cutaneous SSc. Proximal muscle weakness can occur and may represent either a bland myopathy or a possible overlap with inflammatory myositis. Treatment of the musculoskeletal complaints of these patients involves analgesia for arthralgia/arthritis, physical and occupational therapy to avoid flexion contractures, and immunosuppression for inflammatory joint or muscle involvement.

Questions

1. Patients with limited cutaneous SSc are most likely to have which of the following positive tests?

    (A) Rheumatoid factor (RF)
    (B) Anti-SCL-70 antibody
    (C) Anti-RNA polymerase III antibody
    (D) Anti-centromere antibody

2. Which of the following about RNA III polymerase antibodies is true?

    (A) Associated with a higher risk of developing scleroderma renal crisis
    (B) Presence of this antibody is thought to increase risk for developing interstitial lung disease
    (C) Presence of this antibody is thought to reduce the risk of developing interstitial lung disease
    (D) Both A & C

3. Which one of the following is more of a risk factor for developing scleroderma renal crisis?

    (A) Having the limited variant of SSc
    (B) +Anti-nuclear antibody
    (C) Having the diffuse variant of SSc
    (D) Raynaud phenomenon

4. Which finding would establish that a patient has diffuse cutaneous SSc?

    (A) Skin thickening proximal to the elbows or knees
    (B) Telangiectasias
    (C) Interstitial lung disease on HRCT of the chest
    (D) +RNP antibody

5. Which disease can mimic SSc and may also be associated with multiple myeloma?

    (A) Eosinophilic fasciitis
    (B) Morphea
    (C) Scleromyxedema
    (D) Scleredema

6. The leading cause of mortality in patients with SSc is?

    (A) Raynaud phenomenon
    (B) Renal Crisis
    (C) Calcinosis
    (D) Pulmonary disease

7. All of the following are characteristics of scleroderma renal crisis except:

   (A) Macrocytic anemia
   (B) Thrombocytopenia
   (C) Schistocytes on peripheral blood smear
   (D) Proteinuria

8. Which pulmonary function test suggests that a patient has pulmonary arterial hypertension?

   (A) Reduced FVC
   (B) Reduced diffusion capacity
   (C) Increased diffusion capacity
   (D) Increased FEV1/FVC ratio

9. A groove sign would be a feature of which scleroderma mimicking disease?

   (A) Morphea
   (B) Nephrogenic Systemic Fibrosis
   (C) Eosinophilic fasciitis
   (D) Scleredema

10. Tendon friction rubs would be most likely found in a patient with?

    (A) Limited cutaneous SSc
    (B) Eosinophilic fasciitis
    (C) Diffuse cutaneous SSc
    (D) Morphea

Answers Key: 1 (D), 2 (D), 3 (C), 4 (A), 5 (C), 6 (D), 7 (A), 8 (B), 9 (C), 10 (C).

References

1. Steen VD, Powell DL, Medsger Jr TA. Clinical correlations and prognosis based on serum autoantibodies in patients with systemic sclerosis. Arthritis Rheum. 1988;31(2):196–203.
2. Masi AT, Rodnan GP, Medsger Jr TA, et al. Preliminary criteria for the classification of systemic sclerosis (scleroderma). Arthritis Rheum. 1980;23:581–90.
3. Blockmans D, Beyens G, Verhaeghe R. Predictive value of nailfold capillaroscopy in the diagnosis of connective tissue diseases. Clin Rheum. 1996;15(2):148–53.
4. Reimer G, et al. Correlates between autoantibodies to nucleolar antigens and clinical features in patients with systemic sclerosis (scleroderma). Arthritis Rheum. 1988;31(4):525–32.
5. Steen VD, et al. Severe restrictive lung disease in systemic sclerosis. Arthritis Rheum. 1994;37(9):1283–9.
6. Steen VD, Medsger Jr TA. Case-control study of corticosteroids and other drugs that either precipitate or protect from the development of scleroderma renal crisis. Arthritis Rheum. 1998;41:1613–9.
7. Taylor MH, McFadden JA, Bolster MB, Silver R. Ulnar Artery Involvement in Systemic Sclerosis (scleroderma). J Rheumatol. 2002;29(1):102–6.

8. Catterall M, Rowell NR. Respiratory function in progressive systemic sclerosis. Thorax. 1963;18:10–5.
9. Galie N, Hoeper MM, Humbert M, et al. Guidelines for the diagnosis and treatment of pulmonary hypertension. Eur Respir J. 2009;34:1219.
10. Clements PJ, Becvar R, Drosos AA, et al. Assessment of gastrointestinal involvement. Clin Exp Rheumatol. 2003;21:S15–18.
11. Steen VD, Medsger Jr TA. Severe organ involvement in systemic sclerosis with diffuse scleroderma. Arthritis Rheum. 2000;43:2437–44.
12. Steen VD, et al. Factors predicting development of renal involvement in progressive systemic sclerosis. Am J Med. 1984;76:779–86.

Part III
Inflammatory and Metabolic Diseases of the Immune System

Chapter 9
Polymyositis

Uma Thanarajasingam and Floranne Ernste

Abstract Polymyositis (PM) is an inflammatory myopathy characterized by symmetric proximal muscle weakness with CD8+ T cells invading non-necrotic muscle fibers. Myositis-specific antibodies may serve as markers of clinical phenotype and treatment response. Statin use has been associated with precipitating an immune-mediated, necrotizing myositis. Herein, we present two cases that were challenging in diagnosis, treatment, and follow-up.

Keywords Idiopathic inflammatory myopathies • Polymyositis • Myositis-specific autoantibodies • Statin-induced myositis

Case 1

Our patient is a 39 year old Caucasian female who presented in 2010 for treatment recommendations for myositis. Her symptoms began in 2002 with an insidious onset of myalgias involving the neck, bilateral shoulders and flanks. Within six months, she developed severe proximal muscle weakness resulting in significant functional limitations with an inability to get out of bed and arise from a seated position. She had elevated a creatine kinase (CK) of 8,325 U/L (38–176 U/L) and an aldolase of 81.2 U/L (normal is <7.7 U/L). An electromyogram (EMG) revealed short duration, low amplitude myopathic motor unit potentials, particularly in the biceps, triceps, and left vastus lateralis. Magnetic resonance imaging (MRI) of the left shoulder demonstrated muscle edema in the supraspinatus, infraspinatus, biceps, and subscapularis musculature. A muscle biopsy of the left deltoid revealed necrotic

U. Thanarajasingam, M.D., Ph.D. (✉) • F. Ernste, M.D.
Division of Rheumatology, Department of Internal Medicine, Mayo Clinic Rochester, 200 First Street SW, Rochester, MN 55905, USA
e-mail: thanarajasingam.uma@mayo.edu; ernste.floranne@mayo.edu

M. Mahmoudi (ed.), *Challenging Cases in Rheumatology and Diseases of the Immune System*, DOI 10.1007/978-1-4614-5088-7_9,
© Springer Science+Business Media, LLC 2013

and regenerating fibers in muscle fascicles and a moderate inflammatory exudate indicative of an active inflammatory myopathy. There were not enough fibers to classify the infiltrate in a perimysial or perivascular distribution. There was no perifascicular atrophy. There were no congophilic deposits.

She was treated initially with intravenous steroids in high doses, and then switched to high doses of prednisone. In addition, she started oral methotrexate that was later changed to the subcutaneous route due to gastrointestinal side effects. After a year, the patient had persistently elevated muscle enzymes and an inability to reduce the steroid dose; therefore, she was switched to cyclosporine. This medication proved to be ineffective and therefore intravenous immunoglobulin was started on a monthly basis over 2 days before she came to see us.

Past medical history. Her past medical history was remarkable for a benign thyroid nodule and untreated hyperlipidemia.

Family and social history. Her family history was notable for early coronary artery disease in her father and a sister who had a myocardial infarction at age 30. Her mother died of metastatic ovarian cancer. One sister had breast cancer. The patient was married with four children, all daughters, who were healthy. She denied smoking, illicit drug, or alcohol use.

Review of systems. Occasional dry cough and shortness of breath. There were no fevers, chills, weight loss, or rash. She denied photosensitivity, malar rash, discoid rash, alopecia, sicca, Raynaud's phenomenon, inflammatory arthritis, serositis, or kidney disease.

Physical examination. This was a youthful-appearing female, well-nourished, and in no apparent distress. Vitals: Height: 165.0 cm; Weight: 67.7 kg; Blood pressure: 98/70 mmHg; Pulse: 85 beats per minute and regular. HEENT: Normocephalic, atraumatic, extra-ocular muscles intact. Skin: No heliotrope rash, shawl sign, Gottron's papules, livedo reticularis, sclerodactyly, or vasculitic lesions. No periungual erythema, telangiectasias, or mechanic's hands. Heart: Regular in rate and rhythm without murmurs, rubs, or gallops. Lungs: clear bilaterally without dullness to percussion. Abdomen: Soft and benign without organomegaly. Joints: No synovitis of the upper and lower extremities including hands, wrists, elbows, knees, ankles, or feet bilaterally. Neurologic: Mental status and cranial nerves were normal. She had significant loss of strength in the proximal muscles bilaterally. She had moderate neck flexor weakness and an inability to rise from a seated position with her arms crossed in front of her chest. There was no muscle atrophy. Sensory examination was normal. Reflexes were normal.

Data

Her laboratory studies at the time of our evaluation were remarkable for an elevated creatine kinase level; the highest value was 5,077 U/L (38–176 U/L). Other elevated muscle enzymes included an aldolase of 81.1 U/L (normal is <7.7 U/L); AST of 176 U/L (8–43 U/L); ALT of 213 U/L (7–45 U/L). She had an elevated anti-nuclear antibody by enzyme-linked immunosorbent assay (ELISA) testing of 6.9 U (normal is 1.0 U). Other autoantibodies were negative including DNA double-stranded antibody, anti-SS-A antibody, anti-SS-B, anti-Smith, anti-Jo-1 antibody, anti-U1-RNP antibody, and SCL-70 antibody. However, an anti-SRP antibody returned as positive. An electromyogram (EMG) showed a moderate to severe active inflammatory myopathy. A midstream urinalysis was unremarkable.

With Presented Data, What Is Your Working Diagnosis?

This is a 39 year old female with severe proximal muscle weakness, significantly elevated muscle enzymes, a positive ANA, positive anti-SRP antibody, an EMG that shows severe inflammatory myopathy, and a muscle biopsy that had a moderate inflammatory exudate indicative of an active inflammatory myopathy. The presented data and exam led us to the diagnosis of a severe polymyositis with a positive myositis-specific autoantibody refractory to standard treatment.

Differential diagnosis. The differential diagnosis includes systemic lupus erythematosus, dermatomyositis, cancer-associated myositis, inclusion body myositis, anti-synthetase syndrome, and polymyositis with a positive myositis-specific autoantibody.

Workup

Computed tomography (CT) scans of the chest, abdomen, and pelvis were negative for lymphadenopathy, malignancy, or any other abnormality. A pelvic ultrasound was negative for ovarian tumors or endometrial abnormalities. A mammogram was unremarkable. A colonoscopy revealed a medium-sized rectal polyp and a small sigmoid polyp, both of which were treated and pathology revealed fragments of a villous adenoma and an inflammatory polyp. An echocardiogram revealed normal ejection fraction, chamber sizes, valves and pressures. Pulmonary function testing was within normal limits.

What Is Your Diagnosis and Why?

Systemic lupus erythematosus (SLE). Although the patient had a positive ANA, she did not have the typical clinical features of SLE such as photosensitivity, malar rash, discoid rash, inflammatory arthritis, serositis, or kidney disease. The midstream urinalysis did not reveal active sediment. Moreover, she did not have positive antibodies to double-stranded DNA or Smith which are specific for a diagnosis of SLE.

Dermatomyositis. Although the patient had features classic for an inflammatory myopathy with proximal muscle weakness, elevated muscle enzymes, and myopathic motor unit action potentials on the EMG, the patient did not have the classic rash of dermatomyositis described on exam such as a heliotrope rash, Gottron's sign or Gottron's papules, periungual erythema and/or telangiectasias, or a shawl sign. Moreover, the muscle biopsy of the left deltoid was not specific for features of an inflammatory infiltrate located in a perivascular and/or perifascicular distribution, nor was there perifascicular atrophy.

Cancer-associated myositis. Although the patient had a severe myopathy as can be seen in most cancer-associated cases, her extensive workup did not reveal a malignancy.

Sporadic inclusion body myositis (sIBM). Although the patient had a myositis refractory to standard treatment as can be seen in patients with sIBM, our patient did not have the typical clinical characteristics of distal muscle weakness with atrophy of the forearm flexors, intrinsic muscles of the hands, or quadriceps. In addition, the muscle biopsy did not reveal congophilic deposits or rimmed vacuoles which are classic histopathologic findings of IBM.

Anti-synthetase syndrome. The patient did not have the classic clinical features of anti-synthetase syndrome which are inflammatory arthritis, interstitial lung disease, Raynaud's phenomenon, and a positive anti-synthetase antibody.

Our patient did have a positive anti-SRP antibody in the context of polymyositis, which was refractory to standard treatment. She had marked elevation of the muscle enzymes and significant muscle weakness despite conventional therapy with methotrexate, cyclosporine, intravenous immunoglobulins, and high-dose steroids. Lack of an expected response to standard immune suppressant therapy should prompt a workup into checking for myositis-specific autoantibodies such as the anti-SRP antibody.

Plan. Our patient was switched to mycophenolate mofetil in addition to intravenous immunoglobulin at a dose of 0.4 g/kg twice weekly for approximately 6 weeks which was subsequently reduced to 0.4 g/kg once weekly for an additional 8 weeks. Over the course of 1 year, she was pulsed intermittently with methylprednisolone when symptoms of worsening dysphagia or proximal muscle weakness, 1 g daily, for 3 days in a row. This was followed by high dose prednisone at 80 mg daily with subsequent reduction by 5–10 mg every 2–4 weeks. The patient responded gradually over 1.5 years with improved CPK levels and muscle strength. At the time of last follow-up which was May 2011, the CK level had improved to 633 U/L (38–176 U/L) and the aldolase had improved to 9.1 U/L (normal is <7.7 U/L). Muscle strength was trending back toward her baseline, and she denied significant dysphagia. She was on mycophenolate mofetil at 2,500 mg daily and prednisone at 15 mg daily.

Discussion

Polymyositis (PM) is an autoimmune inflammatory myopathy that develops over weeks to months and it is characterized by symmetric proximal muscle weakness, elevated serum muscle enzymes, and EMG evidence of muscle inflammation and

Table 9.1 Myositis-specific autoantibodies in adult idiopathic inflammatory myopathies (IIM)

Autoantibody	Antigen	Clinical features	Frequency
Anti-synthetase	Aminoacyl-tRNA synthetase	Antisynthetase syndrome	25–30%
Jo-1	Histidyl-tRNA synthetase		
PL-7	Threonyl-tRNA synthetase		
PL-12	Alanyl-tRNA synthetase		
OJ	Isoleucyl-tRNA synthetase		
EJ	Glycyl-tRNA synthetase		
KS	Asparaginyl-tRNA synthetase		
Ha	Tyrosyl-tRNA synthetase		
Zo	Phenylalanyl-tRNA synthetase		
P155/140	Transcriptional intermediary	Malignancy	13–20% factor-1 (TIF1-γ)
Anti-Mi2	Nuclear helicase	Mild myositis Classic DM skin features	<10%
Anti-SRP	Signal recognition particle	Necrotizing myositis	5–10%
Anti-CADM-140	MDA5	ILD in Asians	50–75%

ILD interstitial lung disease; *DM* dermatomyositis; *RP* Raynaud's phenomenon. *MDA5* melanoma differentiation-association gene
Adapted from Chiu and Co [7]

damage. Unlike dermatomyositis, patients do not present with a rash. There is not a family history of myositis such as can be seen with muscular dystrophy or limb-girdle dystrophy. PM is often an exclusionary diagnosis as the phenotype may be nonspecific with features shared with other inflammatory myopathies, leading some experts to believe that it may be over-diagnosed [1, 2].

Myositis-specific autoantibodies (MSA) are found in the serum of patients with inflammatory myopathies and are directed toward specific proteins in the nucleus and cytoplasm. They are associated with specific clinical phenotypes and disease prognosis, but their relationship to pathogenesis is unknown at this time (Please see Table 9.1). The myositis-specific autoantibodies are categorized into three main groups: anti-synthetases, anti-SRP, and anti-Mi2 autoantibodies. The most common are a family of antibodies directed against aminoacyl-tRNA synthetases which are enzymes that catalyze the binding of amino acids to specific tRNAs and characterize the so-called "anti-synthetase syndrome." There are many autoantigens involved: Jo-1, PL-7, PL-12, OJ, EJ, KS, Ha, and Zo. The anti-Jo-1 antibody is the most common, occurring in about 15–20% of adult myositis patients. The clinical manifestations of anti-synthetase syndrome are fever, mechanic's hands (hyperkeratosis along the lateral edges of fingers), Raynaud's phenomenon, myositis, interstitial lung disease, and a mild inflammatory arthritis. The anti-Mi2 is directed against the 218 kDa nuclear protein which is a helicase involved in transcriptional activation. Patients with anti-Mi2 autoantibodies may have the classical cutaneous features including Gottron's papules, shawl sign, cuticle overgrowth, V-sign, and a heliotrope rash. These patients often have a milder myositis course. The anti-SRP is directed against the signal recognition particle; it is a 6 polypeptide protein complex that escorts newly synthesized proteins from the cytoplasm to the endoplasmic reticulum. The clinical manifestations of patients with the anti-SRP antibody are a severe myositis of acute onset with features of a necrotizing myopathy on biopsy, occasional cardiac involvement, and poor survival. Other autoantibodies include the anti-transcriptional intermediary factor 1-γ (also known as p155/140 doublet kilodalton protein), and anti-melanoma differentiation-association gene 5 autoantibodies. The p155/140 doublet protein has been highly associated with cancer-associated myositis (CAM) and severe skin disease. The anti-MDA5 antibody has been linked to rapid onset of interstitial lung disease in the Asian population. The MSAs may just be markers of disease, although recent studies have suggested that certain MSAs, such as Jo-1, may act as endogenous type 1 interferon inducers by peripheral blood mononuclear cells in vitro, possibly contributing to disease pathogenesis [3–6].

Pathophysiology. Muscle biopsies typically show an endomysial inflammatory infiltrate composed of cytotoxic, CD8+ T-cells surrounding and invading normal muscle fibers expressing up-regulated major histocompatibility class I (MHC-1) leading to muscle fiber necrosis via the perforin pathway. Genetic and environmental factors may play a role in triggering PM. Certain haplotypes such HLA-DRB1*03, DQA1*05, DQA1*0301, and DQB1*02 are thought to be genetic risk factors in Caucasians from the United Kingdom. Other populations such as Asians and Native Americans have differing haplotypes conferring risk for PM development. Environmental risk factors include ultraviolet light, certain latitudes, and viral infections [6–8].

Workup. The workup for PM begins with a detailed history about recent infections, medication use (such as a statin), features concerning for a malignancy, and high-risk activities such as intravenous drug use and/or sexual behavior. The examination should include a detailed strength examination of the major proximal and distal muscles. Laboratory investigations should include a complete blood count (CBC), erythrocyte sedimentation rate (ESR), C-reactive protein (CRP), creatinine, lactate dehydrogenase (LDH), AST, ALT, creatine kinase (CK), aldolase, and serum myoglobin. HIV testing should be done to exclude an HIV-associated myopathy. In addition, a urinalysis with myoglobin should be obtained to check for myoglobulinuria. Basic serum chemistries should include a sodium, potassium, bicarbonate, blood urea nitrogen, fasting calcium, phosphorous, magnesium, and a fasting glucose and lipid panel. In addition, autoantibodies such as an anti-nuclear antibody (ANA) and antibodies to the extractable nuclear antigens (ENA) such as anti-SS-A, anti-SS-B, anti-Smith, anti-RNP, anti-Scl-70, and anti-centromere are important to check to determine if the myositis may be secondary to a connective tissue disease. An electrocardiogram (ECG) should be obtained to ensure no electrical abnormalities such as conductance system disturbances or chamber hypertrophy are present.

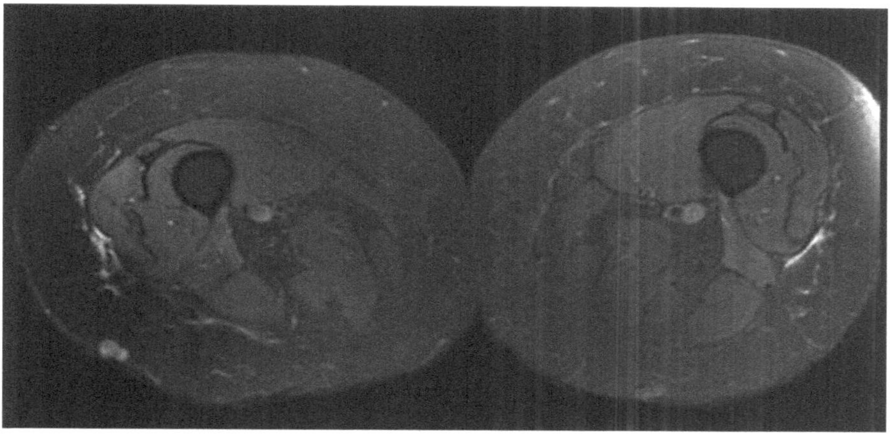

Fig. 9.1 Magnetic resonance imaging of the bilateral thighs without intravenous gadolinium in a patient with anti-synthetase syndrome revealing increased T2 signal within the anterior aspect of the short head of the biceps femoris muscles, bilaterally

An EMG will determine whether there is electrophysiologic evidence of polyphasic motor unit action potentials of short duration and low amplitude with increased insertional and spontaneous activity in the form of fibrillation potentials, sharp waves, or repetitive discharges. Finally, a muscle biopsy is important to confirm the diagnosis. Histopathologic features diagnostic for PM are an endomysial inflammatory infiltrate surrounding and invading non-necrotic fibers [1–4].

Imaging studies. Occasionally, a magnetic resonance image (MRI) is obtained of the affected proximal musculature such as the deltoids, biceps femoris, or quadriceps muscles to determine whether there is muscle inflammation and/or edema (See Fig. 9.1).

Treatment. The treatment begins with high-dose corticosteroids intravenously for 3–5 days such as 500–1,000 mg of methylprednisolone if there is severe dysphagia and/or weakness. For outpatient treatment, begin oral prednisone at 60–80 mg daily (1 mg/kg/day) as a single dose for 2–4 weeks followed by 40 mg daily for 2–4 weeks and then tapering by 10 mg every 2–4 weeks until down to 20 mg daily. Once the patient is at 20 mg daily, then the steroid taper should by slowed by 2.5 mg every 2 weeks until completed. At the same time that the patient begins steroids, an immunosuppressive agent should be started. Standard agents used are methotrexate, azathioprine, and mycophenolate mofetil (off-label). Steroid and immunosuppressant doses should be titrated according to patient response and/or side effects encountered.

Summary and conclusion. PM is an inflammatory muscle disease that presents with symmetric, proximal muscle weakness without a rash, and elevated muscle enzymes, an abnormal EMG, and distinct histopathologic features involving an endomysial inflammatory infiltrate composed of cytotoxic CD8+ cells invading non-necrotic fibers on muscle biopsy. Myositis-specific autoantibodies are important for defining clinical phenotypes and determining prognosis. Treatment involves high-dose corticosteroids with a taper and an immunosuppressant agent with doses adjusted according to patient response.

Case 2

Our patient is a 64 year lady who presented to us in March 2010 with myalgias and severe proximal muscle weakness. Her symptoms began in the fall of 2009 with shooting axial muscle pains, and an inability to get out of bed and arise from low chairs. She had developed proximal limb weakness as well as cramps in the calves, and the muscle enzymes were significantly elevated beyond 2× the upper limits of normal. An EMG showed polyphasic motor unit potentials and decreased amplitude in the right deltoid and right triceps with increased insertional activity and fibrillations. The patient began high dose prednisone of 40 mg daily with a rapid taper over 2 weeks.

Past medical history. She had essential hypertension and hyperlipidemia. Approximately six months prior to her acute presentation, she had started a statin medication which was subsequently discontinued.

Family and social history. The patient was married with adult children who were healthy. She denied smoking, illicit drug, or alcohol use. Her father had died of smoking-related lung cancer.

Review of systems. She had an occasional dry cough and dyspnea on exertion. There was also dysphagia and a twenty pound weight loss in the last three months. There were no fevers or chills. She denied a rash. She denied photosensitivity, malar rash, discoid rash, alopecia, sicca, Raynaud's phenomenon, inflammatory arthritis, serositis, or kidney disease.

Physical examination. This was a pleasant female, well-nourished, and in no apparent distress. Vitals: Height: 159.8 cm; Weight: 73.4 kg; Blood pressure: 116/76 mmHg; Pulse: 117 beats per minute. Skin: No heliotrope rash, no shawl sign, no Gottron's papules, no livedo reticularis, no sclerodactyly, no telangiectasias, no vasculitic lesions. No periungual erythema or mechanic's hands. Heart: Tachycardic without murmurs or rubs. Lungs: Mild, Velcro-sounding crackles in bases bilaterally. Lymph: No cervical or supraclavicular lymphadenopathy. Abdomen: Soft and benign with organomegaly. Joints: A few metacarpophalangeal (MCP) joints were swollen bilaterally with tenderness with slight swelling of a few proximal interphalangeal (PIP) joints bilaterally. The rest of the joint examination was unremarkable. Neurologic: Mental status and cranial nerves were normal. There was moderate, symmetric weakness of the neck flexors, external rotators, deltoids, triceps, biceps, and supinators. Strength in the other upper extremity muscles was otherwise normal. In the lower extremities, she had severe, symmetric weakness of the iliopsoas, thigh adductors, abductors, and mild-to-moderate weakness of the quadriceps and hamstrings. No muscle atrophy. Sensory examination was normal. Reflexes were normal. Her gait was mildly waddling, and she had difficulty arising from the chair without arm rail support.

Table 9.2 Abnormal laboratory findings in a female patient with myositis

Test	Abnormal results	Range
WBC 10^3 per mm	19.2 H	3.5–10.5
Platelets 10^3 per mm	483 H	150–450
AST (SGOT) U/L	262 H	8–43
ALT (SGPT) U/L	392 H	7–45
Creatine kinase U/L	5,423 H	38–176
Aldolase	60.5 H	<7.7
C-reactive protein (mg/L)	17.4 H	<8.0
Urine analysis	Cloudy, protein, moderate hemoglobin, WBC, bacteria	Clear negative

Data

The abnormal lab results are presented in Table 9.2. The ANA, extractable nuclear antigens (ENA), rheumatoid factor, and anti-CCP antibodies were negative. A mid-stream urinalysis showed a moderate amount of hemoglobin, but no active sediment, and bacteriuria. A muscle biopsy of the left thigh was obtained and revealed scattered necrotic and regenerating fibers with a focal collection of rare mononuclear cells with an absence of significant muscle inflammation.

With Presented Data, What Is Your Working Diagnosis?

This is a 64-year old lady with subacute onset of severe, symmetric proximal muscle weakness in the upper and lower extremities, elevated muscle enzymes, an EMG with findings of an active myopathy, and a muscle biopsy of the quadriceps revealing a necrotizing myopathy. The presented data and examination led us to the diagnosis of a severe, non-inflammatory, necrotizing myopathy with a possible association with recent statin use.

Differential diagnosis. The differential diagnosis includes dermatomyositis, cancer-associated myositis, inclusion body myositis, and anti-synthetase syndrome.

Workup

A computed tomography of the chest was remarkable for bilateral reticular opacities suggestive of interstitial fibrosis without honeycombing. Pulmonary function testing revealed mild restriction with a total lung capacity (TLC) of 3.47 L (72% of predicted) and a diffusing lung capacity (DLCO) of 11.6 L (57% of predicted). There was decreased maximal expiratory pressure suggestive of neuromuscular weakness. A barium-double contrast esophagram revealed markedly decreased primary peristalsis in the skeletal muscle upper third of the esophagus. A transvaginal ultrasound showed a normal-appearing uterus; there were no adnexal masses. A colonoscopy was unremarkable except for internal hemorrhoids. A mammogram was normal. An echocardiogram was essential normal with a normal ejection fraction, right ventricular systolic pressures, and no pericardial effusion.

What Is Your Diagnosis and Why?

Dermatomyositis. Although the patient had features classic for DM with proximal muscle weakness, elevated muscle enzymes, and myopathic motor unit action potentials on EMG, she did not have the classic rash of dermatomyositis such as a heliotrope rash, Gottron's sign or Gottron's papules, periungual erythema and/or telangiectasias, or a shawl sign. Moreover, the muscle biopsy of the left quadriceps was not specific for features of DM.

Cancer-associated myositis. Although she had a severe myopathy as can be seen in cancer-associated cases, her extensive workup did not reveal a malignancy.

Sporadic inclusion body myositis (sIBM). Our patient did not have the typical clinical characteristics of distal muscle weakness with atrophy of the forearm flexors, intrinsic muscles of the hands, or quadriceps. In addition, the muscle biopsy did not reveal congophilic deposits or rimmed vacuoles which are classic, histopathologic findings of sIBM.

Anti-synthetase syndrome. Although the patient seemed to have pulmonary findings concerning for the development of early interstitial lung disease, she did not have the classic clinical features of anti-synthetase syndrome which are mechanic's hands, Raynaud's phenomenon, a positive anti-synthetase antibody, and an inflammatory myopathy.

Our patient had a unique presentation of a necrotizing myopathy that had subacutely developed in the context of recent statin use. The duration of exposure to the statin was approximately six months prior to onset of myalgias, weakness, and elevated muscle enzymes. The statin was stopped. She has been treated with immune suppressants and is currently in remission.

Discussion

Statin therapy has been associated with various forms of myotoxicity, ranging from asymptomatic elevation of the creatine kinase, myalgias and muscle cramps, to necrotizing myopathy and frank rhabdomyolysis. Statin-induced toxicity is often defined as myalgias or muscle weakness with CK levels greater than ten times the upper limit of normal. Statin myopathy is often dose-dependent as well as higher levels result in greater toxicity. Statin-induced toxicity often resolves within several weeks to months after discontinuation. However, statins have been associated with necrotizing autoimmune myopathy (NAM) that may progress even after the drug is removed. The histopathologic findings are necrotizing and regenerating muscle fibers with major histocompatibility class I expression (MHC-1) on the sarcolemma of non-necrotic fibers, but NAM is unique in that there is an absence of a prominent inflammatory infiltrate and it is typically composed of macrophages [9–11].

Several risk factors have been associated with statin-induced myotoxicity. These include a personal or family history of muscle cramps, hypothyroidism, and elevated baseline creatine kinase levels. Patient-related risk factors are female gender, concomitant treatment with cytochrome P450 inhibitors such as fibrates and antifungals, elderly patients, renal and/or hepatic impairment [11].

Pathophysiology. The exact pathophysiology of stain-induced myopathy is largely unknown; however, several hypothetical mechanisms have been proposed based upon statin function. Statins are selective 3-hydroxy-3-methylglutaryl coenzyme A (HMG-CoA) reductase inhibitors. HMG-CoA reductase catalyzes the conversion of HMG-CoA to mevalonate, a precursor of cholesterol, coenzyme Q (CoQ10), and isoprenoid intermediary metabolites. Adequate stores of the latter are necessary for appropriate cell signaling and regulation of apoptosis [11, 12].

Deficiencies of cholesterol precursors may result in impairment at the cellular level that could lead to myotoxicity. Cholesterol is a crucial component of cell walls as it helps modulate fluidity in tissues including skeletal muscle. Impairment in fluidity across cell membranes may affect the function of certain ion channels. CoQ10 is an important antioxidant in mitochondria and cell membranes, thus its depletion in the mitochondria of myocytes may result in myotoxicity [12].

Statin-associated NAM is presumed to have an autoimmune basis, but the exact pathogenesis is unknown. Autoantibodies identified as the 200/100 kDa proteins against the 3-hydroxy-3-methylglutaryl-coenzyme A reductase protein have been found to be elevated in patients with NAM who have been exposed to statins. Unlike most statin-induced myopathies which tend to resolve upon discontinuation of the statin, statin-associated NAM has been observed to progress despite statin cessation [13].

Workup. As yet, there are no tests to definitively prove the diagnosis of statin-induced myotoxicity. The diagnosis is based on a comprehensive history, examination, and laboratory findings. Basic laboratory evaluation should include a serum CK and TSH level. Ultimately, a muscle biopsy may be required to determine whether there is evidence of NAM.

Treatment. The first step is discontinuation of statins. Recovery is usually seen within weeks to months after stopping statins. Lowering the dose of statins, reducing the dosing interval (e.g., to alternate-day dosing), or switching to a water-soluble statin may prevent recurrence of statin myotoxicity, although outcomes vary among patients.

For treatment of statin-associated NAM, prednisone may be used initially, especially if there is an inflammatory infiltrate on muscle biopsy. For patients refractory to prednisone alone, a steroid-sparing agent may be added such as methotrexate or azathioprine.

Summary and conclusion. Statin therapy has been associated with myotoxicity, ranging from asymptomatic elevation of the CK level to necrotizing autoimmune myopathy, and it typically occurs in a dose-dependent manner. The pathophysiology remains largely unknown, but upregulation of HMG CoA reductase enzyme levels with subsequent autoantibody formation against that target antigen in NAM is probably one pathogenic mechanism. The initial step in treatment is discontinuation of the statin. Recovery is expected within weeks to months of discontinuation. In NAM, immune suppression with steroids and steroid-sparing agents have shown efficacy; however, further investigation into treatments are needed.

Questions

1. What is the common clinical presentation of polymyositis?
   (a) Asymmetric proximal and distal muscle weakness with atrophy of the forearm flexors, finger flexors, and quadriceps
   (b) Symmetric, proximal muscle weakness with elevated serum muscle enzymes
   (c) Normal muscle strength with elevated muscle enzymes
   (d) Symmetric, proximal muscle weakness with constitutional symptoms of fevers, sweats, and abnormal weight loss
   (e) Symmetric, proximal muscle weakness with Gottron's papules and heliotrope rash
2. Which myositis-specific autoantibody is associated with the anti-synthetase syndrome?
   (a) Anti-SRP
   (b) Anti-Mi2
   (c) Anti p155/140
   (d) Anti-CADM-140
   (e) Anti-Jo-1
3. Which of the following statements is true regarding the diagnosis of polymyositis?
   (a) Elevated muscle enzymes, motor unit action potentials of short duration and small amplitude with fibrillations, endomysial inflammatory muscle infiltrate
   (b) Elevated muscle enzymes, motor unit action potentials of long duration and large amplitude with fibrillations, endomysial inflammatory muscle infiltrate
   (c) Elevated muscle enzymes, motor unit action potentials of short duration and small amplitude with fibrillations, perimysial inflammatory muscle infiltrate
   (d) Normal muscle enzymes, motor unit action potentials of short duration and small amplitude with fibrillations, endomysial inflammatory muscle infiltrate
   (e) Elevated muscle enzymes, motor unit action potentials of short duration and small amplitude with fibrillations, endomysial inflammatory muscle infiltrate with rimmed vacuoles

4. What myositis-specific autoantibody would you expect to see with severe necrotizing myopathy and a poor response to standard therapy?

   (a) Anti-Zo
   (b) Anti-SRP
   (c) Anti p155/140
   (d) Anti-Mi2
   (e) Anti-CADM-140

5. Which of the following regimens is standard of care for initial treatment of inflammatory myositis patients?

   (a) Low-dose corticosteroids and immunosuppressant
   (b) High-dose corticosteroids alone
   (c) High-dose corticosteroids followed by a steroid taper plus immunosuppressant
   (d) Low-dose corticosteroids alone
   (e) None of the above

6. What is the clinical presentation of statin-induced myotoxicity?

   (a) Elevated creatine kinase level
   (b) Muscle cramps
   (c) Rhabdomyolysis
   (d) Symmetric, proximal muscle limb weakness in the upper and lower extremities
   (e) All of the above

7. Statin-induced necrotizing autoimmune myopathy (NAM) may be due to what cause?

   (a) Viral trigger
   (b) Autoantibody against HMG-CoA reductase enzyme
   (c) Thyroid disorder
   (d) Malignancy
   (e) Connective tissue disease

8. What are the typical, histopathologic findings of NAM on muscle biopsy?

   (a) Necrotic and regenerating muscle fibers with minimal inflammatory infiltrate
   (b) Endomysial inflammatory infiltrate composed of cytotoxic CD8+ T-cells
   (c) Perimysial inflammatory infiltrate composed of CD4+T cells
   (d) Endomysial inflammatory infiltrate and congophilic inclusion deposits
   (e) Non-necrotic muscle fibers without an inflammatory infiltrate

9. What is the initial treatment of statin-induced myotoxicity?

   (a) Prednisone
   (b) Methotrexate
   (c) Stop statin
   (d) Prednisone and methotrexate
   (e) Azathioprine

10. What is the commonly expected duration of time to recover from symptoms of statin-induced myotoxicity after discontinuation?

    (a) Immediately
    (b) Several days
    (c) Several weeks to several months
    (d) Years
    (e) There is no recovery time

Answer key: 1. (b), 2. (e), 3. (a), 4. (b), 5. (c). 6. (e), 7. (b), 8. (a), 9. (c), 10. (c).

References

1. Bohan A, Peter JB. Polymyositis and dermatomyositis (first of two parts). N Engl J Med. 1975;292(7):344–7.
2. Dalakas MC, Hohlfeld R. Polymyositis and dermatomyositis. Lancet. 2003;362:971–82.
3. Gunawardena H, Betteridge Z, McHugh N. Newly identified autoantibodies: relationship to idiopathic inflammatory myopathy subsets and pathogenesis. Curr Opin Rheumatol. 2008;20:675–80.
4. Targoff IN. Myositis specific autoantibodies. Curr Rheumatol Rep. 2006;8:196–203.
5. Chiu YE, Co DO. Juvenile dermatomyositis: immunopathogenesis, role of myositis-specific autoantibodies, and review of rituximab use. Pediatr Dermatol. 2011;28:357–67.
6. Love LA, Leff RL, Fraser DD, Targoff IN, Dalakas M, Plotz PH, Miller FW. A new approach to the classification of idiopathic inflammatory myopathy: myositis-specific autoantibodies define useful homogenous patient groups. Medicine (Baltimore). 1991;70:360–74.
7. Dalakas MC, Sivakumar K. The immunopathologic and inflammatory differences between dermatomyositis, polymyositis, and sporadic inclusion body myositis. Curr Opin Neurol. 1996;9:235–9.
8. Engel AG, Arahata K, Emslie-Smith A. Immune effector mechanisms in inflammatory myopathies. Res Publ Assoc Res Nerv Ment Dis. 1990;68:141–57.
9. Mammen AL, Chung T, Christopher-Stine L, Rosen P, Rosen A, Doering KR, Casiola-Rosen LA. Autoantibodies against 3-hydroxy-3-methylglutaryl-coenzyme A reductase in patients with statin-associated autoimmune myopathy. Arthritis Rheum. 2011;63:713–21.
10. Joy TR, Hegele R. Narrative review: statin-related myopathy. Ann Intern Med. 2009;150:858–68.
11. Liang C, Needham M. Necrotizing autoimmune myopathy. Curr Opin Rheumatol. 2011;23:612–9.
12. Jacobson TA. Toward "pain-free" statin prescribing; clinical algorithm for diagnosis and management of myalgia. Mayo Clin Proc. 2008;83:687–700.
13. Sirvent P, Mercier J, Lacampagne A. New insights into mechanism of statin-associated myotoxicity. Curr Opin Pharmacol. 2008;8:333–8.

Chapter 10
Dermatomyositis

Elena Schiopu and Heather Gladue

Abstract Dermatomyositis is an inflammatory myopathy associated with a variety of skin manifestations, has an association to malignancy, and usually presents with symmetric proximal muscle weakness. The manifestations vary dramatically between patients. Here, we present two challenging cases of amyopathic dermatomyositis and anti-synthetase syndrome.

Keywords Inflammatory myopathies • Amyopathicdermatomyositis • Anti-synthetase syndrome

Case 1

Our patient is a 64-year-old female who was referred to us by her primary care physician for evaluation of a generalized skin rash. She had been healthy until 18 months prior when she noticed a pruritic rash on her upper back, which subsequently extended to involve her chest, face and knuckles. She had a punch biopsy one month prior to seeing us with findings consistent with dermatomyositis (DM). She was started on a high dose prednisone taper for almost a year and was off prednisone at time of our visit. She also had a short trial of hydroxychloroquine, but the

E. Schiopu, M.D.
Division of Rheumatology, Scleroderma Program, University of Michigan,
24 Frank Lloyd Wright Drive, Lobby M, Suite 2500, SPC 5753, P.O. Box 481,
Ann Arbor, MI 48106, USA
e-mail: eschiopu@umich.edu

H. Gladue, D.O. (✉)
Division of Rheumatology, University of Michigan, 24 Frank Lloyd Wright
Drive, Lobby M, Suite 2500, SPC 5753, P.O. Box 481, Ann Arbor, MI 48106, USA
e-mail: hgladue@med.umich.edu

M. Mahmoudi (ed.), *Challenging Cases in Rheumatology and Diseases of the Immune System*, DOI 10.1007/978-1-4614-5088-7_10,
© Springer Science+Business Media, LLC 2013

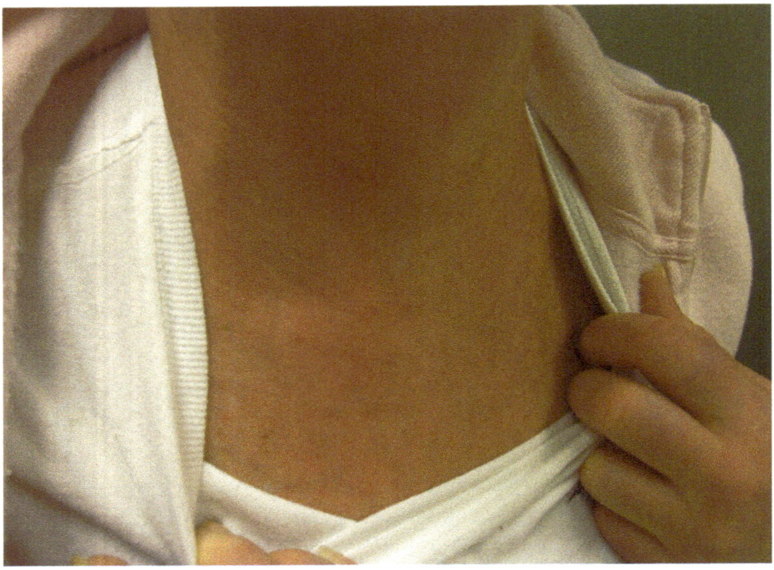

Fig. 10.1 Characteristic erythematous rash on the upper chest, known as the shawl sign

rash persisted despite the oral therapy. She denied symptoms such as Raynaud's phenomenon, shortness of breath, mouth or nose ulcers, dry mouth or eyes, and muscle weakness.

Her past medical history included a benign spinal tumor removed 10 years ago.

Social history. She admits to having used tobacco in the past, ½ pack per day for 20 years, but quit 15 years prior to the clinic visit; she denies alcohol or drug use and is a retired teacher.

Physical Examination. She was a pleasant but anxious female. Vitals: Height 66 in., Weight 131 kg, blood pressure 124/70 mmHg, pulse 74, temperature 37° C. HEENT: neck muscles were well preserved. Heart had regular rate and rhythm with no murmur. Auscultation of chest was clear. Neuro: Muscle strength was 5/5 both distally and proximally in bilateral upper and lower extremities. Skin exam showed an extensive erythematous macular rash present on her face, scalp, back of her neck, upper chest (Fig. 10.1), and most predominant over her upper back. She had classic Gottron's papules (Fig. 10.2). Skin was atrophic with multiple excoriations. She had no evidence of mechanic hands, Raynaud's phenomenon, or digital ulcers; however, the nailfold capillaroscopy showed dilatation and distortion of the capillaries (Fig. 10.3). Her scalp was erythematous and there were fine scales intermixed with excoriations. The remainder of the exam was within normal limits.

Diagnostic Testing: Our patient had a previous electromyogram (EMG) which showed focal abnormal spontaneous activity in the left biceps and deltoid, possible myopathy with no definite evidence of left cervical radiculopathy. Her serum creatine phosphokinase (CK) was mildly elevated (495 IU/L) and the serum aldolase

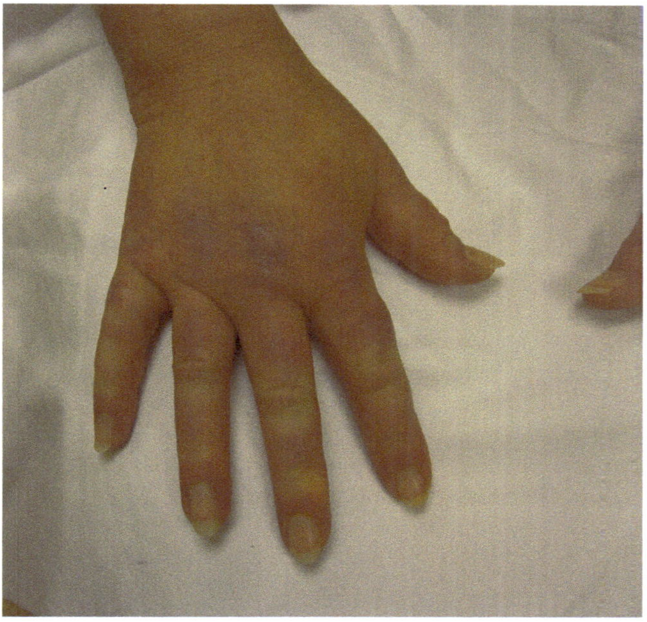

Fig. 10.2 Periungeal erythema, diffuse digital swelling and metatarso-phalangeal and proximal inter-phalangeal papules (Gottron's sign), which are typically seen in dermatomyositis

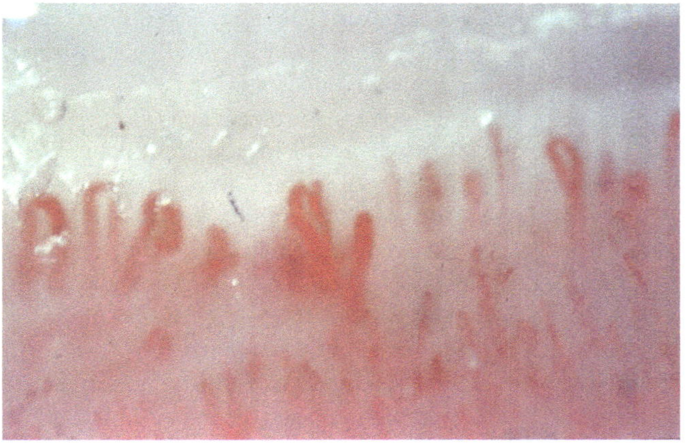

Fig. 10.3 Nailfold capillaroscopic changes: distorted capillaries and dilatation, with signs of neo-vascularization

was normal. The liver function tests (AST and ALT) were mildly elevated: 59 and 44 IU/L, respectively, with a negative Hepatitis profile. Her autoantibodies profile revealed a positive anti-nuclear antibody with a titer of 1:1,280 and a speckled titer, and the serum immunoglobulins were normal. She has had chest imaging that showed nodular changes in the right apex and low attenuation changes in her liver but the subsequent chest computed tomography (CT) showed no changes in the nodule size.

With the Presenting Data What Is Your Working Diagnosis?

Sixty-four-year-old female with refractory, pruritic rash, mildly elevated CK with no associated muscle weakness and mildly abnormal EMG suggesting myopathy. Working diagnosis is DM sine (without) myositis.

Workup. She had a muscle biopsy of her left biceps which showed some intermixture of neuromuscular trophic forms intermixed with scattered normal forms, and no inflammation; no evidence of perifascicular atrophy, perivascular cuffing or vaculitis.

Plan: Hydroxyzine 50 mg PO three times a day for symptomatic control; however, her symptoms persisted, so Methotrexate was initiated at a starting dose of 25 mg SQ weekly. After 6 weeks of methotrexate her rash-related pruritus increased, so the hydroxyzine dose was increased to 100 mg PO three times a day as needed. At this time she also admitted to mild Raynaud's phenomenon with biphasic color changes.

Six months later she developed severe muscle weakness, and was unable to lift objects or rise from a seated position, so a diagnosis of DM was confirmed. At this time we discussed enrollment in the Rituximab in Inflammatory Myopathy (RIM) clinical trial. She subsequently received infusion of rituximab, a CD20 monoclonal antibody, 1 g IV X 2 spaced 2 weeks apart. Three months after rituximab infusions her muscle weakness was essentially gone, the rash dramatically improved and the pruritus subsided so she no longer needed hydroxyzine.

The next month she had a chest computed tomography for the nodule follow-up which showed a right upper lobe nodule which increased in size, along with new development of ground glass appearance in the lower lung. Two months later she noticed worsening periungual erythema, worsening erythematous rash over face, neck, upper chest, upper back, antecubital area, upper arm, and fingers. Muscle strength was 5/5 in deltoids, biceps, triceps, knee flexion, knee extension. Muscle strength was 3/5 on both hipflexors.

Two months later she underwent right lower lobe wedge resection and the lung histopathological examination revealed a tumor size of 2 cm, with an adenocarcinoma pattern, described to be moderate to well differentiated. Four months later her erythematous rash over forearms, upper chest, and upper back had stabilized and improved.

What Is Your Diagnosis and Why?

Paraneoplastic Syndrome. At the initial evaluation, this patient had an erythematous pruritic rash, which did not respond to steroids. The chest imaging failed to reveal evidence of tumors, and her cancer screening was negative to that date. She had no other complains, such as myalgia/arthralgias, and in the absence of a neoplastic process, a diagnosis of paraneoplastic process was excluded. However, the patient developed lung adenocarcinoma 2 years after the initial diagnosis of DM; while it is difficult to assess the presence of the lung tumor preceding the DM diagnosis, based on the available initial testing, this patient did not have a cancer diagnosis.

Inclusion Body Myositis. Although commonly thought of as a differential diagnosis for patients presenting with proximal symmetrical muscle weakness, this diagnosis is mainly based on presence of inclusion bodies in the muscle biopsy slides.

Hypothryoidism. Although the presentation of hypothyroidism could be multi-systemic, this patient had normal thyroid hormone levels.

Systemic Lupus Erythematus. The rash and the positive ANA could suggest a diagnosis of SLE, but this patient did not present with a malar distribution of the rash, and she did not meet other SLE classification criteria.

Dermatomyositis. This patient presented with a refractory erythematous generalized rash which later progressed to involve specific areas of the body such as the upper chest and back (shawl sign), periungal areas, knuckles (Gottron's papules). She also had abnormal nail fold capillary changes and later developed elevation in the serum muscle enzymes, along with symmetrical proximal muscle weakness which are usually completing the clinical picture of a diagnosis of inflammatory myopathy, in this case starting as amyopathic dermatomyositis.

Discussion

Dermatomyositis is a distinct clinical entity characterized by specific cutaneous manifestation, proximal muscle weakness and elevated muscle enzymes. Estimated incidence is 10 per 1,000,000 people/year [1]. DM occurs more commonly in the fourth and fifth decade of life and tends to affect women and men in a 2:1 ratio. Classically, the diagnosis of DM is made based on the Bohan and Peter criteria for idiopathic inflammatory myopathies (IIM) [2, 3]: symmetric proximal muscle weakness, typical DM rash (including Gottron's papules, heliotrope rash, shawl and V sign, erythroderma, ucleration, scalp psoriasiform changes), elevated muscle enzymes, myopathic changes on electromyography and characteristic muscle biopsy abnormalities in the absence of histo-pathological signs of other myopathies. The classification of IIM has been refined since to include the following entities [4]:

- Inclusion body myositis
- Definite/probable polymyositis
- Definite/probable DM
- Amyopathic DM (DM sine dermatitis)

The pathogenesis of DM is still not completely understood; however, it is different from the one of other inflammatory myopathies. Although it is characterized by muscle fiber necrosis, degeneration/regeneration and inflammatory infiltrates, DM is fundamentally driven by perivascular inflammatory infiltrates, mostly CD4+, and complement-related vasculopathy [5]. The muscle biopsy in DM is characterized by perifascicular atrophy and muscle infarcts secondary to capillary necrosis. The pathophysiology of amyopathic DM, characterized by lack of significant muscle manifestations, but classic cutaneous findings is less understood. Our patient presented with greater than a 2 year history of cutaneous manifestations prior to having any muscle involvement; it is interesting that she eventually developed mildly inflammatory myopathy to complement her dermatological findings. The construct amyopathic DM describes patients with amyopathic DM and those with hypomyopathic DM, as having no muscular clinical features but some evidence of muscle inflammation on muscle biopsy, imaging or lab findings [6]. It is estimated that approximately 20 % of DM cases are clinically amyopathic dermatomyositis [1].

A systematic review showed that patients with clinically amyopathic DM are still at risk of developing interstitial lung disease and internal malignancy [6], which makes them clinically similar to the classic DM patients.

Factors suggestive of poor prognosis in DM and polymyositis include older age, lung or cardiac involvement, dysphagia, and cancer [7]. The overall mortality in inflammatory myopathies at 5 years ranges from 5 % to 37 % [8].

The initial treatment of DM involves high dose steroids (1 mg/kg) for up to 3 months, followed by a slow taper, and depending on response methotrexate or azathiprine is often added. A recent analysis of predictors of survival in patients with inflammatory myopathies showed that the initial exposure to intravenous steroids was associated with higher mortality, likely related to disease severity, but the exposure to methotrexate versus azathioprine seemed to be similar [9]. Patients who are refractory to the steroids/methotrexate combination can be exposed to intravenous immunoglobulin (IVIG); however, the results of this therapy are still controversial. Additional therapies to be considered in resistant cases include mycophenolate-mofetil and rituximab [10]. A randomized, double-blind, placebo-controlled (8 weeks) study or rituximab in a cohort of patients with inflammatory myopathies refractory to classic therapies (the RIM study) showed that 83 % of the patients met definition of improvement of the end of the study period of 1 year [11].

In conclusion, the DM patients present with various physical complaints and organ involvement, but a high index of suspicion should be maintained regarding the presence of malignancy, and careful distinction between subgroups of DM should be made.

Case 2

Our patient is a 55-year-old gentleman with a previous diagnosis of rheumatoid arthritis related interstitial lung disease, whom we were asked to evaluate for a second opinion. Based on his description, approximately three months prior to our visit, he woke up short of breath and unable to move his hands. He was evaluated by his primary care physician who initially suspected acute coronary syndrome but the workup was negative. The patient further recalls joint stiffness for approximately one year prior to this event, which progressed from a few minutes to a few hours over the past three months. He also noticed swelling over his knuckles and became increasingly anxious since he could not perform his job as an international pilot. At the time of our evaluation he had been on a steroid taper (currently on 20 mg prednisone daily) and he had started subcutaneous etanercept weekly 5 weeks prior. He noticed mild improvement in the stiffness and swelling of his hands and wrists, but he admitted to severe weakness and inability to lift his arms or get up from a chair. He was very concerned about his shortness of breath, and was evaluated by a pulmonary specialist who diagnosed with mild obstructive sleep apnea and initiated on continuous positive airway pressure (CPAP) therapy. Because he did not improve as expected, he recently underwent a bronchoscopy with trans-bronchial biopsy showing parenchymal lung tissue with mild septal fibrosis and chronic inflammation without evidence of granulomas or malignancy.

On further evaluation of his systems, he did not notice any type of rash, triphasic Raynaud's phenomenon or digital ulcerations, but admits to his fingers cracking a lot without any particular exposure to household chemicals, or any other types of skin irritants. He did not notice mouth or nose ulcers, mouth or eye dryness, chest pain, palpitations, or abnormal infections.

Social history: history of moderate tobacco exposure (10 pack years), quit over one year prior, no exposure to silica dust or chemicals, and social alcohol use.

Physical Exam: slightly overweight male in mild respiratory distress, weight was 233 pounds, height 63 in., blood pressure 111/62 mmHg, pulse 75/min and respiratory rate of 18/min. HEENT: no parotid enlargement, no pharyngeal erythema, tongue was well papillated with good salivary pool, good dentition, no oral ulcerations, no cervical lymphadenopathy. Skin: no rashes; he had mild cracking around his fingers (Fig. 10.3), no nail fold capillary changes, no sclerodactyly, no digital pitting scars or Gottron's papules. Cardiovascular examination: S1, S2 present, no murmurs. Lungs: end-inspiratory rales at both bases. Abdomen: soft, nontender, no organomegaly.

Musculo-skeletal examination: synovial thickening was present on his 2nd and 3rd metacarpo-phalangeal (MCP) joints, positive MCP squeeze; mild swelling of his 2nd and 3rd proximal inter-phalangeal (PIP) joints and bilateral wrists; marked decrease flexion and extension of his wrists. Elbows, shoulders, hips, knees and metatarso-phalangeal (MTP) joint squeeze were negative for tenderness. His muscles seemed to be of normal bulk, although during the examination the patients voiced concerns about the muscle mass decreasing significantly over the past few months. There was tenderness over the proximal arms' and thigh' muscles. The muscle strength was decreased in the proximal muscle groups to 4/5 bilaterally and symmetrically, with significant involvement of the gluteus maximus. Neurological examination: cognition was intact.

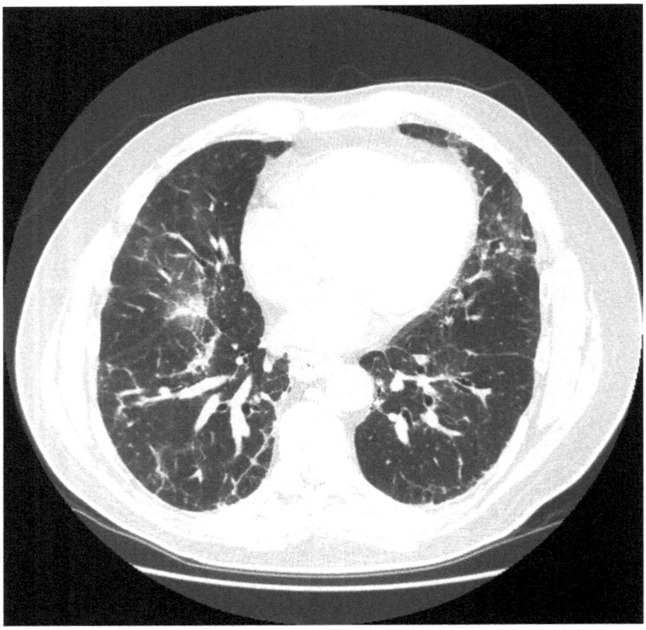

Fig. 10.4 High resolution computed tomography of the chest showing signs of nonspecific interstitial pneumonitis

Diagnostic Testing

Laboratory values: ALT 50 IU/l (normal range 7–35), AST 43 IU/l (normal range 8–30), creatine phosphokinase (CK) was 280 IU/l (normal range 38–240), aldolase was 12 IU/l (normal range 1–7), angiotensin converting enzyme and thyroid stimulating hormone were normal, Hepatitis B and C serology was negative, serum level of C-reactive protein was 0.3 mg/dl (normal range 0.0–0.6). As far as various serologies, the results are as follows: rheumatoid factor (RF)was negative, the anti-cyclic citrullinated peptide (CCP) antibody was negative, the anti-nuclear antibody (ANA) was negative, and the rapid plasma regain (RPR) was negative. The only other positive finding was the anti-Jo-1 antibody.

Imaging studies: plain radiographs of the patient's bilateral hands and wrists did not reveal any erosions or signs of inflammatory arthritis aside from peri-articular osteopenia.

Thoracic computed tomography (Fig. 10.4): subtle ground glass opacities in the mid and lower lungs; lower lobe predominant ground glass opacities associated with septal thickening and mild bronchiectasis, without evidence of honeycombing; multiple lymph nodes within the mediastinum most likely reactive. The overall conclusion of the chest imaging was that the patient had interstitial lung disease (ILD), the nonspecific interstitial pneumonitis type, most likely in the setting of a connective tissue disease.

With the Presented Data, What Is Your Working Diagnosis?

This is a 55-year-old man with history of symmetrical, proximal muscle weakness, acute onset of shortness of breath and symmetrical small joint inflammatory changes. A key element in his history is the cracks on the lateral aspect of his fingers, called "mechanic's hands," which is pathognomonic for a subgroup of inflammatory myopathies called anti-synthetase syndrome, characterized by inflammatory myopathy, ILD, and presence of anti-Jo-1 antibody.

Workup

The patient's initial pulmonary function test showed significant restrictive defect (forced vital capacity (FVC) of 55 % of predicted, total lung capacity (TLC) of 65 % of predicted and carbon monoxide diffusion capacity (DLco) of 64 % of predicted). A 6 min walk test revealed that the baseline pulse oximetry of 94 %, dropped to 88 % during his walk. His cancer screening was up to date and revealed no suspicion of neoplasm.

Based on the new diagnosis of anti-synthetase syndrome and ILD, a decision was made to stop the etanercept, continue the prednisone, and add mycophenolate-mofetil in an effort to address the lung involvement. The patient was later exposed to a rituximab treatment, and was able to completely wean the steroids and to improve his vital capacity by 20 %. Subsequently though he noticed worsening of his breathing and increased arthralgias, so a moderate dose of steroids (prednisone 0.5 mg/kg) was used to control his symptoms.

What Is Your Diagnosis and Why?

Rheumatoid Arthritis with ILD. This patient presented with a mix of musculoskeletaland respiratory complaints. Although ILD is not uncommon in rheumatoid arthritis, it tends to occur later in the disease, and it rarely is the presenting complaint. Aside from that, the patient did not meet the classification criteria for rheumatoid arthritis which includes postive RF or anti-CCp antibody.

Idiopathic Pulmonary Fibrosis. Since the presenting complaint was shortness of breath, and the chest tomography undoubtedly showed the presence of ILD, IPF should have been high in the differential. Recently, it has been observed that a lot of the diagnoses of IPF are actually being challenged and changed into ILD in the setting of a connective tissue disorder, which is particularly true in our case. Our patient had other systemic complaints, and clear signs of inflammatory muscle disease, which places him outside the IPF spectrum of disorders.

Anti-synthetase syndrome. The characteristic combination of inflammatory myopathy, ILD, mechanics' hands, inflammatory myopathy and presence of anti-Jo-1 antibody leaves no doubt about the diagnosis of our patient.

Discussion

The anti-synthetase syndrome gets its name from the presence of autoantibodies to eight of the aminoacyl-transfer RNA synthetases, of which the most recognized is the anti-histidyl-tRNA synthetase (Jo-1) [12]. Since first identified in 1976 in a patient (John P) who had polymyositis and ILD [13], the anti-synthetase syndrome has been described to involve production of anti-Jo-1 antibodies, ILD, inflammatory myopathy, polyarthritis, fever, Raynaud's phenomenon and thick cracked skin on fingers (mechanic's hands); ILD is seen in as many as 86 % of patients with anti-Jo-1 positive patients [14], and the most common pattern is NSIP.

The clinical manifestations of anti-synthetase syndrome vary from patient to patient. Myositis may present years after the onset of disease, and is common in patients with Anti-Jo-1 (78–91 %). Mechanics hands are located on the palmar surface of the hands and fingers and consist of scaling and fissuring of the skin. Mechanics hands can also be seen in DM associated with other autoantibodies. Arthritis is more common in patients with positive anti-synthetase antibodies occurring in (64–83 %) versus 18 % in those who are serologically negative. The arthritis can be deforming, non-deforming, erosive or non-erosive. Interstitial lung disease is the major contributor to morbidity and mortality in these patients [12].

Treatment depends on the symptomatology. In those with seropositive ILD, especially NSIP, there is a favorable response to steroids with a prolonged taper. Other cytotoxic agents are often used as steroid sparing therapy, such as cyclophosphamide, azathioprine, mycophenolate mofetil, cyclosporine, tacrolimus, intravenous immunoglobulin and rituximab [12]. A recent retrospective series of seven patients showed improvement in lung volumes (FVC, DLCO) and decreased use of steroids, in patients with anti-synthetase syndrome-related refractory ILD treated with rituximab [15].

In conclusion, the anti-synthetase syndrome is a clinically unique form of DM characterized by presence of ani-Jo-1 antibody, mechanic's hands, ILD and polyarthritis. It is important to rule out other connective tissue diseases such as rheumatoid arthritis or systemic sclerosis since the respiratory symptoms could be the very initial presentation.

Questions

1. What is the classic muscle biopsy description in dermatomyositis?

   (A) Perifascicular atrophy, muscle infarcts and capillary necrosis
   (B) Vaculoar degeneration
   (C) Inflammatory infiltrates with normal blood vessels
   (D) Invasion of nonnecrotic muscle cells by CD8+ cytotoxic t-cells
   (E) Necrotic myopathy

2. What antibody is most commonly associated with anti-synthetase syndrome?

   (A) Anti-dsDNA
   (B) Anti-Jo-1 antibody
   (C) AntiMi-2 antibody
   (D) SRP antibody

3. What are the classic skin findings in dermatomyositis?

   (A) Gottron's Papules
   (B) Periungual Erythema
   (C) Heliotrope Rash
   (D) Shawl sign
   (E) All of the Above

4. Which is not included in the diagnostic criteria for Dermatomyositis?

   (A) Myopathic changes on EMG
   (B) Typical Rash including Gottron's papules, shawl sign
   (C) Underlying malignancy
   (D) Elevated serum muscle enzymes
   (E) Symmetric proximal muscle weakness

5. Approximately what percentage of patients with Dermatomyositis have a positive Antinuclear antibody (ANA)?

   (A) 80 %
   (B) 10 %
   (C) 20 %
   (D) 50 %

6. What is the first line treatment for Dermatomyositis?

   (A) Plasmapheresis
   (B) Intravenous immunoglobulin
   (C) High dose steroids
   (D) Rituximab
   (E) Azathioprine

7. What is the approximate percentage of developing or having a coexisting malignancy in dermatomyositis?

   (A) 80 %
   (B) 50 %
   (C) 30 %
   (D) 15 %
   (E) 0 %

8. Which cancer is most commonly known to be increased in dermatomyositis?

    (A) Ovarian Cancer
    (B) Skin Cancer
    (C) Colon Cancer
    (D) Pheochromocytoma

9. What do patients with dermatomyositis have most difficulty doing?

    (A) Grasping a cup
    (B) Rising from a chair
    (C) Walking on tiptoe
    (D) Using a remote control

10. What is the most common pattern of ILD in anti-synthetase syndrome?

    (A) Bronchial obliterans organizing pneumonitis (BOOP)
    (B) Usual interstitial pneumonitis (UIP)
    (C) Nonspecific interstitial pneumonitis (NSIP)
    (D) Lymphocytic interstitial pneumonitis (LIP)
    (E) Desquamative interstitial pneumonitis (DIP)

Answer key: 1. (A), 2. (B), 3. (E), 4. (C), 5. (A), 6. (C), 7. (C), 8. (A), 9. (B), 10. (C).

References

1. Bendewald MJ, Wetter DA, Li X, Davis MD. Incidence of dermatomyositis and clinically amyopathic dermatomyositis: a population-based study in Olmsted County, Minnesota. Arch Dermatol. 2010;146(1):26–30.
2. Bohan A, Peter J. Polymyositis and dermatomyositis (first of two parts). New Engl J Med. 1975;292(7):344–7.
3. Bohan A, Peter J. Polymyositis and dermatomyositis (second of two parts). New Engl J Med. 1975;292(8):403–7.
4. Hoogendijk J, Amato A, Lecky B, Choy E, Lundberg I, Rose M, et al. 119th ENMC international workshop: trial design in adult idiopathic inflammatory myopathies, with the exception of inclusion body myositis, 10–12 Oct 2003, Naarden, The Netherlands. Neuromuscular Disorders. 2004 2003;14(5):337.
5. Kissel J, Mendell J, Rammohan K. Microvascular deposition of complement membrane attack complex in dermatomyositis. New Engl J Med. 1986;314(6):329.
6. Gerami P, Schope JM, McDonald L, Walling HW, Sontheimer RD. A systematic review of adult-onset clinically amyopathic dermatomyositis (dermatomyositis sine myositis): a missing link within the spectrum of the idiopathic inflammatory myopathies. J Am Acad Dermatol. 2006;54(4):597–613.
7. Marie I. Morbidity and mortality in adult polymyositis and dermatomyositis. Curr Rheumatol Rep. 2012; Jun; 14(3): 275–85

8. Rider L, Lachenbruch P, Monroe J, Ravelli A, Cabalar I, Feldman B, et al. Damage extent and predictors in adult and juvenile dermatomyositis and polymyositis as determined with the myositis damage index. Arthritis Rheum. 2009;60(11):4325–35.
9. Schiopu E, Phillips K, Macdonald P, Crofford L, Somers E. Predictors of survival in a cohort of patients with polymyositis and dermatomyositis: effect of corticosteroids, methotrexate and azathioprine. Arthritis Res Ther. 2012;14(1):R22.
10. Marie I, Mouthon L. Therapy of polymyositis and dermatomyositis. Autoimmun Rev. 2011;11(1):6–13.
11. Oddis C, Reed A, Aggarwal R, Ascherman D, Barohn R, Feldman B et al. Rituximab in the treatment of refractory adult and juvenile dermatomyositis (DM) and adult polymyositis (PM)—the RIM study. Arthritis RRS. 2010; 62 suppl. 12:3844
12. Katzap E, Barilla-LaBarca M, Marder G. Antisynthetase syndrome. Curr Rheumatol Rep. 2011;13(3):175–81.
13. Imbert-Masseau A, Hamidou M, Agard C, Grolleau J, Chérin P. Antisynthetase syndrome. Joint Bone Spine: Revue du Rhumatisme. 2003;70(3):161–8.
14. Richards T, Eggebeen A, Gibson K, Yousem S, Fuhrman C, Gochuico B, et al. Characterization and peripheral blood biomarker assessment of anti-Jo-1 antibody-positive interstitial lung disease. Arthritis Rheum. 2009;60(7):2183–92.
15. Marie I, Dominique S, Janvresse A, Levesque H, Menard J. Rituximab therapy for refractory interstitial lung disease related to antisynthetase syndrome. Respir Med. 2012;106(4):581–7

Part IV
Vasculitis

Chapter 11
Wegener's Granulomatosis

Kartik V. Shenoy, Jennifer Sloane, and Gilbert D'Alonzo

Abstract Granulomatosis with Polyangiitis (GPA), formerly known as Wegener's Granulomatosis, is a multisystem disease that predominantly involves the respiratory tract and the kidneys. The pathological hallmarks are necrotizing granulomatous lesions and vasculitis of small and/or medium vessels. It is difficult to diagnose because its presentation is similar to many common diseases such as upper respiratory tract infections, pneumonia, and asthma. Understanding the signs and symptoms, laboratory findings, and biopsy results are key to making the diagnosis of Granulomatosis with Polyangiitis. A heightened degree of clinical suspicion for this rare disease will often lead to the correct diagnosis.

Keywords Wegener's • Granulomatosis with polyangiitis • Vasculitis • ANCA

Case 1

A 39-year-old woman presents with cough productive of mucous and blood for approximately 1 month. She also reports episodes of dyspnea, fevers, and night sweats. Recently she has experienced fatigue which limits her activity during the day and there has been a significant weight loss of nearly 15 pounds over the past month. Diffuse pain throughout her body, especially myalgias and arthralgias of her lower extremities, has reduced her ambulatory function.

K.V. Shenoy, M.D. (✉) • G. D'Alonzo, D.O
Department of Pulmonary and Critical Care, Temple University School of Medicine, 3401 N. Broad Street Suite 710 C, Philadelphia, PA 19140, USA
e-mail: kartik.shenoy@tuhs.temple.edu

J. Sloane M.D.
Department of Rheumatology, Thomas Jefferson University Hospital, 211 S 9th Street, Room 215, Philadelphia, PA 19140, USA
e-mail: Jennifer.Sloane@jefferson.edu

M. Mahmoudi (ed.), *Challenging Cases in Rheumatology and Diseases of the Immune System*, DOI 10.1007/978-1-4614-5088-7_11,
© Springer Science+Business Media, LLC 2013

Past Medical History

She has a history of sinusitis requiring sinus surgery.

Family and Social History

She is a lifelong nonsmoker, uses alcohol socially, but has never used illicit drugs. She is a homemaker who has numerous pets including, a dog, cat, snake, and fish. She does not have a family history of rheumatologic disease.

Medication and Allergies

Oxycodone with acetaminophen has been prescribed for cough and pain by her primary care provider. No other medications are being used and she denies medication and environmental allergies.

Physical Exam

Temperature 98.2°F, Blood pressure 101/63 mmHg, heart rate 68 beats/min, respiratory rate 16 breaths/min, and weight 122 pounds. She appears to be in no acute distress but has scant dried blood in her nostrils. There are no oral lesions. Lymphadenopathy was not found. Her lungs are clear to auscultation with normal breath sounds and her cardiovascular examination was normal. There is no tenderness to palpation of her elbows, wrists or small joints of the hands. Knees, ankles, and feet are normal. There is no evidence of foot drop. She has normal strength and function in all extremities.

Data

Complete blood count shows a white blood cell count of 10.8 g/dl (4.1–10.7 g/dl), a hematocrit of 23.4% (36.0–47.0%), and platelet count of 541 K/μl (150–400 K/μl). She has a normal creatinine of 0.79 mg/dl (0.52–1.04 mg/dl) without any red blood cell casts or active urine sediment seen. Her chest CT scan shows multiple nodular ground-glass opacities in a centrolobular distribution (Fig. 11.1).

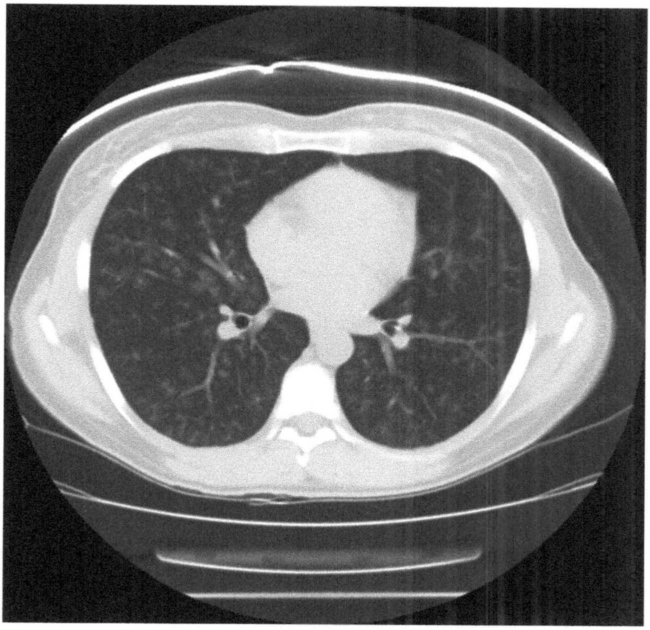

Fig. 11.1 Multiple nodular ground glass opacities in a centrolobular distribution

Impression

With the Presented Data What Is Your Working Diagnosis?

The patient's history, physical examination, laboratory, and chest CT scan findings point to an inflammatory-immunologic disorder. She has sinus disease, abnormal CT chest findings, and signs of a rheumatological process given her history of myalgias, arthralgias, and weight loss.

Differential Diagnosis

However, the diagnosis is not established without further workup. In the differential includes, crack induced lung disease, lymphomatoid granulomatosis, rheumatoid lung disease, Churg–Strauss syndrome, sarcoidosis and microscopic polyangiitis. Granulomatosis with Polyangiitis is also in the differential given the sinopulmonary findings along with her systemic symptoms.

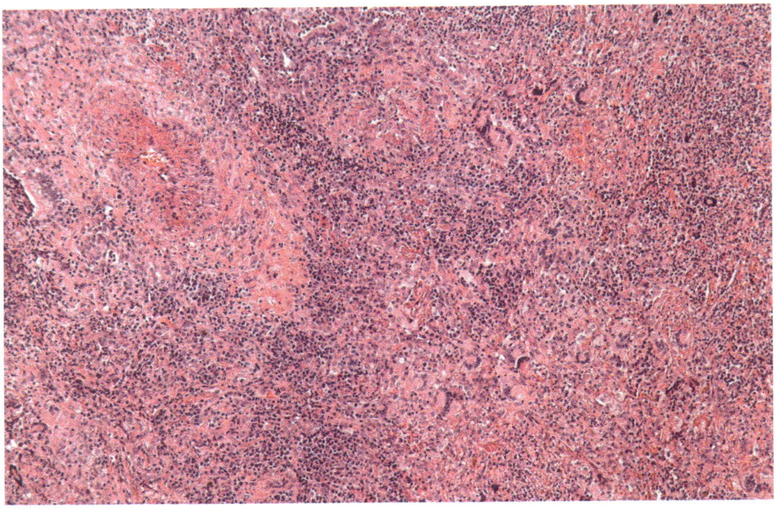

Fig. 11.2 Pathology with peribronchial and vascular granulomatous inflammation (reprinted with permission: http://commons.wikimedia.org/wiki/User:Nephron)

Workup

Further testing reveals her antineutrophilic cytoplasmic antibodies (ANCA) are positive for p-ANCA, and MPO-ANCA and negative for c-ANCA and PR-3-ANCA. She has a positive rheumatoid factor of 229 U with a negative anti-cyclic citrullinated peptide (anti-CCP) and, an elevated CRP of 3.19 mg/dl (0.08–0.8 mg/dl). Liver function blood values are normal. Her sinus CT displays mild mucosal wall thickening within the anterior left ethmoid sinuses. A Video Assisted Thoracoscopic Surgical (VATS) lung biopsy was performed and the pathology revealed peribronchial and vascular granulomatous inflammation with neutrophils, lymphocytes, and macrophages (Fig. 11.2).

What Is the Diagnosis and Why?

Granulomatosis with Polyangiitis. This patient's presentation fits three out of four American College of Rheumatology criteria for the diagnosis of Granulomatosis with Polyangiitis [1]. Her blood testing shows a positive p-ANCA/MPO. While c-ANCA/PR3 is more common in Granulomatosis with Polyangiitis, up to 20% of Wegener's cases can have positive p-ANCA/MPO instead of c-ANCA [2]. Furthermore, since she has granulomatous inflammation on her biopsy, the diagnosis is consistent with Granulomatosis with Polyangiitis.

Case 2

A 22-year-old African American man presents with a 1 year history of a chronic ulcer on his left calf. For the last month his ulcer has been growing in size. He also has developed upper respiratory tract symptoms of sinus headache and congestion. His headache involves frontal and parietal pain. The pain is worse at night when he lies down to go to sleep. His primary care physician prescribed nasal corticosteroids and an oral antibiotic which he cannot recall. He also has systemic symptoms of weight loss, chills, night sweats, and generalized arthralgias.

Past Medical History

The past medical history only consisted of the lower extremity ulcer. He denies any previous surgical history

Family and Social History

He works for a steam cleaning company and smokes two packs of cigarettes per week. He also admits to smoking marijuana regularly and heavy alcohol use. There is no family history of rheumatological disease.

Medications

He denies any medication or environmental allergies. His only medication is daily fluticasone nasal spray.

Physical Examination

Temperature 101.3°F, blood pressure 136/80 mmHg, heart rate 112 beats/min, and respiratory rate 16 breaths/min. He appears to be in no distress. Examination of his nares reveals intranasal exudative ulcers. There are no oral lesions. Lymphadenopathy was not found. His lungs are clear to auscultation with normal breath sounds and his cardiovascular examination was also normal. There is no tenderness to palpation of his elbows, wrists or small joints of the hands. Knees, ankles, and feet are normal. There is mild weakness found in the flexor and extensor muscles of left ankle. There are also two leg ulcers approximately 2 cm in diameter with some purulent discharge.

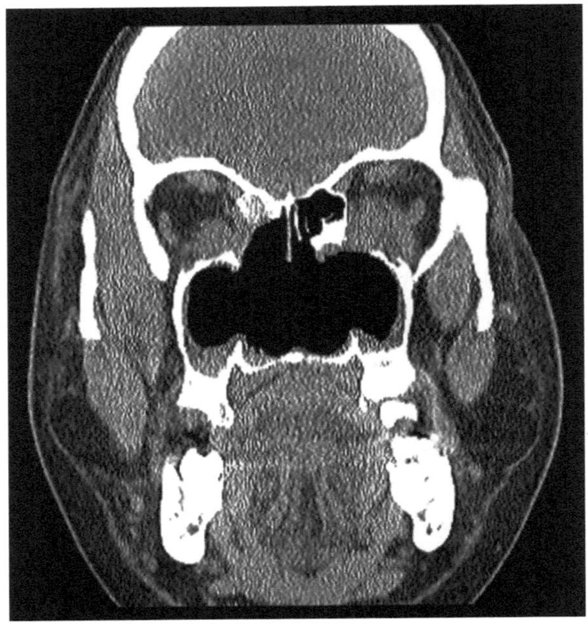

Fig. 11.3 CT sinus with large nasal septal defect

Data

Complete blood count shows a white blood cell count of 12.5 cells/dl (4.1–10.7 cells/dl), a hematocrit of 38.8% (41–52%), and platelet count of 660 K/μl (150–400 K/μl). He has a normal serum creatinine of 0.9 mg/dl and urinalysis is without any red blood cell casts or active urine sediment. He has normal liver function testing. He has an erythrocyte sedimentation rate of 81 mm/h (0–10 mm/h). His sinus CT shows a large nasal septal defect with large air filled maxillary sinuses with absent medial antral walls and turbinates likely related to necrosis (Fig. 11.3).

Impression

With the Presented Data What Is Your Working Diagnosis?

The patient's history, physical examination, laboratory, and sinus CT findings leave us with a broad differential diagnosis. Though an inflammatory-immunological disorder could cause all of the patient's symptoms, ruling out a necrotizing infection is of considerable importance.

Differential Diagnosis

The inflammatory/immunological differential includes: crack induced nasal destruction, Churg–Strauss syndrome, sarcoidosis, and relapsing polychondritis. Granulomatosis with Polyangiitis is again in the differential given the sinopulmonary findings, along with systemic symptoms. The infectious differential includes histoplasmaosis, coccidiomycosis, blastomycosis, mucormycosis, and mycobacterial diseases. Syphilis at any age or stage can cause intranasal disease. A variety of malignancies also cause this degree of nasal destruction including: lymphomas, adenocarcinomas, and squamous cell cancer.

Workup

Further blood testing reveals that his ANCA is positive for c-ANCA and PR-3-ANCA and negative for p-ANCA, and MPO-ANCA. He has a negative rheumatoid factor with a negative anti-CCP, but an elevated CRP of 10.8 mg/dl (0.08–0.8 mg/dl). His white blood cell differential from the CBC shows 55% segmented neutrophils (50–75%), 29% lymphocytes (20–44%), and 10% eosinophils (2–5%) Liver function blood values are normal. Culture of leg and sinus discharge grows staphylococcus Aureus. Urine drug screen was negative. A CT thorax revealed multiple circular lucent lesions with dense borders seen in the right perihilar regions (Fig. 11.4). Finally, nasal and sinus biopsies were performed under general anesthesia. There was large posterior septal perforation. There was evidence of devitalized tissue within nearly the entire nasal cavity. Multiple biopsies were taken. Biopsies revealed extensive necrotic tissue with necrotic granulomas and severe vasculitis.

What Is the Diagnosis and Why?

Granulomatosis with Polyangiitis. This patient's presentation fits three out of four American College of Rheumatology criteria for the diagnosis of Granulomatosis with Polyangiitis [1]. His case presentation is considerably different from the patient in Case 1. Both represent the variable presentation of Granulomatosis with Polyangiitis. His blood testing, unlike the first case, was positive for the c-ANCA/PR3 which is more common in Granulomatosis with Polyangiitis. The granulomatous inflammation on his biopsy is also consistent with Granulomatosis with Polyangiitis. Complicating his case is the positive sinus culture with Staphylococcus Aureus and peripheral eosinophilia. Peripheral eosinophilia can indicate other immune disorders such as Churg–Strauss or fungal infection. His ANCA testing was more consistent with Granulomatosis with Polyangiitis. Also, his biopsy did not have eosinophils along with vasculitis which would be seen in Churg–Strauss

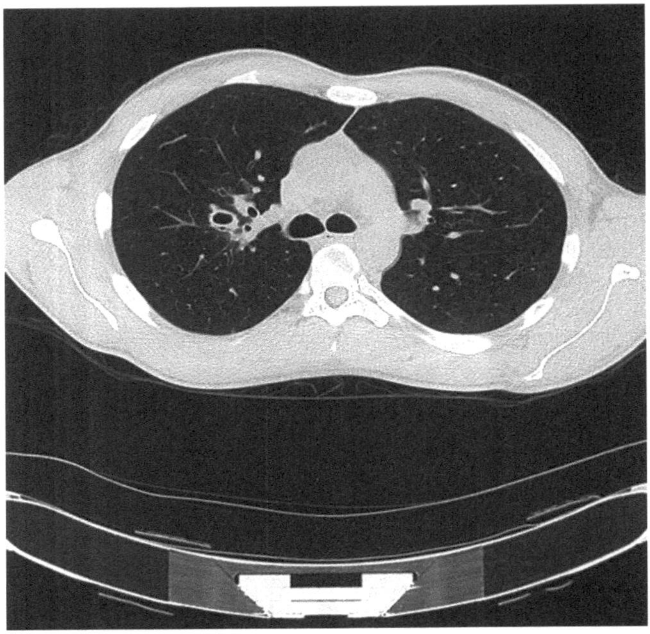

Fig. 11.4 CT chest with circular lucent lesions with dense borders in the right perihilar region

disease. Also, his cultures did not grow fungal pathogens. The Staphylococcus is likely chronic nasal carriage and is implicated in the pathogenesis and relapse of Granulomatosis with Polyangiitis.

Discussion

Granulomatosis with Polyangiitis is a multisystem disease that predominantly affects the respiratory tract and the kidneys. Originally described by Dr. Friedrich Wegener, its histological hallmark is the combination of granulomas and vasculitis [3]. Granulomatosis with Polyangiitis generally affects individuals in the fourth and fifth decade of life; however, it can affect both younger and older patients. Women and men are affected equally. There is a predilection for Caucasians and cases of this disease are rare in African Americans. Granulomatosis with Polyangiitis has a 1 year mortality rate approaching 90% without treatment. With recent treatment strategies, the 5 year survival has improved to 87% [4].

Given its grave prognosis without treatment, clinicians need to be aware of Granulomatosis with Polyangiitis; however, initial signs and symptoms can be variable and may involve almost every organ system. Ocular involvement may include scleritis, conjunctivitis, uveitis, and episcleritis [3]. Many patients present initially with some form of rhinitis or nasal pain, bleeding, and crusting. In more severe forms, a saddle nose deformity can develop secondary to a perforated septum. Sinus involvement is also common [3]. Oral cavity and auditory symptoms may also be present. Patients may have a conductive hearing loss from auditory tube dysfunction while others may present with sensory-neuronal hearing loss. Patients can also have bony destruction with loosening of the teeth and gingivitis. Involvement of the trachea with subsequent subglottic stenosis may occur. Arthritis and purpuric skin lesions may also occur. The vasculitis often involves the vasa vasorum of nerves resulting in a sensory neuropathy or mononeuritis multiplex. Lung involvement is common, with many features including multiple pulmonary nodules, infiltrates that mimic pneumonia, cavitary lesions, and pulmonary hemorrhage [5]. Kidney involvement can range from microhematuria with red cell casts to rapidly progressive glomeurolonephritis leading to chronic renal failure. The gastrointestinal tract and heart may also be involved.

There are two main diagnostic criteria. The American College of Rheumatology initially established guidelines for diagnosis in 1990 [1]. These guidelines involve four "traditional" symptoms of: nasal or oral inflammation, abnormal chest radiograph, active urinary sediment, and granulomatous inflammation on biopsy. If a patient has at least two of these four criteria, there is a diagnostic sensitivity of 88% and a specificity of 92%. Nasal or oral inflammation is defined as having painful or painless oral ulcers or purulent or bloody nasal discharge. Abnormal chest radiograph means there is either the presence of nodules, fixed lung infiltrates, or cavities. Positive urinary sediment consists of either microhematuria (>5 red blood cells per high power field) or red cell casts. Biopsy results should show the histological findings of granulomatous inflammation within the wall of an artery or within the perivascular or extravascular area.

The Chapel Hill Consensus Guidelines bases its classification on a biopsy result showing vasculitis of small and medium sized arteries and granulomatous inflammation within the respiratory tract [6].

Biopsy is the "gold standard" for diagnosis and should be pursued if possible [6]. The skin and kidney are the easiest sites to biopsy and often provide the diagnosis. Nasal biopsies show a diagnostic utility in only ~50% of patients. Neural biopsy has an even lower yield. If skin or kidney is not available for biopsy, a lung biopsy is often needed. While transbronchial biopsies are less invasive and have less anesthesia risk compared to open thoracotomy or VATS, the diagnostic yield of transbronchial biopsy is low. Thoracotomy or VATS biopsy usually provides enough tissue for the diagnosis of Granulomatosis with Polyangiitis.

ANCA are another tool in the diagnosis of Granulomatosis with Polyangiitis [7]. A fluorescent assay and an ELISA are the two different assays that are currently used. In the fluorescent assay, the patient's serum is incubated with ethanol fixed neutrophils on a glass slide. If ANCA are present in the patient's serum, they will bind to the neutrophils on the slide. An additional anti-human fluorescent antibody is then used to label the bound antibody. The illuminated neutrophil is then examined by microscopy. A test result with fluorescent granules scattered in the cytoplasm of the neutrophil is considered positive for cytoplasmic ANCA (c-ANCA) (Fig. 11.5). A test with fluorescent granules near the nucleus is considered positive

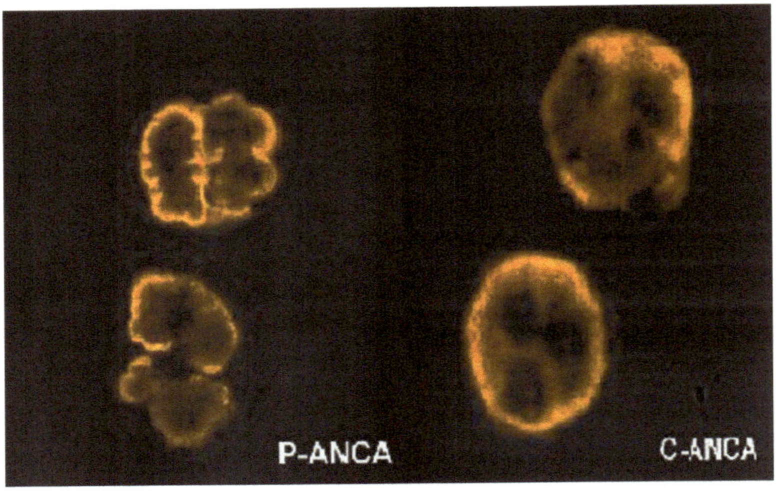

Fig. 11.5 Immunofluorescence stain for antineutrophilic cytoplasmic antibody (ANCA). Fluorescent granules scattered in the cytoplasm of the neutrophil is positive c-ANCA. A test with fluorescent granules near the nucleus is considered positive for p-ANCA (reprinted with permission: http://en.wikipedia.org/wiki/File:P_anca.jpg)

for perinuclear ANCA (p-ANCA). Another method of ANCA testing is the use of antigen-specific enzyme-linked immunosorbent assay (ELISA). The specific antigens tested are proteinase 3 (PR-3) and myeloperoxidase (MPO). PR3 is associated with c-ANCA and MPO is associated with p-ANCA. Although most patients with Granulomatosis with Polyangiitis have a positive c-ANCA/PR-3, it is not uncommon to have p-ANCA/MPO or be seronegative. The sensitivity of ANCA testing for Wegener's is related to the extent, severity, and disease activity at the time of testing. The sensitivity of c-ANCA testing for Wegener's ranges from 34 to 92% and the specificity ranges from 88 to 100% [7].

Other disease processes to consider in the differential are other ANCA-associated vasculitides such as Churg–Strauss Syndrome and Microscopic Polyangiitis (Table 11.1) [2]. Churg–Strauss Syndrome can occur between 14 and 75 years of age with a mean age of 50. There are no clear gender differences, however; some studies show a slight predilection for males. Churg–Strauss Syndrome can involve the upper and lower airways; however, different than Granulomatosis with Polyangiitis, patients with Churg–Strauss Syndrome usually have a long history of asthma that has become refractory to treatment. Patients with Churg–Strauss Syndrome also has high eosinophil counts and may have infiltrates in the lung or other organs such as the gastrointestinal tract, heart, skin and nervous system. As the disease progresses, the patients develop constitutional symptoms such as weight loss, fever, and malaise. It may take years for the diagnosis to be made. Pathological findings of Churg–Strauss syndrome are similar to Granulomatosis with Polyangiitis; however, in addition to vasculitis, there is eosinophilic infiltration.

Table 11.1 Differential diagnosis of granulomatous polyangiitis

	Granulomatosis with polyangiitis (Wegener's)	Churg–Strauss	Microscopic polyangiitis	Lymphomatoid
Lung/upper respiratory	Yes	Yes	Yes (but less common)	Yes
ANCA	c-ANCA	p-ANCA	p-ANCA	No
Blood eosinophils	No	Yes	No	No
Necrotizing granulomas	Yes	Yes	No	No
Vasculitis	Neutrophilic	Neutrophilic with background of eosinophils	Neutrophilic	Lymphocytic

There is also an association with p-ANCA and MPO. Microscopic Polyangiitis is similar to the other ANCA-associated vasculitides in its signs and symptoms. Patients usually have rapidly progressive glomerulonephritis but may also have involvement of the lung, skin, nervous system, gastrointestinal tract and numerous other organs. They also usually have constitutional symptoms and are more likely to have p-ANCA/MPO positivity than c-ANCA/PR3 positivity. Biopsy results show intense small to medium vessel vasculitis without the characteristic granuloma of Granulomatosis with Polyangiitis and without the eosinophilia of Churg–Strauss Syndrome.

Lymphomatoid granulomatosis, anti-glomerular basement membrane disease (Anti-GBM), and cocaine-induced vasculitis are other diseases that can mimic Granulomatosis with Polyangiitis. Lymphomatoid granulomatosis is a disorder of T-lymphocytes that can progress to lymphoma. It generally presents with cough, dyspnea, and chest pain. It can also involve the skin, kidney, central and peripheral nervous system, and upper respiratory tract. Patients with Lymphomatoid granulomatosis do not have ANCA; furthermore, the biopsy does not show vasculitis. Biopsies of lymphomatoid granulomatosis show invasion of small arteries and veins by lymphocytes with resultant luminal obliteration. Anti-GBM is a disease defined by the presence of autoantibodies directed at specific antigen targets in the gloumerular and pulmonary basement membranes [8]. Malaise, weight loss, fever, and arthralgias may be the initial symptoms in Anti-GBM disease [8]. Pulmonary hemorrhage is the most common feature occurring in approximately 70% of cases. Renal disease can occur in isolation or in conjunction with pulmonary hemorrhage. Microscopic hematuria is present with red cell casts formation as disease progresses. Progressive renal failure can develop leading to oliguria. Diagnosis is made with clinical symptoms and the presence of Anti-GBM antibodies either in circulation or in kidney tissue. Cocaine-induced vasculitis can mimic the symptoms and serological findings of Granulomatosis with Polyangiitis causing significant nasal deformities and has positive ANCA studies. However, biopsy results are not consistent with the granulomatous vasculitis seen in Granulomatosis with Polyangiitis.

Although steroids can help control some of the manifestations of Granulomatosis with Polyangiitis, steroids alone are an ineffective long-term treatment strategy[9]. Patients who only receive steroids have an increased mortality compared to those who receive immunosuppressive medications. The classic medication, in concert with steroids, used to induce a remission of Granulomatosis with Polyangiitis is cyclophosphamide. It can be given orally or intravenously usually for 3–6 months [10]. Studies have suggested that patients with Granulomatosis with Polyangiitis who receive oral Cyclophosphamide have a lower rate of relapse compared to those who receive intravenous administration; however, patients who take oral cyclophosphamide may have more adverse effects from the medication. Adverse effects include infertility, bone marrow suppression, hemorrhagic cystitis, and increased risk of cancer. Once the patient has achieved remission with cyclophosphamide, patients are switched to either azothioprine or methotrexate as maintenance treatment. Steroids are usually tapered to a low dose at 3 months and then slowly reduced further. Rituximab is a new option recently approved for initial treatment of ANCA associated vasculitis [9]. While the data suggest rituximab is not inferior to induction of remission of ANCA associated vasculitis, long term data regarding relapse is not yet available. Patients who have less severe disease or "Limited Granulomatosis with Polyangiitis" (without kidney involvement) may receive less toxic drugs for induction such as methotrexate. However, use of methotrexate may be associated with a higher relapse rates. Trimethoprim/sulfamethoxazole twice daily can also be used as an adjunct therapy to the immunosuppressive medications. As all of these immunosuppressive medications have adverse effects, patients need consistent reevaluation and monitoring by their physician.

Questions

1. Which of the below are symptoms seen in Granulomatosis with Polyangiitis
   (a) Hemoptysis
   (b) Hematuria
   (c) Rhinitis
   (d) Arthritis
   (e) All of the above
2. Which laboratory results are most consistent with Granulomatosis with Polyangiitis
   (a) Positive PR3/c-ANCA
   (b) Positive MPO/p-ANCA
   (c) Peripheral Eosinophilia
   (d) Positive Rheumatoid factor
3. Which treatment option is NOT recommended for Granulomatosis with Polyangiitis
   (a) Cyclophosphamide with corticosteroids
   (b) Methotrexate with corticosteroids
   (c) Corticosteroids alone
   (d) Antithymocyte globulin
4. This biopsy result is consistent with Granulomatosis with Polyangiitis
   (a) Necrotizing granulomas, vasculitis, with eosinophilic infiltrates
   (b) Lymphocytic vasculitis
   (c) Necrotizing granuloma with vasculitis
   (d) Small vessel vasculitis

5. These three organ systems are most commonly involved in Granulomatosis with Polyangiitis
   (a) Heart, Lung, Kidney
   (b) Upper Airway, Kidney, Lung
   (c) GI tract, Heart, Bone
   (d) Lung, Liver, Kidney
6. What is the best method of diagnosis for Granulomatosis with Polyangiitis.
   (a) Clinical diagnosis alone
   (b) Clinical, laboratory, and radiological findings are sufficient to make diagnosis.
   (c) Clinical, laboratory, and radiological findings are not sufficient to make diagnosis. Biopsy procedure is necessary.
   (d) Positive PR3/c-ANCA makes the diagnosis
7. This pathogen has been implicated in the pathogenesis and relapse of Granulomatosis with Polyangitis.
   (a) Streptococcus
   (b) Staphylococcus Auras
   (c) Pseudomonas
   (d) Klebsiella
8. This is the classic medication used to induce remission in Granulomatosis with Polyangiitis
   (a) Methotrexate
   (b) Steroids
   (c) Cyclophosphamide
   (d) IVIG
9. This illicit drug can mimic Granulomatosis with Polyangiitis
   (a) Heroin
   (b) Marijuana
   (c) Methamphetamine
   (d) Cocaine
10. This is a side effect of cyclophosphamide
   (a) Infertility
   (b) Bone marrow suppression
   (c) Hemorrhagic cystitis
   (d) Increased risk of cancer
   (e) All of the above

Answers: 1(e), 2(a), 3(c), 4(c), 5(b), 6(c), 7(b), 8(c), 9(d), 10(e).

References

1. Leavitt RY, et al. The American College of Rheumatology 1990 criteria for the classification of Wegener's granulomatosis. Arthritis Rheum. 1990;33(8):1101–7.
2. Savige J, et al. Antineutrophil cytoplasmic antibodies and associated diseases: a review of the clinical and laboratory features. Kidney Int. 2000;57(3):846–62.
3. Jennings C, Jones N, Dugar J, et al. Wegener's granulomatosis—a review of diagnosis and treatment in 53 subjects. Rhinology. 1998;36:189–91.
4. Hoffman GS, et al. Wegener granulomatosis: an analysis of 158 patients. Ann Intern Med. 1992;116(6):488.
5. Lohrmann C, et al. Pulmonary manifestations of Wegener granulomatosis: CT findings in 57 patients and a review of the literature. Eur J Radiol. 2005;53(3):471–7.
6. Jeannette C, Falk R, Andrassy K, et al. Nomenclature of systemic vasculitides. Arthritis Rheum. 1994;37(2):187–92.
7. Rao JK, Weinberger M. The role of antineutrophil cytoplasmic antibody (c-ANCA). Ann Intern Med. 1995;123(12):925–932.
8. Matthay R, bromberg S, Putman C. Pulmonary renal syndromes—a review. Yale J Biol Med. 1980;53(6):497–523.
9. Reinhold-Keller E, et al. An interdisciplinary approach to the care of patients with Wegener's granulomatosis: long-term outcome in 155 patients. Arthritis Rheum. 2000;43(5):1021–32.
10. Groot K, Dwomoa A, Savage O. The value of pulse cychophosphamide in ANCA-associated vasculitis: meta analysis and critical review. Nephrol Dial Transplant. 2001;16(1):2018–27.

Chapter 12
Churg–Strauss Syndrome

Paul Hoffman and Michael Schivo

Abstract Of all the vasculitides, Churg–Strauss Syndrome (CSS) is one of the least common. Though regarded as an ANCA-associated vasculitis, serologies may be negative in a high proportion of patients. As a systemic disorder, disease presentation may be highly variable. Here we discuss two challenging cases of CSS.

Keywords Vasculitis • Pulmonary eosinophilia • Asthma • Churg–Strauss syndrome

Case 1

A 50-year-old Caucasian male prisoner is brought in to the hospital with a complaint of shortness of breath and fever. He reports last feeling well about 6 months ago, but he has since developed a nonproductive cough, fatigue, and malaise. He denies wheezing or hemoptysis. He has experienced intermittent nonradiating anterior chest tightness associated with his cough which is neither exertional nor positional. His past medical history is notable for severe persistent asthma which was first diagnosed at age 34 and complicated by multiple hospitalizations for acute exacerbations. Whereas control of his asthma had previously required daily corticosteroids, these have been weaned off and there have been no requirements for steroid burst for the past 4 years. Over the past week he has experienced progressively worsening shortness of breath, initially with moderate exertion but now with simple activity such as walking to the prison cafeteria. He first noted fevers 1 week

P. Hoffman, M.D. (✉) • M. Schivo, M.D., MAS
Division of Pulmonary, Critical Care & Sleep Medicine, Department of Internal Medicine, UC Davis Medical Center and UC Davis Asthma Network (UCAN),
4150 V Street, Suite 3400, Sacramento, CA 95835, USA
e-mail: paul.hoffman@ucdmc.ucdavis.edu; mschivo@ucdavis.edu

M. Mahmoudi (ed.), *Challenging Cases in Rheumatology and Diseases of the Immune System*, DOI 10.1007/978-1-4614-5088-7_12,
© Springer Science+Business Media, LLC 2013

ago when he was seen in the infirmary. He was prescribed an oral macrolide at that visit without any symptomatic improvement. A CT scan of the chest was also performed 4 weeks prior to rule out a pulmonary embolism.

Past medical history. Asthma, diagnosed at age 34. Hepatitis C, genotype 1a, for which he had not undergone any prior treatment. Dyslipidemia. GERD. Chronic rhinosinusitis. Coronary artery disease for which he is status post coronary artery bypass graft surgery at age 48.

Medications. budesonide, salmeterol, pantoprazole, simvastatin, intranasal fluticasone, aspirin, metoprolol

Drug allergies. None

Family History. His father is deceased at age 52 of a myocardial infarction, preceding medical problems had included type 2 diabetes mellitus and hypertension. His mother is deceased at age 64 of breast cancer, with a past history significant for cerebrovascular accident at age 61, hypertension, and rheumatoid arthritis. He has one sibling, a younger brother in his late 40s with no known medical problems.

Social history. He is a former smoker, with a 15 pack year history. He has been imprisoned on multiple occasions for drug-related offenses, including a current stay of just over 3 years. He has a history of polysubstance abuse, including alcohol, marijuana, and intravenous heroin. He reports last recreational drug use just prior to his most recent incarceration. He is originally from southern California but moved to the northern central California region at age 5 and has resided there ever since. He has never traveled outside of California. He dropped out of school in the eleventh grade to apprentice as a plumber, and he has intermittently worked as an assistant within his family's plumbing business.

Review of systems. Notable for an unintentional weight loss of 15 pounds over the past 6 months, arthralgias of the knees and wrists, and occasional postprandial nausea.

Physical Examination. Vitals: Temperature 99.6 F, pulse of 98, blood pressure 152/88 mmHg, respirations 22 breaths per minute, pulse oximetry of 96% on room air, height of 5 feet-10 inch, weight of 165 pounds. In general, he is a thin male who appears older than his stated age who is speaking in 8–10 word sentences. HEENT: normocephalic. Sclera are normal. Pupils equal, round, reactive to light. Nasal polyps present bilaterally. Neck: No jugular venous pulsation noted. Chest auscultation reveals occasional rhonchi, greatest in the right mid posterior lung fields and the bibasilar regions. The heart rate is regular with normal heart sounds and no appreciable murmur or gallop. PMI is nondisplaced. Abdominal exam is normal. There is no clubbing, cyanosis or edema noted within the peripheral extremities. There are several tender subcutaneous nodules on the dorsum of the right elbow. Musculoskeletal exam reveals no evidence of ulnar deviation, synovitis, or joint effusions.

Data and diagnostic testing. Initial labs are presented in Table 12.1. This is most significant for 18% eosinophils on manual differential and an absolute eosinophil count of 1,746 cells/mm^3 (normal 100–300 cells/mm^3). ECG reveals normal sinus rhythm with q-waves in leads III and aVF which is unchanged from prior. BNP is normal. Transthoracic echocardiogram shows normal LV function with an ejection

Table 12.1 Initial laboratory findings

Parameter	Value	Normal range
Sodium (mEq/L)	137	135–145
Potassium (mEq/L)	4.3	3.3–5
Chloride (mEq/L)	107	95–110
Bicarbonate (mEq/L)	26	24–32
BUN (mg/dL)	20	8–22
Serum creatinine (mg/dL)	0.6	0.44–1.27
Serum calcium (mg/dL)	8.8	8.6–10.5
WBC (10^3 per mm^3)	9.7	4.5–11
Hemoglobin (g/dL)	11.8 L	12–16
Platelet count (10^3 per mm^3)	294	130–400
MCV (fL)	88	80–100
Neutrophil (%)	74	
Neutrophils absolute (10^3 per mm^3)	7.12	1.8–7.7
Lymphocytes (%)	8	
Lymphocytes absolute (10^3 per mm^3)	0.78 L	1–4.8
Eosinophils (%)	18 H	
Eosinophils absolute (10^3 per mm^3)	1.75 H	0.1–0.3
Albumin (g/dL)	3.6	3.2–4.6
Total protein (g/dL)	7.1	6.3–8.3
INR	0.94	0.87–1.13
AST (U/L)	32	15–43
ALT (U/L)	28	5–54
Alkaline phosphatase (U/L)	94	35–115
Total bilirubin (mg/dL)	0.6	0.3–1.3
Urinalysis	Clear appearance, no protein, 0 wbc, 2 rbc, no casts	Clear appearance, negative (protein, rbc, wbc, casts)

fraction of 55%, estimated right ventricular systolic pressure of 28 mmhg, and no valvular or wall motion abnormalities. CT imaging of the chest from 4 weeks prior shows no evidence of pulmonary embolism but is notable for patchy air-space opacities involving the left upper lobe with lesser involvement of the right upper, middle, and lower lobes. A representative image is shown in Fig. 12.1.

Impression. A middle-aged male with coronary artery disease and previously severe adult onset asthma now presenting with dyspnea on exertion and nonproductive cough, who is found to have peripheral eosinophilia and pulmonary infiltrates.

Clinical course. He is initially hospitalized on the general medicine service where he is treated for pneumonia with broad spectrum antibiotics. After several days without symptomatic improvement, his supplemental oxygen requirement increases. A repeat CT scan of the chest is obtained which demonstrates significant clearing of the left upper lobe opacities, but worsening ground glass opacities of the right upper, middle, and lower lobes. Figure 12.2 depicts a representative image

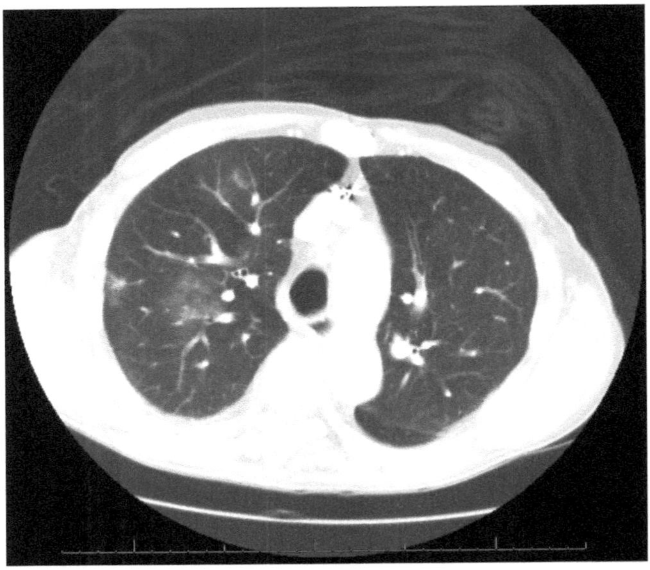

Fig. 12.1 CT of the Chest. Patchy air space opacities are seen predominantly within the *left upper lobe* with lesser involvement of the *right upper*, *middle*, and *lower lobes*

corresponding to a similar anatomic section as that shown in Fig. 12.1, taken less than 5 weeks prior. He subsequently develops hypoxemic respiratory failure requiring mechanical ventilation and is transferred to the medical intensive care unit (MICU).

With Presented Data, What Is Your Working Diagnosis?

This 50-year-old male with coronary artery disease, adult onset asthma, and recurrent rhinosinusitis presents with acute respiratory failure and chronic weight loss, fatigue, malaise, and arthralgias. Exam is significant for nasal polyposis and tender nodules on the extensor surface of the right upper extremity. Laboratory studies demonstrate peripheral eosinophilia, and chest imaging is remarkable for migratory pulmonary infiltrates. Based on this information, a diagnosis of Churg–Strauss Syndrome (CSS) is strongly suspected.

Differential Diagnosis. The differential diagnosis includes CSS, acute eosinophilic pneumonia (AEP), chronic eosinophilic pneumonia (CEP), infection (helminthic and nonhelminthic), allergic bronchopulmonary aspergillosis (ABPA), medication/toxin exposure, malignancy, hypersensitivity pneumonitis (HP), granulomatosis with polyangiitis (GPA), microscopic polyangiitis (MPA), and the hypereosinophilic syndrome (HES).

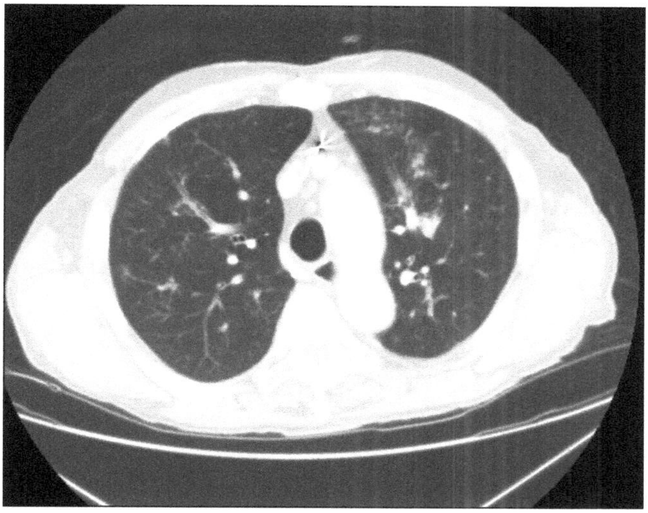

Fig. 12.2 Repeat CT of the Chest. Follow-up CT imaging 5 weeks later at a similar anatomic level showed interval improvement of *left upper lobe* disease with worsened ground glass opacities in the *right upper*, *middle*, and *lower lobes*

Workup

ANA returned negative. However, ANCA serology returned positive with an anti-MPO pattern. Serum IgE returned elevated at 567 kU/L. Stool studies for ova and parasites were negative. *Coccidioides* serology was negative (by complement fixation and immunodiffusion). *Aspergillus spp* antibodies were negative (IgE and IgG). PPD and quantiferon gold both returned negative. BAL was performed during the patient's stay in the MICU and was significant for 35% eosinophils on cell count. BAL bacterial, fungal, and viral cultures were all negative. Biopsy of the upper extremity extensor nodules was performed, but no eosinophilic infiltrate or leukocytoclastic vasculitis was identified. Thoracic surgery was then consulted, and the patient was taken for a surgical lung biopsy. On pathologic review, numerous alveolar macrophages are seen forming multinucleated giant cell granulomas surrounding necrotic eosinophils. Numerous eosinophils are seen in the extravascular space near the pulmonary capillaries with evidence of vasculitis.

What Is Your Diagnosis and Why?

Infection. The patient's history of imprisonment presenting with chronic weight loss, fever, and pulmonary infiltrates raises the possibility of infectious etiology. However, he has not improved despite multiple courses of antibiotics. Pulmonary infectious and helminthic infectious workup was also unrevealing. PPD and quantiferon gold were negative, and *coccidioides* serologies were negative, making mycobacterial or coccidioidal infection less likely.

ABPA. In an individual with a prior diagnosis of difficult to control asthma, peripheral eosinophilia and elevated IgE, a diagnosis of ABPA should be considered. However, CT scan would be expected to show bronchiectasis, bronchial wall thickening, and evidence of mucus plugging. Without characteristic radiographic findings or evidence of *Aspergillus spp* seropositivity, a diagnosis of ABPA is unlikely.

Medication/toxin exposure. Our patient had recently been empirically treated with azithromycin. While there are rare case reports of pulmonary eosinophilia and vasculitis associated with this macrolide, his symptoms and radiographic abnormality had predated this medication. Both metoprolol and simvastatin have been associated with pneumotoxicity, but neither typical of the pattern seen in our patient. Various toxin exposures have been associated with pulmonary eosinophilia, including inhaled recreational drugs, smoke, and occupational inhalation (sulfites, metals, organic chemicals, dusts). Although this patient has a history of intravenous drug abuse, his history of inhaled toxins is relatively minimal and is not the most likely etiology.

Malignancy. Although uncommon, certain leukemias, lymphomas, lung carcinomas, and other malignancies have been associated with pulmonary eosinophilia. Constitutional symptoms such as fever, weight loss, and fatigue are common. However, positive ANCA serologies and biopsy demonstrating evidence of vasculitis would not be expected in these conditions.

Hypersensitivity pneumonitis. HP can have acute, subacute, or chronic presentations and results in pulmonary parenchymal damage as a result of immunologic reactions to numerous inhaled agents, especially organic antigens. Subacute or chronic presentations may manifest as the gradual onset of cough, dyspnea, fever, fatigue, and weight loss in the absence of identifiable acute attacks. CT most often shows ground-glass or nodular opacities in a mid-to-upper zone predominance. BAL cell counts usually show lymphocytosis, but eosinophilia can be seen. However, poorly formed noncaseating granulomas would be expected on histopathology, not evidence of eosinophilic vasculitis.

GPA/MPA. Presentation with several months of constitutional symptoms such as fever, weight loss, and arthralgias is common with both GPA and MPA, as was seen in our patient. Sinus symptoms are more common in GPA patients, but can be seen in GPA, MPA, and CSS. Pulmonary symptoms are also common, and patchy opacities can be seen in all three. Cutaneous lesions are frequent, especially leukocytoclastic vasculitis, though tender nodules also occur in all ANCA associated vasculitis. However, whereas our patient was ANCA positive with an anti-MPO pattern, GPA is usually associated with an anti-PR3 pattern. And, neither GPA nor MPA is strongly associated with late-onset asthma or eosinophilia.

HES. Diagnosis of HES requires the presence of peripheral eosinophilia for >6 months, signs/symptoms of eosinophilic organ infiltration, and an absence of any other cause for the eosinophilia. The duration of this patient's eosinophilia was not known. Moreover, asthma is rare in HES and features of vasculitis would not be expected on biopsy.

AEP/CEP. AEP is an exceedingly rare cause of pulmonary eosinophilia. Patients usually present with fever, shortness of breath, and nonproductive cough of less than 1–3 weeks duration and often progress to respiratory failure. If done, CT scans of the chest often show bilateral patchy ground glass opacities, as were seen in our patient. An eosinophil count of >25% on BAL, also seen in our patient, is common. However, lung biopsy would be expected to show a diffuse alveolar damage pattern with evidence of eosinophilic infiltrate but without overt vasculitis. And while our patient had a clear decline over the prior week, a diagnosis of AEP would not satisfactorily explain his 6 months of preceding symptoms. CEP also results from a pathologic accumulation of eosinophils in the lung. Like our patient, the presentation is typically subacute and often consists of fever, weight loss, night sweats, cough, and progressive dyspnea. Asthma and peripheral eosinophilia are common. Peripheral pulmonary infiltrates in a pattern described as the photonegative of pulmonary edema is pathognomonic but uncommon. Multinucleated giant cells and eosinophilic infiltration are most frequently seen on biopsy. However, the cutaneous and musculoskeletal symptoms present in this patient as well as a finding of ANCA positivity and vasculitis on biopsy would not be supported by a diagnosis of CEP. The time course of our patient's presentation, in combination with his symptoms, history of late onset asthma, peripheral eosinophilia, migratory pulmonary infiltrates, anti-MPO ANCA positivity and lung biopsy showing eosinophilic infiltration with vasculitic features make CSS the most likely diagnosis.

Case 2

A 76-year-old female is referred to an asthma specialist for evaluation of asthma and radiographic infiltrates. She was diagnosed with asthma in her late 50s, which was often difficult to control. She also had recurrent episodes of sinusitis for several years. Over the past 3 months she has noted progressively worsening dyspnea on exertion and severely decreased exercise tolerance such that she can no longer walk across the room without becoming dyspneic. This resulted in a recent hospitalization at which time she was diagnosed with new onset congestive heart failure. At that same stay, both plain radiography and a CT scan of the chest showed bilateral pulmonary infiltrates.

Past medical history. Asthma diagnosed at the age of 59, which has been periodically difficult-to-control. Breast cancer, status-post lumpectomy and adjuvant radiation therapy 15 years ago. A right-sided hemorrhagic cerebrovascular accident 10 years prior. Her post-CVA course was complicated by seizure disorder. She had previously made a full recovery without sensorimotor deficits until development of lower extremity peripheral neuropathy approximately 5 years ago. Other comorbidities have included allergic rhinitis as well as recurrent episodes of sinusitis.

Medications. Aspirin, carbamazepine, salmeterol/fluticasone, montelukast, amitriptyline

Drug allergies. Cephalexin with unknown reaction.

Family history. Her parents are deceased, both at an age of late 80s. Their medical history is otherwise unknown. She has two siblings, ages 84 and 87, who are believed to be in good health.

Social history. She is a lifetime nonsmoker. There is no other history of past or present alcohol or recreational drug use. She is widowed for the past 2 years. She has resided in the Northern Central Valley region of California for her entire life. A retired travel agent, she had previous extensive work related travel to both urban and rural locations throughout Europe, Africa, Asia and South America. She has not traveled outside of the United States within the past 8 years. She does not have a hot tub, swamp cooler, or any pets at home.

Review of systems. Notable for an unintentional weight loss of 25 pounds over the preceding 12 months, worsening numbness of the right foot, right greater than left lower extremity weakness, and recurrent bouts of nonbloody diarrhea over the past several months.

Physical examination. Vitals: Temperature 96.1 F, pulse of 107 beats per minute, blood pressure 114/77 mmHg, respirations 18 breaths per minute, pulse oximetry of 97% on room air, height of 5 feet-4 inches, weight of 90.6 pounds. In general, she is a cachectic chronically ill appearing female who looks older than her stated age. HEENT: there is temporal wasting. Sclera are normal. Pupils equal, round, reactive to light. There are no obvious nasal polyps. Neck: jugular venous pulsations are estimated at 10 cm H_2O. Chest auscultation reveals fine bibasilar late inspiratory crackles. The heart rate is regular with normal heart sounds and no appreciable murmur or gallop. There is lateral displacement of the PMI. Abdominal exam is normal. Extensive ecchymoses are noted on the bilateral lower extremities. There is trace pitting pedal edema. Neurologic exam reveals 1 out of 5 strength on dorsiflexion of the right foot, 3 out of 5 on dorsiflexion of the left foot. There is reduced sensation to pinprick of both feet.

Data and diagnostic testing. Initial labs are shown in Table 12.2. Most notable for leukocytosis to 27,000 with the differential revealing 46% eosinophils (normal leukocyte count 4,500–11,000; normal eosinophil count 100–300). Review of past hemograms had also demonstrated marked eosinophilia. Cardiac catheterization revealed globally hypokinetic left ventricular function with an estimated ejection fraction of 30–35%, but no angiographic evidence of significant coronary artery disease. Esophagogastroduodenoscopy shows mild nonerosive gastritis and duodenitis. Gastric and esophageal biopsies are consistent with mild inflammation, but neither demonstrated tissue eosinophil infiltration. Representative images from her inpatient CT scan of the chest are shown in Fig 12.3. Imaging from 3 years prior revealed mild bronchiectasis. However, compared with the prior study, there has been interval development of a pericardial effusion, bilateral pleural effusions, and bilateral diffuse reticulonodular infiltrates.

Impression. Subacute presentation of a patient with severe late onset asthma now found to have nonischemic cardiomyopathy, diffuse reticulonodular pulmonary infiltrates, peripheral neuropathy, and peripheral eosinophilia.

Clinical course. The patient is simultaneously referred to the Hematology/Oncology clinic where a bone marrow biopsy is obtained. A Pulmonary consultation recommends additional serologic and laboratory tests including outpatient bronchos-

Table 12.2 Initial laboratory findings

Parameter	Value	Normal range
Sodium (mEq/L)	134 L	135–145
Potassium (mEq/L)	3.5	3.3–5
Chloride (mEq/L)	101	95–110
Bicarbonate (mEq/L)	27	24–32
BUN (mg/dL)	12	8–22
Serum creatinine (mg/dL)	0.7	0.44–1.27
Serum calcium (mg/dL)	10	8.6–10.5
WBC (10^3 per mm^3)	27.1 H	4.5–11
Hemoglobin (g/dL)	10 L	12–16
Platelet count (10^3 per mm^3)	322	130–400
MCV (fL)	93	80–100
Neutrophil (%)	29	
Neutrophils absolute (10^3 per mm^3)	7.86 H	1.8–7.7
Lymphocytes (%)	2	
Lymphocytes absolute (10^3 per mm^3)	0.54 L	1–4.8
Eosinophils (%)	46 H	
Eosinophils absolute (10^3 per mm^3)	12.5 H	0.1–0.3
Albumin (g/dL)	1.7 L	3.2–4.6
Total protein (g/dL)	5.1 L	6.3–8.3
INR	1.03	0.87–1.13
AST (U/L)	43	15–43
ALT (U/L)	37	5–54
Alkaline phosphatase (U/L)	146 H	35–115
Total bilirubin (mg/dL)	0.7	0.3–1.3
C-reactive protein (mg/dL)	3.6 H	0–0.8
ESR	32 H	0–30
Urinalysis	Amber appearance, trace protein, 1 wbc, 4 rbc, no casts	Clear appearance, negative (protein, rbc, wbc, casts)

copy with bronchoalveolar lavage (BAL) and sural nerve biopsy. However, the patient's condition continues to deteriorate and she is rehospitalized on the Coronary Care Unit service with decompensated heart failure, non-ST elevation myocardial infarction and a B-type natriuretic peptide level of 975 pg/mL (reference range 0–100). She appears nearly moribund. Interestingly, her readmission plain chest radiography demonstrates improvement of bilateral upper lobe pulmonary disease.

With Presented Data, What Is Your Working Diagnosis?

This 76-year-old female with late-onset asthma and recurrent sinusitis presents with a subacute course of dyspnea and is found to have a severe nonischemic

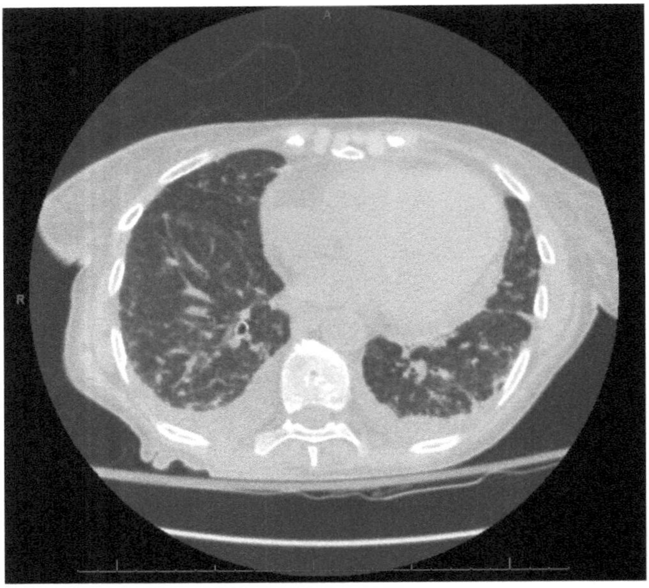

Fig. 12.3 CT of the Chest. Prior imaging 15 months prior revealed mild bilateral lower lobe bronchiectasis. The current study shown above demonstrated no adenopathy in mediastinal windows, pericardial and bilateral pleural effusions were noted. Lung windows revealed bronchiectasis with diffuse bilateral reticulonodular infiltrates and interlobular septal thickening

cardiomyopathy. Exam demonstrates a lower extremity peripheral neuropathy and extensive ecchymoses. Chest imaging is significant for diffuse bilateral reticulonodular infiltrates, pericardial effusion, and bilateral pleural effusions. Review of her medical records reveals a chronic severe peripheral eosinophilia. Based on this information, the multisystem nature of her disease, and the severity of presentation, a diagnosis of CSS is made.

Differential Diagnosis. The differential diagnosis includes CSS, HES, helminthic/nonhelminthic infections, CEP, malignancy, medications/toxins, systemic mastocytosis, ABPA, and sarcoidosis.

Workup

ANA, c-ANCA, and p-ANCA were all negative. Serum IgE was elevated at 387 kU/L. Tryptase and vitamin B12 levels were normal. Fluorescence in situ hybridization (FISH) analysis for chromosome 4q12 anomalies (FIP1LI/PDGFRα, PDGFRβ) was negative. Stool examination for ova and parasites was negative. *Aspergillus spp* antibodies and *coccidioidesmycosis* serologies were negative. EMG studies confirmed mononeuritis multiplex. The bone marrow biopsy returned normal. Flow cytometry studies showed no evidence of a clonal proliferative process. Sural nerve biopsy and diagnostic flexible fiber-optic bronchoscopy with transbronchial biopsy were planned; however, the patient's decompensated heart failure precluded these procedures in the short-run. Ultimately, outpatient bronchoscopy with endobronchial and transbronchial biopsies was performed, and was unrevealing.

What Is Your Diagnosis and Why?

Infectious. The patient's history of extensive travel now presenting with peripheral eosinophilia and pulmonary infiltrates raises the possibility of helminthic infection (including Loeffler's syndrome). However, stool cultures for ova and parasite were negative. *Coccidioides* infection can cause nonhelminthic infection presenting with pulmonary infiltrates and peripheral eosinophilia. However, serologies for this were checked and negative

Chronic eosinophilic pneumonia. This most often presents as a subacute illness with cough, progressive dyspnea, wheezing, and constitutional symptoms such as fever, weight loss, and night sweats. Asthma may precede illness in up to 50% of patients. CEP is an idiopathic disorder resulting from eosinophil accumulation within the lungs. Interestingly, cases have been described following radiation therapy for breast cancer. However, our patient's treatment was 15 years prior. Although uncommon, CEP classically presents with bilateral peripheral pulmonary infiltrates on chest xray, a pattern that has been described as the photographic negative of pulmonary edema. A diagnosis of CEP would not explain our patient's worsening neuropathy, gastrointestinal symptoms, or heart failure.

Malignancy. Neoplastic processes are rare causes of pulmonary eosinophilia, but important diagnoses to exclude. These can include acute eosinophilic leukemia, chronic eosinophilic leukemia, and lymphoma. Pulmonary eosinophilia associated with undifferentiated lung carcinoma or lung metastases from primary cervical, squamous carcinoma (skin, nasopharynx, vagina, and penis), gastrointestinal adenocarcinomas, and bladder cancer is rare, but have all been described. In this case, bone marrow biopsy, flow cytometry, and gastrointestinal workup were all unrevealing.

Systemic mastocytosis. This comprises a rare disorder of mast cells. Symptoms can arise from organ infiltration as well as mast cell mediator release. It is typically associated with flushing, pruritus, and gastrointestinal complaints (abdominal pain, nausea, vomiting, and diarrhea). However, extracutaneous involvement can occur and usually involves the bone marrow, skeletal system, GI tract, liver, spleen, and lymph nodes. Eosinophilia is common. Elevations in tryptase are common. Comorbid asthma is common. While this diagnosis might explain our patient's chronic diarrhea, weight loss, and eosinophilia, her primary pulmonary and cardiac processes would not be expected in systemic mastocytosis. It is ruled out by the absence of increased mast cells on bone marrow biopsy and normal tryptase levels.

Medication/toxin. Numerous medications have been associated with pulmonary eosinophilia, most commonly NSAIDs and antimicrobials, but also including multiple anticonvulsants, antidepressants, beta blockers, sulfas, and ACE inhibitors. A breadth of various toxin exposures have been associated with this diagnosis as well. These include inhaled recreational drugs (heroine, crack), smoke, occupational inhalational exposures (sulfites, metals, organic chemicals, dust), as well as ingestions (rapeseed oil, L-tryptophan). This patient was on carbamazepine, which has been associated with both pneumotoxicity as well as fatal eosinophilic myocarditis. The latter described in a singular case report within several months of starting the medication. At least one case of granulomatous necrotizing angiitis secondary to carbamazepine has also been reported. In spite of the absence of any temporal relationship to her eosinophilia or symptoms, her carbamazepine was discontinued at her initial hospitalization without improvement in her eosinophilia or clinical symptoms. There was no identifiable toxin exposure.

ABPA. Prior imaging demonstrated mild bronchiectasis. In a patient with a prior diagnosis of asthma and elevated IgE, a diagnosis of ABPA might explain her radiographic findings but it does not account for her multisystem organ involvement. The diagnosis is also refuted by negative *Aspergillus spp* antibodies.

Sarcoidosis. This multisystem disorder, more prevalent in African Americans, involves the lung in over 90% of patients with symptoms often including cough, dyspnea, as well as constitutional symptoms such as fever, fatigue and weight loss. Rhinosinusitis is not uncommon. Cardiac involvement can lead to conduction abnormalities, and right ventricular failure can occur as a result of the development of pulmonary hypertension and cor pulmonale. However, left ventricular dysfunction, as seen in our patient, is not common. Neurologic involvement is also infrequent, occurring in about 5% of patients. Although radiographic findings can be variable, hilar adenopathy is most common. While bronchiectasis and nodular infiltrates, similar to that seen in this patient, can occur, they most commonly involve the mid to upper lung zones. Airway disease is most commonly restrictive. Neither this patient's history of marked eosinophilia nor severe asthma is characteristic of sarcoidosis. The absence of granulomas on transbronchial biopsies makes this diagnosis unlikely.

Churg–Strauss Syndrome/Hypereosinophilic Syndrome

Our patient with adult onset asthma and recurrent sinusitis presents with chronic eosinophilia, weight loss, weakness, and worsening dyspnea, who is found to have diffuse pulmonary infiltrates, nonischemic cardiomyopathy, and mononeuritis multiplex. This clinical presentation is consistent with systemic disease which was most concerning for CSS or HES. There can be considerable overlap between these two entities and distinguishing between them is often challenging.

A diagnosis of HES requires the satisfaction of three criteria, (1) Peripheral eosinophilia >1,500cells/μL for >6 months, (2) signs/symptoms indicative of eosinophilic organ infiltration, and (3) absence of another known cause. Contrary to CSS, organ dysfunction from HES is the sole result of eosinophilic tissue infiltration, small vessel vasculitis is always absent on tissue biopsy. Cardiac manifestations due to eosinophilic myocarditis are common. This progresses to a thrombotic then fibrotic phase resulting in restrictive cardiomyopathy, although dilated cardiomyopathy can be seen. Cardioembolic disease can result in CVA. Like CSS, sensorimotor peripheral neuropathies are common. Pulmonary infiltrates are present in up to one third of patients, but eosinophilic pleural effusions are rare. Diarrhea is present in 20%. Cutaneous manifestations are common, particularly urticaria, angioedema, and pruritic erythematous papules/nodules.

Several subtypes of HES have been described. These were previously characterized as myeloproliferative (mHES), lymphocytic (lHES), familial, undefined, overlap, and associated variants. The mHES variant was present in a 9:1 male-to-female predominance and strongly associated with chromosome 4q12 mutations. These mutations result in the generation of an FIP1L1/PDGFRα fusion protein product with tyrosine kinase activity. These patients were also noted to have a higher incidence of elevations in serum B12 and tryptase. They were the most likely to have cardiac involvement. Whereas those with the lHES variant were typified by a similar male-to-female ratio, clonal T-cell populations on flow cytometry, elevated IgE levels, atopic disease, and cutaneous symptoms. Cardiac involvement was rare in the lHES group. Recently, *The Year 2011 Working Conference on Eosinophil Disorders and Syndromes* proposed a more unified classification schema for the HES, and these variant subtypes may ultimately be abandoned. While our patient did not exhibit characteristics of either the mHES or lHES variants, this is an important distinction to make as those with FIP1L1/PDGFRα mutations can be treated with great efficacy with imatinib (Gleevec), a tyrosine kinase inhibitor.

Distinguishing between HES and CSS, particularly ANCA negative CSS as in this patient, can be very challenging. Unlike in CSS, a prodromal asthmatic phase is absent in HES. While pulmonary infiltrates are common in HES, breathlessness is typically associated with the development of heart failure. Pulmonary symptoms are actually much rarer than in CSS and absent altogether in up to 60% of HES patients.

Therefore, based on the presentation and subsequent workup, the most likely diagnosis is CSS.

Discussion

History and Epidemiology

In 1951 Jacob Churg and Lotte Strauss described the CSS in a series of 13 patients who died of status asthmaticus in Mount Sinai Hospital, New York [1]. In addition to fatal asthma, these patients shared characteristics of "fever and hypereosinophilia, symptoms of cardiac failure, renal damage, and peripheral neuropathy resulting from vascular embarrassment in various systems of organs." CSS is recognized as a systemic inflammatory disease with multi-organ involvement. It classically presents as refractory (oral corticosteroid-requiring) asthma, allergic rhinosinusitis, pulmonary infiltrates, and peripheral eosinophilia. Often antineutrophil cytoplasmic antibodies (ANCA) are found thereby classifying CSS as one of the ANCA-associated vasculitides along with MPA and GPA (formerly called Wegener's). Overall CSS is uncommon making up only 10% of all vasculitides and the minority of patients with an ANCA-associated vasculitis. The mean age of onset is 40, and CSS uncommonly affects adults older than 65 or children where other vasculitides are more common. CSS affects men and women with equal frequency, and there does not appear to be a geographic or ethnobiologic predilection.

Presentation, Prognosis and Diagnosis

CSS classically presents as above with severe asthma, allergic rhinosinus disease, peripheral eosinophilia, and ANCA positivity. In reality, though, CSS often has a variable presentation and the limited number of cases, frequent use of steroids before diagnosis, prolonged time course of the disease, and varying degrees of organ system involvement confound a "classic" presentation. Also, as there are three phases to CSS, presentation will depend on the phase. The first phase is the *prodromal* phase which occurs in the second to third decades of life and is characterized by any combination of allergic rhinitis, asthma, and allergic dermatitis or eczema. Often the asthma is severe and requires frequent bursts of oral corticosteroids. Next is the *eosinophilic* phase marked by eosinophilic infiltration of any organ, most commonly the lungs and gastrointestinal tracts. Often eosinophilia is >1,500 cells/microL or >10% of the total leukocyte count, and lung involvement results in patchy and fleeting infiltrates on plain chest radiography. The *vasculitic* phase carries the highest morbidity/mortality and is marked by a small- and medium-sized vessel vasculitis. Patients present in this phase during the third and fourth decades of life with symptoms of fatigue, fever, anorexia, weight loss, abdominal pain, shortness of breath, and a number of other complaints depending on the organs involved. Patients commonly show subcutaneous nodules, peripheral neuropathy, nasal polyps, ANCA-positivity, and an elevated IgE on exam and laboratory testing. Interestingly, asthma tends to improve during the vasculitic phase. Though the symptoms and organ systems listed above represent the more common findings in CSS, any organ system may be involved as detailed in Table 12.3, relative frequencies are noted when available [2].

Some cases of CSS present after the initiation of medications or the use of inhaled toxicants. CSS may manifest when patients with severe asthma are treated with oral corticosteroid-sparing agents such as high-dose inhaled corticosteroids (ICS) or leukotriene modifying agents (LTMAs). In these cases it is believed that initiating ICS or LTMAs unmask CSS by allowing patients to reduce their oral corticosteroids, which are necessary to control the CSS. A similar rationale is used for omalizumab,

Table 12.3 Organ systems which may be involved in the Churg-Strauss syndrome (relative frequencies noted, when available)

Pulmonary	Neurologic
Asthma ~95%	Peripheral neuropathy (mononeuritis multiplex, ~75%)
Pulmonary opacities and infiltrates	
Effusions, often exudative and eosinophilic	Subarachnoid or intracranial hemorrhage
Nodules, sometimes cavitating	Stroke, cerebral
Alveolar hemorrhage	Central retinal artery occlusion
Upper airway and ears	Renal (often ANCA-positive)
Allergic rhinosinusitis, >60%	Acute kidney injury (glomerulonephritis)
Recurrent sinusitis	Microscopic hematuria
Nasal obstruction	Proteinuria
Nasal polyposis	Hypertension
Serous otitis media	
Sensoneural hearing loss	
	Gastrointestinal
Cutaneous, 50–66%	Eosinophilic gastroenteritis (abdominal pain, diarrhea, GI bleeding)
Subcutaneous nodules, extensor surfaces	
Palpable purpura	Eosinophilic colitis
Maculopapular rash	
Petechiae and ecchymoses	Musculoskeletal
	Myalgias
Cardiovascular (>50% fatal and often ANCA-negative with high peripheral eosinophils)	Migratory polyarthralgias
	Arthritis
Heart failure	Lymphatics
Myocardial ischemia	Eosinophilic lymphadenopathy
Dysrhythmias and conduction blocks/delays	
Valvulopathies	Others
Pericardial effusions	Constitutional symptoms (fevers, lethargy, weight loss)
Mural thrombi	

a monoclonal anti-IgE antibody. Omalizumab use may enable oral steroid reduction causing an unmasking of CSS. Some data suggests that LTMAs may directly cause a CSS-like syndrome, though sufficient evidence is lacking [3]. Last, the use of free-base cocaine has been associated with a CSS-like vasculitis [4], though a clear association with CSS versus other ANCA-associated vasculitides is not apparent.

Of all the extra-pulmonary manifestations of CSS vasculitis, cardiac, gastrointestinal, renal, and neurologic involvement portend the worst prognosis [5]. The French Vasculitis Group developed a validated five-factor score (FFS) which prognosticates in CSS based on five criteria: gastrointestinal, cardiac, and neurologic involvement as well as a serum creatinine >1.58 mg/dL (>140 μmol/L) and proteinuria >1 g/24 h [5, 6]. Specifically, a FFS score of 1+ compared to 0 conferred a 14% increase in mortality [5].

Of particular interest to one of our cases is cardiac involvement. CSS, like many of the vasculitides, can affect the heart at several different levels. In a nice review by Kane and Keogh, small and medium vessel vasculitis can affect the myocardium, valves, pericardium, and coronary vessels to produce a range of clinical manifestations [7]. Additionally, CSS may induce arrythmias if myocardial inflammation occurs or if coronary ischemia ensues following coronary vasculitis. In CSS the heart is involved in 13–47% of cases. When CSS involves the heart, mortality reaches 50%. Death may occur because of systolic heart failure, myocardial infarction, coronary or intraventricular thrombus formation, or ventricular dysrhythmias.

Diagnosis of CSS is often difficult because of the variable presentation and the multitude of signs and symptoms. The most commonly used diagnostic criteria for CSS is by the American College of Rheumatology (ACR) where at least 4 of 6 criteria are required for a sensitivity of 85% and a specificity of 99.7% [8]. The criteria combine clinical history, exam findings, radiography, laboratory data, and histology owing to the multifaceted and complex nature of CSS. The ACR diagnostic criteria are:

- Asthma (by history or physical exam of wheezing)
- >10% peripheral eosinophils (often >1,500 cells/microL)
- Mononeuropathy or polyneuropathy (commonly mononeuritis multiplex)
- Fleeting pulmonary infiltrates on plain chest radiograph
- Paranasal sinus abnormalities (commonly thickened mucosa on imaging)
- Tissue biopsy containing a blood vessel with perivascular eosinophilic infiltrates

Pathophysiology

The pathophysiology of CSS is not well understood, though recent data has improved our view of the immune system in CSS. In an excellent recent review of CSS pathophysiology, Vaglio et al. highlight that although CSS is considered to be an allergic disease with a Th2 CD4+ predominant response, the immune dysfunction in CSS involves an interplay between Th2, Th1, and Th17 cells as well as eosinophils, endothelial cells, and epithelial cells [3]. Clearly allergic sensitization is critical in CSS as the prodromal phase is characterized by allergic rhinosinusitis, nasal polyposis, and asthma. Genetic studies have identified HLA-DRB1*04, *07, and HLA-DRB4 genes as conferring an increased risk for CSS, and these genes are class II CD4+ restricted indicating an antigen-driven process. Single-nucleotide polymorphism studies have shown that IL-10 producing genes are upregulated in ANCA-negative CSS subjects, and IL10 is a Th2 cytokine. Increased levels of peripheral and tissue CD4+ cells are seen in CSS which secrete Th2 cytokines including IL4 and IL13, both implicated in allergic responses. Serum IL5 is also increased in CSS, though it is unclear if the IL5 emanates from CD4+ cells; IL5 specifically recruits eosinophils from bone marrow. Studies of epithelial and endothelial chemokine production in CSS show a predominant Th2 profile. Eotaxin-3, which recruits eosinophils, and CCL17, which recruits additional Th2 cells, are both found in high concentrations in CSS subjects' serum and lesions compared to controls. Interestingly, unlike atopic asthma the asthma seen in CSS tends to be adult-onset, less associated with skin-prick or radio-allergosorbent (RAST) positivity, and less likely seasonal. According to Vaglio et al., this indicates that the pulmonary and rhinosinus disease seen in CSS may be allergic but not atopic, raising questions about the nature of the allergens.

Though allergy is important in CSS, several lines of evidence support nonallergic propagation of the disease. In addition to CD4+ cells secreting Th2 cytokines, they also secrete Th1 cytokines typically seen in nonallergic vasculitis. High amounts of interferon-γ (IFN-γ) and IL17A are seen from peripheral lymphocytes in CSS, and these cytokines are involved in granuloma-formation and vasculitis, not classic allergic disease. Additionally, studies looking at regulatory T-cells ($CD4+CD25^{high}FoxP3+$, Tregs) found lower numbers and impaired Treg function in CSS compared to controls. Tregs secrete immunomodulating cytokines and preserve a balance between Th2 and Th1 responses. In CSS Tregs have, in part, lost their regulatory abilities.

The humoral immune system is also involved in CSS. Though ANCAs (specifically anti-myeloperoxidase) have long been recognized as associated with CSS during the vasculitic phase, their exact role is uncertain. Newer evidence indicates that the rare subclass of IgG4 is excessively produced in CSS [9]. IgG4 production is associated with a Th2 inflammatory milieu including IL4, IL5, and IL13 production, and it is also associated with B-cell maturation. In essence, elevated IgG4 levels indicate that B-cells are maturing and upregulated in CSS. Other evidence for B-cell involvement in the pathogenesis of CSS is indirect and comes from the use of the B-cell depleting monoclonal antibody rituximab. With rituximab use in refractory CSS, circulating B-cells, eosinophils, and IL5 are reduced [10]. Since IL5 is produced by T-cells exclusively, selectively reducing B-cells and seeing a reduction in a T-cell product indicates significant cross-talk and stimulation between the cellular and humoral immune systems. Further studies are needed to elucidate these interactions.

Eosinophils are clearly both present and participatory in CSS [3]. They are upregulated, activated, and spared from apoptosis by Th2 cytokines, particularly IL5. In a T-cell/eosinophil crosstalk paradigm, eosinophils can induce Th2 cytokine production through IL25, a cytokine produced by eosinophils which binds to IL17RB located on CD4+ cell surfaces. Last, once activated eosinophils are activated and recruited to sites of vascular damage, they release large amounts of eosinophilic cationic protein (ECP) causing tissue injury. This is supported by increased levels of serum and BAL ECP in CSS.

The clinical manifestations of CSS result from allergic disease, eosinophilic tissue infiltration (and tissue damage by ECP), and granulomatous inflammation. In the prodromal phase, signs and symptoms are likely attributed to classic Th2 rhinosinus and pulmonary inflammation. As eosinophils are recruited years later in the eosinophilic phase, eosinophils exert their effect locally through tissue inflammation.

In the vasculitic phase, the Th1 inflammatory response overshadows Th2 inflammation, and systemic symptoms occur. Currently it is unclear if the eosinophils precipitate granuloma formation or if the mechanisms of inflammation differ during the vasculitic phase. In CSS-induced cardiac disease, which generally occurs in the vasculitic phase, tissue injury is due to eosinophilic infiltration, extra-vascular granulomatous inflammation, and vasculitis [7].

In summary, though the pathophysiology of CSS is still largely unknown it is clear that both Th2 and Th1 inflammatory responses exist, that the humoral system is involved and interwoven with the cellular immune system, and that eosinophils are both effector and stimulatory cells. The clinical manifestations result from varying degrees of inflammation.

Workup, Labs, and Diagnostic Procedures

As above, the diagnosis of CSS is made on clinical, radiographic, laboratory and pathologic grounds. In general the workup involves a thorough history with particular attention to timing, duration, and treatment of allergic disease; use of medications including oral steroids, ICS, LTMAs, and omalizumab; and development of systemic and vasculitic symptoms. Prior and current radiography will be particularly helpful especially if infiltrates are fleeting. Prior and current laboratory work will allow identification of trends in eosinophilia. If time permits, accessing tissue for biopsy may confirm the diagnosis, especially if vasculitis with eosinophils, perivascular granulomata, and tissue necrosis are seen. Skin and sural nerve biopsies are particularly accessible if patients present with cutaneous or peripheral nerve symptoms respectively, as lung biopsies are quite invasive. If patients are particularly ill, there may not be time for a biopsy before therapy is required.

For suspected CSS-induced cardiac disease, a few diagnostic modalities are helpful. Most experts recommend beginning with an electrocardiogram (ECG) and transthoracic echocardiogram (TTE) [7]. The ECG is very sensitive for conduction abnormalities, and the TTE is quite sensitive for any myocardial or pericardial dysfunction which may occur with granulomatous or eosinophilic involvement. Both, however, are not specific for CSS. If there are ECG or TTE abnormalities, further testing is warranted. Though endomyocardial biopsy is the gold standard for diagnosing myocardial CSS, it is very insensitive as myocardial inflammation is patchy and a biopsy may miss involved areas. Cardiac MRI with gadolinium enhancement is particularly useful to detect myocardial inflammation. Normally gadolinium washes out of normal myocardium in a predictable time and pattern. If there is delayed washout, particularly in a non-coronary distribution, myocardial inflammation may occur. Still, cardiac MRI with gadolinium is not specific for CSS, but in the right clinical context it may be very useful and avoid endomyocardial biopsy [7].

Specific recommendations for workup are listed below and follow the diagnostic criteria for the ACR [8] and the prognostication based on the FFS [5, 6]. Bolded entries may be particularly useful.

Laboratory testing:	
Peripheral cell count	Gammaglobulins—elevated
Eos—usually 5,000–9,000 cells/μL	Rheumatoid factor—mild elevation
Hgb—normocytic anemia	Complements—Elevated
WBC—leukocytosis	Serum creatinine—may be elevated
ANCA-pANCA or anti-myeloperoxidase	

Imaging:	
Chest X-ray:	High-resolution chest CT:
Transient/patch opacities, 75%	Peribronchial and septal thickening
Pleural effusions, exudates, 30%	Patchy opacities
	Peripheral pulmonary artery enlargement

Pulmonary Function Testing:	
Obstructive—especially early	Reduced DLCO
Restrictive—with vasculitis	Reduced peripheral O_2 saturation
Mixed restrictive and obstructive	

Bronchoscopy:
Often >30% eosinophils on lavage, though this is not specific for CSS

Cardiac Tests:	
ECG—conduction/ischemia	Cardiac MRI with gadolinium:
Transthoracic echocardiography:	Perform if ECG or echo are abnormal
Mural thrombi, wall motion, etc.	Caution in renal dysfunction
Endomyocardial biopsy	Delayed images may show necrosis

Management and Treatment

Conventional

Current treatment guidelines for CSS [3] are largely based on historical glucocorticoid-only strategies and small randomized control trials. Because of this, most CSS cases, regardless of severity, involve glucocorticoids either for induction, maintenance or both. In recent years the French Vasculitis Study Group performed two studies assessing treatment regimens using glucocorticoids alone or with additional immunosuppressants on CSS remission and relapse. CSS inclusion cases had a FFS score of 1 or higher, and the group found that CSS patients with poor prognostic factors often relapsed after glucocorticoid-only regimens were tapered. Additionally, CSS patients with poor prognostic factors did better when they received glucocorticoids plus other immunosuppressants (including azathioprine or cyclophosphamide). Other immunosuppressant therapy used in CSS includes methotrexate, mycophenolate mofetil, and interferon-alpha, though these have not been studied in comparison with corticosteroids and data are limited to very small studies or case series. Studies are underway looking at CSS subjects without poor prognostic factors, though currently little data exists for this population. In total, these data suggest that CSS cases with poor prognostic factors respond better to glucocorticoids plus additional immunosuppressants, though the choice of immunosuppresants is not yet clear. As with all immunosuppressants including glucocorticoids, clinicians must weigh side effect profiles with treatment effects for each patient.

Plasma exchange [11] is another treatment used in severe CSS cases as well as many other severe vasculitides. The idea is that removal of offending antibodies (such as ANCA) may lessen inflammation and tissue destruction. Though successful in many cases, little data exists supporting the use of plasma exchange. Additionally, meta-analyses assessing plasma exchange efficacy in MPA and CSS showed no significant benefit over corticosteroids alone.

Novel

As we begin to understand the CSS pathophysiology on a more sophisticated level, we can look towards more targeted therapeutic interventions. To date published data exists for intravenous immune globulin, hydroxyurea, rituximab (anti-CD20), omalizumab (anti-IgE), and mepolizumab (anti-IL5) [3]. Rituximab is an anti-CD20 monoclonal antibody which selectively depletes B-cell populations. It has been widely used in many neoplastic and rheumatologic diseases, and several case reports and series demonstrate efficacy in CSS. As mentioned above, the efficacy of rituximab in CSS speaks to the humoral system's involvement in the disease progression [3]. Mepolizumab is an anti-IL5 monoclonal antibody which decreases eosinophil recruitment. Several small studies assessing the addition of mepolizumab to steroid agents showed a decrease or cessation of steroids in CSS. Many of these subjects, however, relapsed after stopping mepolizumab, and further studies are needed. Last, omalizumab is an anti-IgE monoclonal antibody with wide use in asthma. Though the role of IgE in CSS is not clear, omalizumab has been effective in some case studies. Its use is controversial, however, as omalizumab has been implicated in worsening CSS, probably due to a steroid-withdrawal effect.

Questions

1. Patients with CSS complicated by cardiomyopathy are most likely to have which of the following findings?

   (a) Positive ANCAs and normal peripheral eosinophil count
   (b) Negative ANCAs and lower peripheral eosinophil count
   (c) Negative ANCAs and higher peripheral eosinophil count
   (d) Positive ANCAs and lower peripheral eosinophil count
   (e) None of the above

2. Chromosome 4q12 anomalies with resultant FIP1L1/PDGFRα gain of function mutations are associated with which of the following?

   (a) CSS
   (b) Sarcoidosis
   (c) Systemic mastocytosis
   (d) HES
   (e) GPA (formerly known as Wegener's)

3. Which of the following has demonstrated efficacy in the treatment of FIP1L1/PDGFRα positive HES?

   (a) Imatinib
   (b) Cytarabine
   (c) Crizotinib
   (d) Hydroxyurea
   (e) None of the above

4. Which of the following conditions is most strongly associated with a preceding diagnosis of asthma?

   (a) ABPA
   (b) HES
   (c) AEP
   (d) CSS
   (e) Both A and D

5. Which of the following conditions are most closely associated with elevated serum tryptase levels?

   (a) CSS
   (b) Systemic Mastocytosis
   (c) HES
   (d) Both B and C, but not A
   (e) Both A and C, but not B

6. Which of the following treatments for the CSS has the *LEAST* amount of support in the literature?

   (a) Oral glucocorticosteroids
   (b) Cyclophosphamide
   (c) Leukotriene modifying agents
   (d) Mepolizumab
   (e) Rituximab

7. Based on current understanding of the CSS, which of the following components of the immune system contribute to the pathophysiology?

   (a) Humoral (B-cells and antibodies)
   (b) Cell-mediated (T-cells)
   (c) Th2 (e.g., allergic)
   (d) Th1 (e.g., autoimmune)
   (e) All the above

8. Which of the following organ systems when involved in the CSS portend a worse prognosis (*choose all that apply*)?

   (a) Cardiac
   (b) Cutaneous/Skin
   (c) Gastrointestinal
   (d) Renal
   (e) Neurologic

9. Which of the following cardiac tests has the highest specificity but low sensitivity for cardiac involvement in CSS?

   (a) Endomyocardial biopsy
   (b) Transthoracic echocardiography (TTE)
   (c) Electrocardiography (ECG)
   (d) Cardiac magnetic resonance imaging (Cardiac MRI)
   (e) Physical Examination

10. In general, which of the following organ systems, when involved in CSS, carries the highest mortality?

    (a) Cutaneous/Skin
    (b) Cardiac
    (c) Pulmonary
    (d) Both A and C
    (e) All the above

Answers: 1. (c), 2. (d), 3. (a), 4. (e), 5. (d), 6. (c), 7. (e), 8. (a, c, d, e), 9. (a), 10. (b).

References

1. Churg J, Strauss L. Allergic granulomatosis, allergic angiitis, and periarteritis nodosa. Am J Pathol. 1951;27(2):277–301.
2. Baldini C, Talarico R, Della Rossa A, Bombardieri S. Clinical manifestations and treatment of Churg-Strauss syndrome. Rheum Dis Clin North Am. 2010;36(3):527–43.
3. Vaglio A, Moosig F, Zwerina J. Churg-Strauss syndrome: update on pathophysiology and treatment. Curr Opin Rheumatol. 2012;24(1):24–30.
4. Orriols R, Munoz X, Ferrer J, Huget P, Morell F. Cocaine-induced Churg-Strauss vasculitis. Eur Respir J. 1996;9(1):175–7.
5. Guillevin L, Lhote F, Gayraud M, et al. Prognostic factors in polyarteritis nodosa and Churg-Strauss syndrome A prospective study in 342 patients. Medicine (Baltimore). 1996;75(1):17–28.
6. Guillevin L, Pagnoux C, Seror R, Mahr A, Mouthon L, Le Toumelin P. The Five-Factor Score revisited: assessment of prognoses of systemic necrotizing vasculitices based on the French Vasculitis Study Group (FVSG) cohort. Medicine (Baltimore). 2011;90(1):19–27.
7. Kane GC, Keogh KA. Involvement of the heart by small and medium vessel vasculitis. Curr Opin Rheumatol. 2009;21(1):29–34.
8. Masi AT, Hunder GG, Lie JT, et al. The American College of Rheumatology 1990 criteria for the classification of Churg-Strauss syndrome (allergic granulomatosis and angiitis). Arthritis Rheum. 1990;33(8):1094–100.
9. Vaglio A, Strehl JD, Manger B, et al. IgG4 immune response in Churg-Strauss syndrome. Ann Rheum Dis. 2012;71(3):390–3.
10. Pepper RJ, Fabre MA, Pavesio C, et al. Rituximab is effective in the treatment of refractory Churg-Strauss syndrome and is associated with diminished T-cell interleukin-5 production. Rheumatology (Oxford). 2008;47(7):1104–5.
11. Casian A, Jayne D. Plasma exchange in the treatment of Wegener's granulomatosis, microscopic polyangiitis, Churg-Strauss syndrome and renal limited vasculitis. Curr Opin Rheumatol. 2011;23(1):12–7.

Chapter 13
Vasculitis: Giant Cell Arteritis

Tanaz A. Kermani and Kenneth J. Warrington

Abstract Giant cell arteritis is a systemic granulomatous large-vessel vasculitis of the aorta and its branches. The inflammatory process in giant cell arteritis may result in large-artery stenosis and tissue ischemia. While this most often involves the upper extremity arteries, in rare cases, lower extremity arterial involvement from giant cell arteritis has also been described. Clinicians should be aware of the different presenting manifestations of large-vessel vasculitis like giant cell arteritis and its evaluation and treatment.

Keywords Giant cell arteritis • Vasculitis • Large-artery stenosis • Claudication

Case 1

A 62-year-old woman presents with arm "fatigue." Over the last 3–4 months, she has developed worsening pain in her left arm with activity. She complains of a dull, achy, feeling. The arm gets "tired" more easily. Symptoms are only present within several minutes of rigorous activity or repetitive movement. They improve with rest. The pain is in the entire left arm. It feels like her muscles are sore. No joint pain. No nocturnal symptoms. Denies neck pain, sharp, shooting pain, numbness or tingling. The left arm seems to change colors on cold exposure and her fingers turn purplish.

T.A. Kermani, M.D., M.S. (✉)
Division of Rheumatology, University of California Los Angeles,
2020 Santa Monica Boulevard, Suite 540, Santa Monica, CA, 90404, USA
e-mail: kermani.tanaz@yahoo.com

K.J. Warrington, M.D.
Division of Rheumatology, Mayo Clinic,
200 First Street SW, Rochester, MN, 55905, USA
e-mail: warrington.kenneth@mayo.edu

M. Mahmoudi (ed.), *Challenging Cases in Rheumatology and Diseases of the Immune System*, DOI 10.1007/978-1-4614-5088-7_13,
© Springer Science+Business Media, LLC 2013

The left hand feels cooler than the right side. Now the right arm is starting to get tired more easily as well. She notes low grade temperatures for several months. Also complains of generalized fatigue and decreased appetite with weight loss of several pounds. She denies headaches, jaw claudication, scalp tenderness, visual symptoms, dizziness, neurologic symptoms, chest pain, pulmonary symptoms, and gastrointestinal symptoms. No rashes, photosensitivity, skin changes, sicca symptoms, mucositis, serositis, history of cytopenias or renal disease. She is a gravida 3, para 3. No history of thromboembolic events.

Past medical history is remarkable only for hypertension for which she takes hydrochlorothiazide. She has had a cholecystectomy for cholelithiasis. She is a never smoker and rarely drinks alcohol.

On examination, she appears well. Vital signs: temperature 37.5° C, pulse 66 and regular, blood pressure 100/76 mmHg in the left arm and 132/78 mmHg in the right arm. Skin examination reveals mild purplish discoloration of the fingers in the left hand which feels cooler than the right. No rashes. Cardiovascular examination is normal. Lung examination is normal. On vessel exam, she is noted to have absent left radial pulse, diminished right radial pulse and a left subclavian bruit. No carotid, abdominal or femoral bruits. Lower extremity pulses are normal. Abdominal examination and neurologic examinations are normal. She has full range of motion of all joints without any swelling or synovitis.

Initial laboratory studies: Hemoglobin 10.2 g/dL (normocytic), white blood count (WBC) normal, platelet count normal. Chemistries including sodium, potassium, calcium, fasting glucose, creatinine, liver enzymes are all normal. Shoulder x-rays are normal. Antinuclear antibody (ANA) is negative.

With the Information Presented, What Is Your Working Diagnosis?

The patient presents with bilateral upper extremity pain with exertion, improvement with rest and temperature changes in the arms. Examination shows a 32 mmHg discrepancy in upper extremity arterial pressures, a left subclavian bruit and diminished/absent pulses. All of these findings are consistent with upper extremity arterial disease. The symptoms are consistent with upper extremity claudication. While rotator cuff disorders are common and also cause pain with movement, the symptoms she describes are atypical since they are diffuse and occur only after a certain amount of exertion. She does not describe pain in the shoulder with movements like abduction or internal rotation, or, nocturnal symptoms which are more common with rotator cuff disease. Since the symptoms are aggravated in the cold, Raynaud's phenomenon would be a possibility. Atypical features for this are the asymmetry in symptoms and arm claudication which suggests involvement of a larger blood vessel than the digital arteries. Patients with secondary Raynaud's (in association with rheumatic diseases) can experience ischemic phenomenon (skin ulcerations, rarely infarcts) but these typically affect the fingers and distal portion of the upper extremity while the patient is describing more diffuse symptoms. Upper extremity claudication is not a feature of Raynaud's. The examination findings also support involvement of a large artery with asymmetric blood pressures, absent pulses and bruits. While lower extremity involvement from peripheral arterial disease is more common, upper extremity arterial disease can also occur. However, apart from hypertension, she has no significant risk factors for peripheral arterial disease. Other possibilities include thoracic outlet syndrome, causes of arterial thrombosis such as antiphospholipid antibody syndrome or vasculitis (Takayasu arteritis or giant cell arteritis). Given the patient's age, giant cell arteritis would be more likely as opposed to Takayasu arteritis which tends to affect young women. Cryoglobulinemia is another possibility but affects the small blood vessels and is unlikely given asymmetry and the examination findings which suggests medium-to-large vessel involvement. Laboratory findings at present are only suggestive of anemia of chronic disease but are otherwise unhelpful in identifying an etiology for the patient's symptoms.

Differential Diagnosis

Thoracic outlet syndrome
Large-vessel vasculitis
Antiphospholipid antibody syndrome (primary or secondary to a connective tissue disease)
Cryoglobulinemia
Atherosclerosis of the subclavian artery

Workup

Additional laboratory studies including erythrocyte sedimentation rate (ESR), c-reactive protein (CRP), hepatitis serologies, cryoglobulins, C3, C4, rheumatoid factor, anticardiolipin antibodies, diluted Russell Viper Venom time (DRVVT), serum protein electrophoresis (Table 13.1) were obtained. Noninvasive arterial Doppler studies of the upper extremity confirmed asymmetric blood pressures and were suggestive of left subclavian occlusive or stenotic disease. A computed tomography angiogram (CTA) of the chest and upper extremities was performed which showed thickening of bilateral subclavian arteries with segmental, diffuse luminal narrowing of the left subclavian and left brachial arteries (Fig. 13.1).

What Is Your Diagnosis and Why?

The symptoms, laboratory studies, and imaging findings are all consistent with upper extremity arterial vasculitis. The markers of inflammation are elevated suggestive an inflammatory process. Additional laboratory studies including serologies

Table 13.1 Additional laboratory studies obtained to evaluate symptoms for Case 1

Laboratory test	Value	Reference value
Erythrocyte sedimentation rate	62 mm/h	0–29 mm/h
C-reactive protein	43 mg/L	<8 mg/L
C3	126 mg/dL	71–141 mg/dL
C4	26 mg/dL	12–34 mg/dL
Hepatitis B surface antigen	Negative	
Hepatitis B surface antibody	Negative	
Hepatitis B core antibody	Negative	
Hepatitis C antibody	Negative	
Cryocrit	Negative	
Diluted Russell Viper venom time	Negative	
IgM anticardiolipin antibody	<12.5 MPL	>20 considered positive
IgG anticardiolipin antibody	<15 GPL	>20 considered positive
Rheumatoid factor	<10 IU/mL	<25 IU/mL
Serum protein electrophoresis	Normal pattern	
Immunofixation	No monoclonal protein detected	

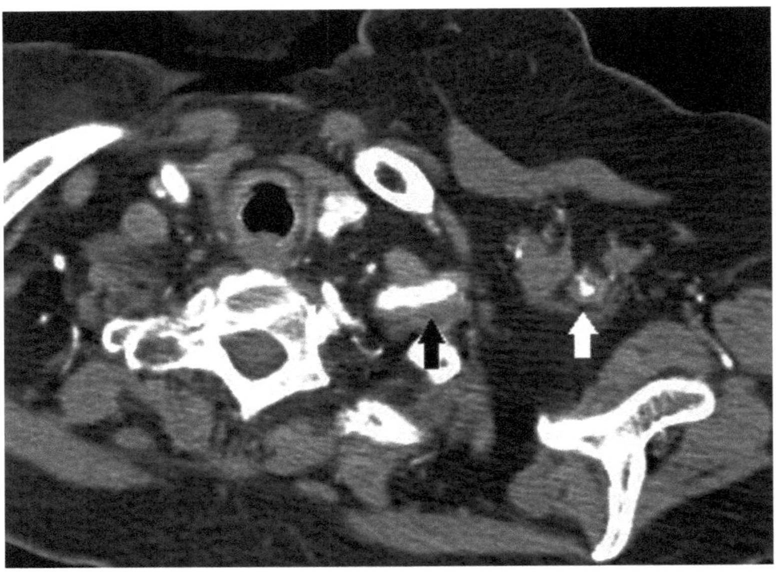

Fig. 13.1 Computed tomography angiography showing thickening of the wall of the left subclavian artery (*arrow*) and, wall thickening and luminal narrowing of the axillary artery (*arrow*) consistent with vasculitis

are normal. Imaging shows wall thickening and stenosis of the subclavian and brachial arteries which would be consistent with vasculitis. Given the distribution, this is a large-vessel vasculitis consistent with Takayasu arteritis or giant cell arteritis.

Given the patient's age, giant cell arteritis is the most likely diagnosis. The patient was started on prednisone 60 mg daily with appropriate bone and *Pneumocystis jiroveci* prophylaxis. This was gradually tapered over the course of the next several months. However, she had recurrent symptoms and elevated markers of inflammation each time prednisone taper below 10 mg daily was attempted. Therefore, methotrexate was added. At 1 year, her upper extremity symptoms had improved and imaging was stable.

Final diagnosis: Giant cell arteritis with upper extremity vasculitis.

Case 2

A 73-year-old woman presents for evaluation of bilateral lower extremity pain. Her symptoms began 6 weeks prior to evaluation when she noticed right leg pain with ambulation. Since that time, her symptoms have been progressive and now affect both legs below the knees. She has cramping and pain in the calves and feet that only occur with movement and resolve with rest or standing still. She is now only able to walk one block without stopping. Right lower extremity symptoms are worse than the left. She also complains of discoloration of the legs and temperature changes with them feeling "cold." No digital ulcerations. No back pain. Leaning forward does not help the symptoms. On systems review, she notes decreased appetite with 10 pound weight loss over the last 2 months. No headaches, scalp tenderness or visual changes. She has noticed pain in her right jaw with chewing food which improves with rest for the last 2 weeks. She has also developed shoulder and hip pain and stiffness over the last 2 months. Symptoms are worse in the morning and improve with activity. She uses ibuprofen with some relief. No other joint pain. No chest pain, dyspnea on exertion, upper extremity claudication, Raynaud's phenomenon, gastrointestinal pain with meals, rashes, numbness or tingling. Past medical history is remarkable only for a history of breast cancer for which she underwent lumpectomy 10 years ago. She is not on any medications. She was a prior smoker (30 pack-years) but quit 10 years ago. On examination, she appears younger than her stated age. Vital signs are as follows: temperature 37.3° C, pulse 78 and regular, blood pressure 130/80 mmHg in the left arm and 132/78 mmHg in the right arm. Skin examination reveals bluish discoloration of the toes, worse on the right than the left. No skin lesions or rashes. Vascular examination reveals normal bilateral temporal artery pulses without nodularity or pain. No carotid or subclavian bruits, absent dorsalis pedis and posterior tibial pulses on the right and diminished pulses on the left. Popliteal pulses are diminished bilaterally. No femoral or abdominal bruits. She has pallor of the right lower extremity with elevation and rubor with dependency. Cardiovascular, pulmonary, gastrointestinal and neurologic examinations are normal. Joint examination reveals limited active abduction of both shoulders and pain with internal rotation. No swelling of the joints. Bilateral hip examination is normal.

Laboratory studies: Hemoglobin 9.9 g/dL (normocytic), WBC normal, platelet count normal. ESR by Westergren method was elevated at 90 mm/h. Chemistries including sodium, potassium, calcium, fasting glucose, creatinine, liver enzymes are all normal. No imaging studies available for review.

With the Information Presented, What Is Your Working Diagnosis?

The patient is an elderly woman who presents with subacute symptoms of bilateral, rapidly progressive, lower extremity claudication. Atypical features include the relatively recent onset of symptoms, their progression within weeks, absence of any significant risk factors associated with peripheral arterial disease (quit smoking many years ago). Additionally, on review of systems, she has had constitutional symptoms, and jaw pain suggestive of jaw claudication with shoulder/hip girdle pain and stiffness consistent with polymyalgia rheumatica. Examination findings confirm this with an abnormal lower extremity vascular examination. There are no findings to suggest critical limb ischemia (no rest pain). Laboratory findings show an inflammatory process with anemia and elevated ESR.

The differential diagnosis at this time is broad and should focus on causes of arterial insufficiency. Atrial fibrillation with embolic phenomenon would be unlikely given the duration of symptoms and the fact that they have been progressive over time rather than an abrupt onset. Additionally, her symptoms are bilateral. Peripheral arterial disease from atherosclerosis also seems unlikely with the above history and absence of significant cardiovascular risk factors. Autoimmune, infectious or paraneoplastic causes need to be considered. Of these, antiphospholipid antibody syndrome, cryoglobulinemia and vasculitis (giant cell arteritis) remain possibilities.

Differential Diagnosis

Large-vessel vasculitis
Atherosclerosis
Cryoglobulinemia
Antiphospholipid antibody syndrome (primary or secondary to connective tissue disease)

Workup

Additional laboratory and imaging workup was pursued to evaluate the patient's symptoms. This included hepatitis serologies, cryoglobulins, C3, C4, rheumatoid factor, anticardiolipin antibodies, DRVVT, serum protein electrophoresis (Table 13.2). To evaluate the lower extremity vasculature, computed tomography angiogram of the abdominal aorta with run offs was obtained and showed severe diffuse segmental tapering of the superficial femoral, popliteal and infrapopliteal vessels with wall thickening consistent with vasculitis (Fig. 13.2). Given the

Table 13.2 Laboratory studies obtained in Case 2

Laboratory test	Value	Reference value
C3	138 mg/dL	71–141 mg/dL
C4	30 mg/dL	12–34 mg/dL
Hepatitis B surface antigen	Negative	
Hepatitis B surface antibody	Negative	
Hepatitis B core antibody	Negative	
Hepatitis C antibody	Negative	
Cryocrit	Negative	
Diluted Russell Viper venom time	Negative	
IgM anticardiolipin antibody	<12.5 MPL	>20 considered positive
IgG anticardiolipin antibody	<15 GPL	>20 considered positive
Rheumatoid factor	<10 IU/mL	<25 IU/mL
Serum protein electrophoresis	Normal pattern	
Immunofixation	No monoclonal protein detected	

symptoms of polymyalgia rheumatica, elevated markers of inflammation and right jaw claudication, right temporal artery biopsy was pursued and showed changes of giant cell arteritis.

What Is Your Diagnosis and Why?

The diagnosis is giant cell arteritis (biopsy proven) with lower extremity arterial vasculitis (extracranial disease). The patient was started on aspirin 81 mg daily, prednisone 60 mg daily with appropriate bone and infectious prophylaxis. Prednisone was gradually tapered. The patient's symptoms remained stable and serial imaging showed stable changes of vasculitis. She never required any vascular intervention for her symptoms.

Final diagnosis: Giant cell arteritis with lower extremity vasculitis.

Discussion

Giant cell arteritis (GCA) is a granulomatous, systemic large-vessel vasculitis. The inflammatory process in GCA has a predilection for the extracranial branches of the carotid artery, but can also affect the aorta and its branches. The estimated annual incidence of GCA is 18.9 per 100,000 people over the age of 50 years [1]. Women are affected two to three times more often than men [2].

Common clinical symptoms include headache (two-thirds of patients), scalp tenderness, jaw claudication, polymyalgia rheumatica (shoulder and hip girdle pain

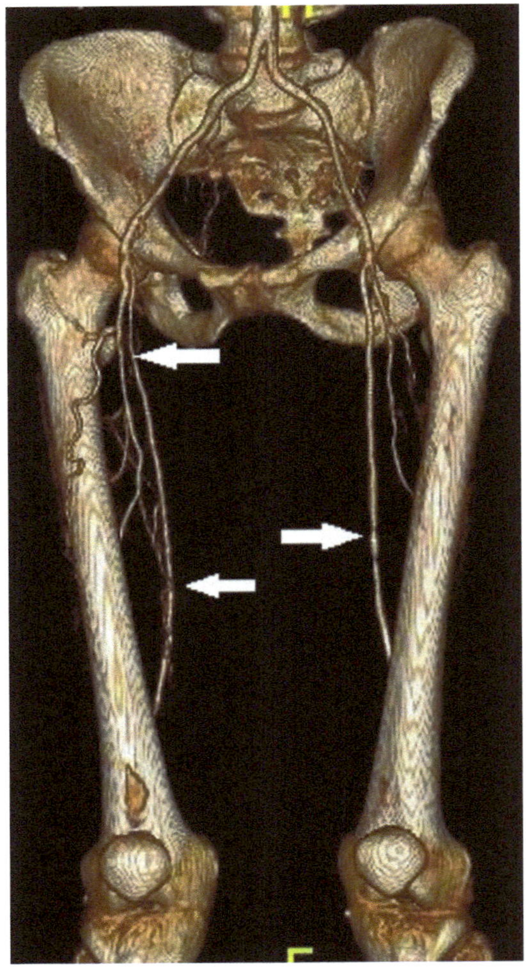

Fig. 13.2 Computed tomography angiography 3D reconstruction image showing segmental smooth, tapered stenosis of the superficial femoral arteries (*arrows*) suggestive of vasculitis

and stiffness), visual symptoms (diplopia, amaurosis fugax, vision loss), and constitutional symptoms like low-grade temperatures, anorexia or weight loss [2]. Vision loss resulting from involvement of the ciliary artery and subsequent ischemia of the optic nerve (arteritic anterior ischemic neuropathy) may occur in 20 % patients and is an ophthalmologic emergency. While cranial manifestations of GCA are well-recognized, patients may present with constitutional symptoms or ischemic manifestations. GCA is should be considered in the differential diagnosis of an elderly patient who presents with constitutional symptoms or fever of unknown origin [2]. Other patients may present with limb ischemia (predominantly upper extremity claudication) due to stenosis of the subclavian, axillary or brachial arteries [2]. Patients with GCA are also at increased risk of aortic aneurysm formation (thoracic and abdominal) [3]. In a population-based study from Olmsted County, Minnesota,

27 % of patients developed large-vessel complications such as aortic aneurysm/dissection or large artery stenoses [4].

The causative agent of GCA remains unknown but genetic and environmental factors are important in disease pathogenesis. Genetic polymorphisms in the HLA-DRB1*04 alleles have been associated with susceptibility [2]. GCA is a T-cell dependent disease [5]. The inflammatory process is thought to begin in the adventitial layer of the artery with activation of dendritic cells via toll-like receptors [5]. Activated dendritic cells in turn provide co-stimulatory signals to activate CD4+ T cells which in turn produce proinflammatory cytokines, particularly interleukin-17 and interferon-gamma (INF-γ). The inflammatory infiltrate in biopsy specimens in patients with GCA consists of CD4+ T-cells and macrophages. The macrophages may coalesce to form multinucleated giant cells. In response to the immunologic injury, the artery releases growth and angiogenic factors such as platelet-derived growth factor (PDGF) and vascular endothelial growth factor (VEGF) that induce migration and proliferation of myofibroblasts, neoangiogenesis, and intimal proliferation [5].

The American College of Rheumatology 1990 classification criteria for GCA [6] are based on the presence of three or more of the following: (1) age 50 years and older, (2) new, localized headache, (3) erythrocyte sedimentation rate greater than or equal to 50 mm/h, (4) abnormal temporal artery examination (tenderness, decreased or absent pulses), (5) abnormal temporal artery biopsy (vasculitis with predominance of mononuclear cell infiltration or granulomatous inflammation). These criteria are helpful in distinguishing GCA from other forms of vasculitis but are not diagnostic criteria. The gold-standard diagnostic study is histopathologic examination of a temporal artery biopsy (TAB). However, in the subset of patients with upper extremity arterial vasculitis, TAB may be negative and diagnosis requires confirmation with imaging studies.

A comprehensive history and physical examination is important in the evaluation of patients with suspected GCA. A systematic review evaluated the value of several clinical features as predictors of a positive TAB for GCA [7]. Presence of any headache has the highest sensitivity (76 %; 95 % CI: 72–79 %). While jaw claudication was only present in 34 % patients with GCA, this clinical feature significantly increased the likelihood of a positive biopsy (positive likelihood ratio (LR) 4.2; 95 % CI: 2.8–6.2). The only other symptom which was associated with increased likelihood of GCA was diplopia (LR 3.4; 95 % CI: 1.3–8.6) [7].

While cranial manifestations of GCA are well-recognized, a subset of patients may present with limb ischemia due to large-artery stenosis related to the vasculitic process. This usually affects the upper extremities and symptomatic lower extremity arterial involvement is rare. In a retrospective study, evaluating 74 patients with angiographic finding suggestive of upper extremity arterial involvement (subclavian, axillary, brachial stenosis) from GCA to 74 patients with biopsy proven GCA, patients with upper extremity stenotic disease were significantly younger at diagnosis and were more frequently female [8]. These patients also had a lower ESR at diagnosis and a longer time from symptom onset to diagnosis than patients with cranial symptoms. Interestingly, a smaller proportion of patients with upper extremity arterial involvement had cranial symptoms (headache, jaw claudication) and visual symptoms compared to those with biopsy-positive GCA. Only 58 % of patients with upper extremity stenotic disease had a positive TAB [8]. In a study using ultrasonography to evaluate the upper extremity arteries in patients with newly diagnosed GCA, upper extremity involvement was observed in 30 % patients [9]. As in the study by Brack et al., a greater proportion of patients with upper extremity vasculitis were women. They also tended to be younger and a smaller percentage had cranial manifestations of GCA. Time to diagnosis was delayed in this study as well which likely reflects failure to recognize this manifestation of GCA compared to patients who present with headaches and other cranial manifestations.

On the other hand, clinically significant symptomatic lower extremity arterial involvement in GCA appears to be rare. In a population-based study only 0.6 % of patients had lower extremity stenotic disease attributed to GCA [4]. However, this complication of GCA is very important to distinguish from the more common atherosclerotic disease given its morbidity and potential improvement with glucocorticoid therapy. The largest clinical series of symptomatic lower extremity involvement from GCA included 19 cases (all women) seen over a 25 year period at a tertiary care institution [10]. Majority (84.2 %) had symptoms of lower extremity claudication as a presenting manifestation that led to the diagnosis of GCA. In most cases, the patients had few to no cardiovascular risk factors and presented with new rapidly progressive claudication. Importantly, approximately 50 % of these patients did not have any cranial symptoms. The diagnosis was made by imaging in all cases with the superficial femoral artery being the most commonly involved. In most cases, bilateral involvement was observed. All patients were treated with corticosteroids but despite therapy, morbidity was high. Two patients required revascularization surgery, two patients underwent limb amputation and one patient underwent toe amputation [10]. While this manifestation is very rare, it is important to consider lower extremity vasculitis in elderly patients with rapidly progressive claudication and few traditional risk factors for atherosclerotic disease.

All patients suspected of having GCA should undergo a comprehensive physical examination with special attention to the vascular examination which should include palpation of the temporal arteries, assessment of peripheral pulses, including radial, carotid, femoral and pedal pulses and auscultation for bruits over carotid, subclavian and femoral arteries. Bilateral upper extremity blood pressures should be obtained. The presence of diminished or absent peripheral pulses, bruits and/or asymmetric blood pressures in the upper extremities may suggest large-artery involvement due to GCA.

Patients with GCA often have evidence of systemic inflammation on laboratory evaluation as evidenced by findings such as anemia, thrombocytosis or elevated acute phase reactants (ESR and CRP). Elevated ESR has been considered a hallmark of this disease with a sensitivity of 96 % (95 % CI: 93–97) in a meta-analysis [7]. However, elevated ESR is nonspecific and can be seen in a variety of autoimmune, infectious, and neoplastic conditions. The sensitivity of CRP is slightly better than that of ESR but there may be clinical utility in obtaining both [11]. In less than 5 % cases, markers of inflammation are normal at diagnosis.

Given the need for prolonged corticosteroid therapy and the morbidity associated with such treatment in GCA, confirmation of the diagnosis should be pursued. Ultrasonography of the temporal arteries is a sensitive imaging modality [12]. The most specific finding is the "halo" sign which is a hypoechoic area surrounding the vessel wall which may represent edema [13]. However, ultrasonography is operator-dependent. At centers with expertise in ultrasonography of the temporal artery, typical findings on ultrasonographic examination may preclude the need for a biopsy. In other cases, histopathologic examination of a TAB specimen remains the diagnostic modality of choice for subjects suspected of having GCA. TAB shows transmural inflammatory infiltrate with mononuclear predominance. Multinucleated giant cells may be absent in 33 % biopsies and are not needed to make a histopathologic diagnosis. Glucocorticoid use for 2–4 weeks does not significantly decrease the yield of TAB and therefore in cases of visual symptoms, treatment should not be delayed while awaiting biopsy [14]. The sensitivity of TAB is estimated at 87 %. In cases of GCA with primarily large-artery stenotic disease (e.g., upper extremity arterial involvement), negative TAB has been reported in up to 42 % [8]. Patients with aortitis and no cranial symptoms may also have a low frequency of TAB positivity. Therefore, in this subset of patients, imaging of the aorta and its branches should be pursued to confirm the diagnosis of GCA.

Modalities such as ultrasonography, magnetic resonance angiography (MRA), computed tomography angiography (CTA), and positron emission tomography (PET) may be useful for evaluation of the aorta and its branches in patients with extracranial manifestations of GCA [12, 15]. Duplex ultrasonography, CTA, and MRA can all provide useful information about the vessel wall and lumen. As in the case of the temporal artery, the most specific sign on ultrasonography of other vessels for involvement by GCA is the "halo." Other findings may include stenosis or occlusion of the vessels. While ultrasonography is useful, it is operator dependent and cannot evaluate the thoracic aorta. Therefore, CTA or MRA may be useful modalities. Findings of vasculitis on CTA or MRA include wall thickening, delayed wall enhancement or long segments of tapered stenoses. PET has been increasingly used in the diagnostic evaluation of patients suspected of having large-vessel vasculitis. Patients with GCA often have increased fluorodeoxyglucose (FDG) uptake in the aorta and major branches (subclavian, carotid, and femoral arteries) [12].

Treatment in GCA consists of high doses of glucocorticoids, typically between 40 and 60 mg prednisone daily. The initial dose is maintained for 2–4 weeks followed by a gradual taper over several months. In cases of visual symptoms, high dose intravenous methylprednisolone (1 g daily for 3 days) is often used followed by high-dose oral prednisone. Addition of low-dose aspirin may be beneficial in reducing the risk of ischemic complications. Relapses may occur during prednisone taper. The typical duration of treatment is 1–2 years. Since glucocorticoid use is associated with adverse side-effects, *P. jiroveci* prophylaxis and bone prophylaxis should be considered where appropriate. In cases where glucocorticoids cannot be successfully tapered due to relapses, methotrexate may be a useful adjunctive agent.

Questions

1. Which of the following IS NOT a clinical feature of GCA?

   (a) Diplopia.
   (b) Fever of unknown origin.
   (c) Limb claudication.
   (d) Hematuria with red blood cell casts.

2. Which of the following genetic polymorphisms has been associated with susceptibility to GCA?

   (a) HLA-B27.
   (b) HLA-DR4.
   (c) HLA-DQ2.

3. Which of the following IS NOT implicated in the pathogenesis of GCA?

   (a) Eosinophils.
   (b) Dendritic cells.
   (c) CD4 T cells.
   (d) Macrophages.

4. Which of the following clinical features is the best predictor of positive temporal artery biopsy?

   (a) Headache.
   (b) Temporal artery abnormality on examination.
   (c) Jaw claudication.
   (d) Polymyalgia rheumatica.

5. Which of the following statements is FALSE?

   (a) Vasculitis in GCA preferentially affects the arteries of the lower extremities.
   (b) Temporal artery biopsy may be negative in up to 42 % of patients with upper extremity vasculitis.
   (c) Diagnosis of GCA in cases of upper extremity arterial involvement tends to be delayed compared to patients with cranial manifestations.

6. Which of the following statements is FALSE?

   (a) Elevated C-reactive protein is a sensitive marker for GCA.
   (b) Elevated sedimentation rate (>30 mm/h) is very specific for the diagnosis of GCA.
   (c) GCA may occur in the setting of normal sedimentation rate and c-reactive protein.

7. All of the following statements are correct EXCEPT

   (a) Ultrasonography of the temporal arteries is a sensitive modality and may preclude the need for a biopsy.
   (b) Temporal artery biopsy may be negative in about 40 % of patients with upper extremity arterial involvement from GCA.
   (c) Treatment with glucocorticoids should not be delayed while awaiting a biopsy.
   (d) Multinucleated giant cells are necessary to make the diagnosis of GCA on histopathology.

8. Which of the following modalities are useful to detect inflammation in the vessel wall in patients with GCA?

   (a) Ultrasonography.
   (b) Computed tomography angiography.
   (c) Magnetic resonance angiography.
   (d) All of the above.

9. Which of the following statements is TRUE?

   (a) There is no role for high dose methylprednisolone in the treatment of GCA.
   (b) Methotrexate may be a useful adjunctive therapy in cases where there is difficulty with tapering prednisone.
   (c) The average length of treatment for GCA is 3 months.
   (d) Prednisone should be rapidly tapered until discontinuation once symptoms improve.

Answer Key: 1(d), 2(b), 3(a), 4(c), 5(a), 6(b), 7(d), 8(d), 9(b).

References

1. Kermani TA, Schafer VS, Crowson CS, Hunder GG, Gabriel SE, Matteson EL, et al. Increase in age at onset of giant cell arteritis: a population-based study. Ann Rheum Dis. 2010;69(4):780–1.
2. Salvarani C, Cantini F, Hunder GG. Polymyalgia rheumatica and giant-cell arteritis. Lancet. 2008;372(9634):234–45.
3. Evans JM, O'Fallon WM, Hunder GG. Increased incidence of aortic aneurysm and dissection in giant cell (temporal) arteritis. A population-based study. Ann Intern Med. 1995;122(7):502–7.
4. Nuenninghoff DM, Hunder GG, Christianson TJ, McClelland RL, Matteson EL. Incidence and predictors of large-artery complication (aortic aneurysm, aortic dissection, and/or large-artery stenosis) in patients with giant cell arteritis: a population-based study over 50 years. Arthritis Rheum. 2003;48(12):3522–31.
5. Weyand CM, Goronzy JJ. Medium- and large-vessel vasculitis. N Engl J Med. 2003;349(2):160–9.

6. Hunder GG, Bloch DA, Michel BA, Stevens MB, Arend WP, Calabrese LH, et al. The American College of Rheumatology 1990 criteria for the classification of giant cell arteritis. Arthritis Rheum. 1990;33(8):1122–8.
7. Smetana GW, Shmerling RH. Does this patient have temporal arteritis? JAMA. 2002;287(1):92–101.
8. Brack A, Martinez-Taboada V, Stanson A, Goronzy JJ, Weyand CM. Disease pattern in cranial and large-vessel giant cell arteritis. Arthritis Rheum. 1999;42(2):311–7.
9. Schmidt WA, Seifert A, Gromnica-Ihle E, Krause A, Natusch A. Ultrasound of proximal upper extremity arteries to increase the diagnostic yield in large-vessel giant cell arteritis. Rheumatology (Oxford). 2008;47(1):96–101.
10. Kermani TA, Matteson EL, Hunder GG, Warrington KJ. Symptomatic lower extremity vasculitis in giant cell arteritis: a case series. J Rheumatol. 2009;36(10):2277–83.
11. Kermani TA, Schmidt J, Crowson CS, Ytterberg SR, Hunder GG, Matteson EL, et al. Utility of erythrocyte sedimentation rate and C-reactive protein for the diagnosis of giant cell arteritis. Semin Arthritis Rheum. 2012;41(6):866–71.
12. Blockmans D, Bley T, Schmidt W. Imaging for large-vessel vasculitis. Curr Opin Rheumatol. 2009;21(1):19–28.
13. Schmidt WA, Kraft HE, Vorpahl K, Volker L, Gromnica-Ihle EJ. Color duplex ultrasonography in the diagnosis of temporal arteritis. N Engl J Med. 1997;337(19):1336–42.
14. Achkar AA, Lie JT, Hunder GG, O'Fallon WM, Gabriel SE. How does previous corticosteroid treatment affect the biopsy findings in giant cell (temporal) arteritis? Ann Intern Med. 1994;120(12):987–92.
15. Pipitone N, Versari A, Salvarani C. Role of imaging studies in the diagnosis and follow-up of large-vessel vasculitis: an update. Rheumatology (Oxford). 2008;47(4):403–8.

Part V
Immunodeficiency

Chapter 14
Primary Immunodeficiency in the Adult Population

Toral A. Kamdar and Leslie C. Grammer

Abstract Primary immunodeficiencies can be clinically important disorders in the adult population and generally present with recurrent, recalcitrant, and/or severe sinopulmonary infections. In particular, common variable immunodeficiency and specific antibody deficiency are relevant. In this chapter, we discuss a common case presentation of each of these immunodeficiencies and include in our discussion the evaluation, differential diagnosis, and treatment.

Keywords Common variable immunodeficiency • Specific antibody deficiency • Recurrent infections

Introduction

Primary immunodeficiency disorders (PIDs) are a heterogeneous group of disorders that can affect the innate or adaptive immune system. They may be genetically determined and can result in an increased risk of infection. The estimated prevalence of PIDs is reported to be at least 1:1,200 of the general population. The "Ten Warning Signs of Primary Immunodeficiency" (http://www.info4pi.org) can be useful benchmarks to guide clinicians as to which patients need an evaluation for PID. In contrast to some causes of secondary immunodeficiency, PIDs are generally not transient; they can be associated with malignancy and/or autoimmunity. Most PIDs are discovered in childhood; however, common variable immunodeficiency (CVID) and specific antibody deficiency (SAD) are two relevant conditions that are often recognized in adulthood.

T.A. Kamdar, M.D. (✉) • L.C. Grammer, M.D.
Division of Allergy/Immunology, Northwestern Memorial Hospital,
Northwestern University, 676 N. St. Chair, 14th floor, Chicago, IL 60657, USA
e-mail: t-kamdar@md.northwestern.edu; l-grammer@northwestern.edu

M. Mahmoudi (ed.), *Challenging Cases in Rheumatology and Diseases of the Immune System*, DOI 10.1007/978-1-4614-5088-7_14,
© Springer Science+Business Media, LLC 2013

CVID is characterized by four criteria: low serum immunoglobulin concentrations, decreased production of specific antibodies after vaccination, increased susceptibility to infection, and absence of any other defined immunodeficiency state. It is a heterogeneous disease and, in some individuals, can be associated with autoimmunity and malignancy. It is the most common clinically relevant primary immunodeficiency. The diagnosis of CVID includes the presence of hypogammaglobulinemia, recurrent sinopulmonary infections, and impaired functional antibody responses. For the most part, the underlying immunopathogenesis of CVID is not fully explained; there are various genetic defects that have been identified in a minority of patients with CVID. The underlying goal of treatment is to decrease the morbidity and mortality associated with recurrent infections; this can be attained with immunoglobulin therapy, by either intravenous or subcutaneous administration.

SAD is characterized by normal serum immunoglobulins with impaired IgG responses to polysaccharide antigens. In general, patients have diminished or absent responses to polysaccharide antigens, as manifested through low titers of *S. pneumoniae* or *H. influenzae* despite vaccination. Patients with this disorder can present with recurrent upper and lower respiratory tract bacterial infections. Treatment ranges from early treatment of infections with antibiotics to antimicrobial prophylaxis and intravenous immunoglobulin (IVIg) therapy.

Case 1

A 28-year-old female presents to the Allergy/Immunology clinic with a history of frequent infections. Her past medical history is significant for a history of asthma, treated with inhaled budesonide, 400 μg/day. She reports that she has had six episodes of sinusitis in the last 2 years as well four episodes of pneumonia. All of these infections required antibiotic therapy. Her most recent infection was bilateral lobar pneumonia that progressed to an empyema; the severity of the illness required inpatient hospitalization, parenteral antibiotic therapy, and chest tube placement. *Pseudomonas aeruginosa* was grown from culture. On a high-resolution computed tomography (CT) scan done while hospitalized, bronchiectasis was visualized in the lower lobes, bilaterally. She denies any history of meningitis, skin abscesses, diarrheal disorders, or recurrent unusual viral infections. She is currently asymptomatic; asthma is well controlled without nighttime symptoms, albuterol use, cough, dyspnea, or wheezing.

On review of systems, she does note morning joint stiffness and occasional edema in her finger digits, bilaterally. Family history is notable for an uncle who passed away in his thirties from infection. There is no significant social history. Environmental history is negative for animal or mold exposure. She has not received a vaccination for pneumococcal pneumonia in the last 10 years.

On physical exam, she is noted to be well appearing and in no acute distress. Her blood pressure is 100/75 with a heart rate of 68 beats per minute. Her height (64 in.)

Table 14.1 Lab results Case 1

Test	Result
CBC	
Hemoglobin	12.6 g/dl
Hematocrit	41.0%
Platelets	350,000 mm^3
WBC	7,200 cells/mm^3
PMNs	55%
Lymphocytes	40%
Monocytes	2%
Eosinophils	1%
Basophils	1%
Quantitative immunoglobulins	
IgG	220 mg/dl (range 700–1,600)
IgA	23 mg/dl (range 70–400)
IgM	42 mg/dl (range 40–230)
Streptococcus pneumonia IgG titers	
Strep Pneum Type 1	0.4 (normal >1.3)
Strep Pneum Type 3	0.8 (normal >1.3)
Strep Pneum Type 4	<0.2 (normal >1.3)
Strep Pneum Type 5	0.3 (normal >1.3)
Strep Pneum Type 6B	0.2 (normal >1.3)
Strep Pneum Type 7F	<0.2 (normal >1.3)
Strep Pneum Type 8	<0.2 (normal >1.3)
Strep Pneum Type 9N	<0.2 (normal >1.3)
Strep Pneum Type 9V	<0.2 (normal >1.3)
Strep Pneum Type 12F	<0.2 (normal >1.3)
Strep Pneum Type 14	5.5 (normal >1.3)
Strep Pneum Type 18C	0.2 (normal >1.3)
Strep Pneum Type 19F	<0.2 (normal >1.3)
Strep Pneum Type 23F	1.2 (normal >1.3)
Quantitative B and T cell analysis	
CD3+	83% (54–84)
CD4+	56% (27–57)
CD8+	18% (12–38)
CD 19+	11% (5–21)
CD 3/16/56+	6% (1–19)
Absolute CD3+	749 mm^3 (629–2,465)
Absolute CD4+	583 mm^3 (500–1,300)
Absolute CD8+	166 mm^3 (93–1,025)

and weight (140 pounds) are unremarkable. The exam is notable for slight synovitis in bilateral metacarpophalangeal (MCP) joints and scant rales in bilateral lung bases. No cervical, axillary, or inguinal lymphadenopathy is detected. The liver and spleen are normal in size. The following laboratory tests were completed (Table 14.1).

With the Presented Data, What Is Your Working Diagnosis?

The history of recurrent infections, combined with the unusual severity of infection (pneumonia progressing to empyema) is concerning for an underlying immunodeficiency. However, immune deficiencies can be primary or secondary—conditions leading to secondary immunodeficiency are more common in adults than an undiagnosed primary immunodeficiency. Some causes of secondary immunodeficiency are HIV, the use of immunosuppressive or immunomodulatory drugs, protein loss, metabolic disease, malnutrition, and malignancy. This patient does not have a history consistent with any of these etiologies of secondary immunodeficiency. Primary immunodeficiency must be considered in an adult presenting with recurrent infections and low immunoglobulins. Based on her laboratory data, both selective IgA deficiency and SAD would be on the differential, along with CVID. Moreover, she has a history of possible bronchiectasis seen on high-resolution CT scan, which can be present in patients with CVID, structural lung disease, or cystic fibrosis. Her history of morning symmetric joint stiffness along with the physical exam findings of synovitis may be related to a rheumatologic disorder; autoimmune diseases are frequently coexistent in many of the PIDs.

Additional Workup

High-resolution CT, vaccination with Pneumovax® 23, and repeat *S. pneumoniae* titers were performed. The high-resolution CT scan revealed a diffuse inflammatory process in the small airways consistent with bronchiectasis. Strep titers (Table 14.2) were drawn 6 weeks after vaccination and revealed minimal improvement in less than 70% of the pre-vaccination titers.

Table 14.2 Lab results Case 1

Test	Result
Streptococcus pneumonia IgG titers	
Strep Pneum Type 1	0.8 (normal >1.3)
Strep Pneum Type 3	0.8 (normal >1.3)
Strep Pneum Type 4	1.4 (normal >1.3)
Strep Pneum Type 5	0.3 (normal >1.3)
Strep Pneum Type 6B	0.5 (normal >1.3)
Strep Pneum Type 7F	<0.2 (normal >1.3)
Strep Pneum Type 8	<0.2 (normal >1.3)
Strep Pneum Type 9N	1.4 (normal >1.3)
Strep Pneum Type 9V	0.6 (normal >1.3)
Strep Pneum Type 12F	<0.2 (normal >1.3)
Strep Pneum Type 14	6.0 (normal >1.3)
Strep Pneum Type 18C	0.4 (normal >1.3)
Strep Pneum Type 19F	<0.2 (normal >1.3)
Strep Pneum Type 23F	1.2 (normal >1.3)

What Is Your Diagnosis and Why?

The patient was diagnosed with CVID. This diagnosis was supported by a history of recurrent severe infections, reduced immunoglobulins, and a defective response to vaccination. Other supporting data includes bronchiectasis, possible autoimmunity, and normal number of B cells on flow cytometry. Treatment involved the initiation of IVIg therapy, antibiotics at the first sign of infection, and frequent follow-up. Six months after the institution of IVIg she has been without upper or lower respiratory infections, and her IgG trough levels are approximately 800 mg/dl.

Discussion

CVID was first reported in 1953 by Janeway in a 39-year old with recurrent sinopulmonary infections, bronchiectasis, and *Haemophilus influenza* meningitis [1]. It is characterized by a disorder of B cell differentiation and maturation, leading to markedly reduced serum IgG (and often IgM and/or IgA levels), impaired specific antibody responses and recurrent infections. In one series of 248 patients with CVID followed for 1–25 years, the most common infections were recurrent bronchitis, sinusitis, otitis media, and pneumonia; a few also had viral hepatitis, severe Herpes zoster infection, and *Giardia* enteritis [2]. Symptoms generally start around age 25 with diagnosis approximately 3 years later, but there is variability in age at presentation, with patients diagnosed from early childhood to later adulthood. In some reported series, the lag time between onset of symptoms and diagnosis has been as long as 10 years. The 20-year survival rate for CVID patients is 64% for males and 67% for females, compared to 92–94% in the general population [3].

CVID has a distinct variability in phenotype, with only about 10–15% of patients having known genetic defects, suggesting that the etiology is multifactorial [4]. Five genetic mutations have been identified to be associated with CVID: TACI (transmembrane activator and calcium-modulator and cyclophilin ligand), Msh5 (a gene encoded in the MHC Class III region), ICOS (inducible co-stimulator of activated T cells), BAFF-R (B cell activating factor of the tumor necrosis factor family receptor). and CD 19 (the B cell surface protein) [5]. As expected, all of these genes are important in B cell differentiation and function. However, it must be acknowledged that TACI and Msh5 mutations have also been found in healthy individuals without an immunodeficiency phenotype, again corroborating that more than one gene is likely responsible for the disease [4]. A familial preponderance of CVID and IgA deficiency in affected patients has been described, implying that genetic factors are likely involved in the pathogenesis [5]. Despite the knowledge that B cell impairment is responsible for CVID phenotypes, T cells have been investigated for their contribution, specifically in regards to B and T cell contact-mediated interaction, which could impact B cell production of immunoglobulins [6]. Half of patients with CVID have some laboratory abnormalities in regards to T cells, including reduced expression of CD40L on activated T cells, decreased lymphocyte proliferation, impaired cytokine production to mitogens and recall-antigens, and changes in CD4/CD8 ratios. Diminished regulatory T cells have also been described in the CVID population [7]. Importantly, poor T cell function at the time of diagnosis of CVID has been associated with a poor prognosis, specifically, early death [2]. One group has even proposed that CD4+ naïve T cell numbers should be incorporated in a parameter to classify CVID [8]. In contrast to CVID, there is no associated autoimmunity or malignancy in patients with X-linked agammaglobulinemia which is a disease that profoundly affects B cell development.

The clinical presentation of CVID can encompass a heterogeneous phenotype, with the potential to affect many different organ systems. Most patients have frequent respiratory tract infections, with more common speciation of encapsulated (*H. influenzae, S. pneumoniae*) and atypical (*Mycoplasma* species) organisms. Severe infections including sepsis, empyema, meningitis, or osteomyelitis have been reported but with less frequency [9]. Repeated episodes of pneumonia can lead to abnormal lung exam and imaging, such as ground-glass attenuation and bronchiectasis. Up to one-half of CVID patients can have gastrointestinal involvement such as chronic diarrhea or malabsorption; superimposed infections with *Camplobacter, Yersinia, or Giardia* species can occur, causing further intestinal damage [3]. Other gastrointestinal diseases such as Crohn's disease, celiac sprue, atrophic gastritis, and intestinal lymphangectasia may coexist at a higher frequency than in the general population. Autoimmune diseases are not uncommon in this patient population; up to 25% of patients will develop or have preexisting evidence of autoimmunity. Autoimmune thrombocytopenic purpura and autoimmune hemolytic anemia, or both (Evans syndrome) are most common, but other diseases such as rheumatoid arthritis, autoimmune thyroiditis, and vitiligo can be seen [10]. Patients may present with hepatosplenomegaly, which can lead to neutropenia and/or thrombocytopenia independent of autoimmunity. A higher incidence of malignancy (approximately 15% of patients) is a concern in these patients, particularly in the fifth and sixth decades of life. The most common malignancies reported are gastric cancers and non-Hodgkin lymphoma, although the incidence of other hematologic and solid tumors is increased in these patients [9, 10]. Granulomatous disease, often mistakenly identified as sarcoidosis, can affect 8–22% of patients with CVID, and more commonly present in the lungs, lymph nodes, and spleen [2, 11, 12]. Interestingly, these subjects with granulomatous disease have a greater incidence of developing autoimmunity as well. On biopsy, the granulomas are well-formed, noncaseating and may contain non-necrotizing epithelioid and giant cells [9].

The diagnosis of CVID is first based on a clinical history of recurrent infections, generally sinopulmonary or involving the gastrointestinal tract. Laboratory tests important for the diagnosis include reduced total serum IgG (two standard deviations below the mean for age) and a reduced serum total IgA and/or IgM (also two standard deviations below the mean for age). These patients also tend to have a reduced or absent response to immunization with polysaccharide vaccines. It is important to rule out causes of secondary immunodeficiency, especially in an adult population with other chronic illnesses requiring multiple medical therapies. If hypogammaglobulinemia is present on initial diagnostic evaluation, then quantitative analysis of T, B, and NK cells should be performed. Evaluation of functional antibody responses to protein antigens (diphtheria toxoid, tetanus toxoid, *Haemophilus influenzae*, isohemmaglutinins) and polysaccharide antigens (*S. pneumoniae* vaccine) is another mainstay in CVID diagnosis. Some authors also suggest analysis for defects in memory B cell and other peripheral B cell subsets to provide further information on the genetic underlay [10].

Alternative diagnoses must be considered in a patient presenting with suspected CVID. Structural anomalies of the lungs and sinuses, as well as an underlying atopic condition such as asthma or allergic rhinitis should be considered, although these can coexist with the diagnosis of CVID. Other types of humoral immunodeficiency can present similarly to CVID; however, the preponderance of these present in childhood and are not necessarily relevant in an adult population. Secondary causes of hypogammaglobulinemia must also be considered, such as protein losing enteropathy, nephrotic syndrome, hematologic malignancies, and the use of immunosuppressive or immunomodulatory drugs [10].

The goal of treatment in CVID is to reduce morbidity and mortality associated with severe and recurrent infections. This is accomplished primarily by immunoglobulin therapy, which is given parenterally, either subcutaneous or intravenous, at a dose of 400–600 mg/kg/month. The replacement of immunoglobulin has been shown to decrease the risk of severe bacterial infections and pneumonia [13]. IVIg is generally well tolerated, but minor reactions including headache, nausea, myalgias, chills, flushing, rash, and low-grade fever can occur. Premedication with acetaminophen and diphenhydramine can help ameliorate these types of reactions. More severe side effects of IVIg are less common, but can include anaphylaxis, stroke, myocardial infarction, and aseptic meningitis, among others. Patients with CVID and IgA deficiency deserve specific mention, as they could be at higher risk for anaphylaxis due to anti-IgA antibodies. If possible, IgA-depleted products should be considered in this patient population. CVID patients should be treated promptly at the first sign of illness, particularly when concerned about upper or lower bacterial respiratory infections. Antimicrobial prophylaxis has been used successfully in some patients who breakthrough IVIg therapy alone, but this has not been validated [14]. Other conditions that coexist in CVID, such as autoimmunity and neoplastic disease, should be treated according to standard protocol.

Case 2

A 44-year-old male presents to the Allergy/Immunology clinic with symptoms of sinus congestion, discolored nasal drainage, and acute cough. His symptoms started 12 days ago with a sore throat and clear rhinorrhea. He does note decreased sense of smell and a low-grade fever. He reports symptoms of allergic rhinitis including nasal congestion and postnasal drip in April and May, and again in the fall. Of note, this is his fourth sinus infection in the past year, and he is concerned, as he has had frequent sinus infections, about 3–5 per year. In addition, in recent years, he reports that antibiotics help his sinus infections, but the infections do not totally resolve. A sinus CT has not yet been obtained. He notes two episodes of pneumonia, about 3 and 7 years ago, respectively. He reports no other infections such as meningitis, diarrheal disorders, skin infections, or abscesses. He has never required hospitalization for any of his infections.

His past medical history is significant for hypertension, treated with hydrochlorothiazide. He denies any past surgical history. There is no family history of frequent infections. Environmental history is negative for animal or mold exposure. There is no significant social history. Review of systems is otherwise negative.

On physical exam, he is noted to be well appearing and in no acute distress. Vital signs are notable for a temperature of 100.7 °F. Physical exam is notable for green mucus in his right nare, edematous and pale nasal turbinates bilaterally, and evidence of cobblestoning in his posterior oropharynx. Lung exam is unremarkable.

The following tests were completed (Table 14.3 and Fig. 14.1).

With the Presented Data What Is Your Working Diagnosis?

Given that the patient presents with anosmia, discolored nasal drainage, and sinus pressure of longer than 10 days duration, he likely has bacterial sinusitis. He does have allergic rhinitis, corroborated by his exam, symptoms during seasons and skin testing; this can predispose patients to be more susceptible to bacterial sinus infections. Furthermore, his CT sinus did show air fluid levels and mucosal thickening, also suggesting a bacterial source of his current symptoms. Importantly, his CT sinus did not show polyps or other structural abnormalities, which could place him at increased risk of sinus disease. He did give a history of infections, both sinonasal and lower respiratory that would be considered more frequent than that of a similar patient in his demographic. In a patient that presents with frequent infections, it is important to evaluate the humoral immune system and screen for conditions such as CVID or SAD, which can occur in the adult population, as well as secondary immunodeficiency. Cystic fibrosis can also predispose patients to experience recurrent sinus infections; given the patient's age, however, this is less likely. Other less

Table 14.3 Skin testing and laboratory data Case 2

Test	Result
Skin test	Positive to: Tree Ragweed Dust mite Negative to: Grass Mold
CBC	
Hemoglobin	13.8 g/dl
Hematocrit	41.0%
Platelets	420,000 mm³
WBC	8,000 cells/mm³
PMNs	52%
Lymphocytes	43%
Monocytes	1%
Eosinophils	2%
Basophils	2%
Quantitative immunoglobulins	
IgG	890 mg/dl (range 700–1,600)
IgA	82 mg/dl (range 70–400)
IgM	45 mg/dl (range 40–230)
Streptococcus pneumonia IgG titers	
Strep Pneum Type 1	0.1 (normal >1.3)
Strep Pneum Type 3	0.5 (normal >1.3)
Strep Pneum Type 4	<0.2 (normal >1.3)
Strep Pneum Type 5	2.2 (normal >1.3)
Strep Pneum Type 6B	0.2 (normal >1.3)
Strep Pneum Type 7F	<0.2 (normal >1.3)
Strep Pneum Type 8	<0.2 (normal >1.3)
Strep Pneum Type 9N	<0.2 (normal >1.3)
Strep Pneum Type 9V	<0.2 (normal >1.3)
Strep Pneum Type 12F	<0.2 (normal >1.3)
Strep Pneum Type 14	1.0 (normal >1.3)
Strep Pneum Type 18C	0.3 (normal >1.3)
Strep Pneum Type 19F	<0.2 (normal >1.3)
Strep Pneum Type 23F	<0.2 (normal >1.3)

common disorders, such as Churg–Strauss disease, should also be considered. Asthma and GERD are conditions that can coexist in patients who present with frequent sinus infections. The patient has no symptoms of reflux, but does have allergic rhinitis and cough which prompts consideration of evaluation for asthma. The patient's immunoglobulins were normal, essentially ruling out CVID. However, he did have decreased *Streptococcus pneumoniae* titers despite likely having been exposed to this bacterium during one of his previous sinus infections.

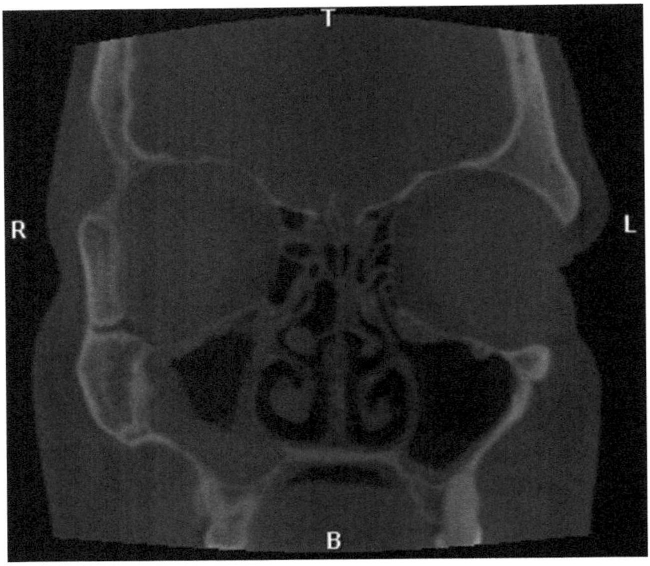

Fig. 14.1 CT of the sinuses

Additional Workup

Pulmonary function tests were performed and essentially normal. T and B cell flow cytometry showed normal quantitative levels and ratios of lymphocytes tested. Sinus culture was positive for *Streptococcus pneumoniae*. Vaccination with Pneumovax® 23 and repeat strep pneumoniae titers were performed, which showed minimal response after 6 weeks. This pneumococcal vaccine is an unconjugated polysaccharide vaccine and adequate responses are indicative of T-cell independent response. A pneumococcal 13-valent conjugate vaccine (Prevnar®) was then administered and repeat titers were again suboptimal. This vaccine is indicative of a functional T-cell dependent response. Notably, current standards for an adequate response are a postimmunization serum antibody concentration of >1.3 μg/ml or at least fourfold over baseline. Expert panels agreed that patients over 5 years of age should be able to response to at least 70% of the serotypes to have an appropriate response [14] (Tables 14.4 and 14.5).

What Is Your Diagnosis and Why?

Given that the patient has had recurrent sinusitis and other infections, without any predisposing etiology such as structural abnormality, and evidence of impaired specific antibody response with administration of both the pneumococcal polysaccharide and conjugate vaccines, the diagnosis is consistent with SAD. The patient

Table 14.4 Case 2

	Pre-bronchodilator	% Predicted	Post-bronchodilator	% Predicted
FVC, L	4.98	93%	4.99	93%
FEV_1, L	3.98	90%	4.01	91%
FEV_1/FVC, %	80%		80%	
FEF_{25-75}% L/s	3.80	82%	3.90	84%
TV, L	0.6	93%		
FRC, L	2.4	94%		
RV, L	1.2	97%		
TLC, L	5.9	98%		
DLCO	26.2	95%		

Table 14.5 Case 2

Test	Result	
Streptococcus pneumonia IgG titers	Post-pneumovax®	Post-prevnar®
Strep Pneum Type 1	0.3 (normal >1.3)	0.3 (normal >1.3)
Strep Pneum Type 3	0.6 (normal >1.3)	0.6 (normal >1.3)
Strep Pneum Type 4	<0.2 (normal >1.3)	1.3 (normal >1.3)
Strep Pneum Type 5	2.4 (normal >1.3)	2.4 (normal >1.3)
Strep Pneum Type 6B	0.2 (normal >1.3)	0.4 (normal >1.3)
Strep Pneum Type 7F	<0.2 (normal >1.3)	<0.2 (normal >1.3)
Strep Pneum Type 8	<0.2 (normal >1.3)	0.4 (normal >1.3)
Strep Pneum Type 9N	<0.2 (normal >1.3)	<0.2 (normal >1.3)
Strep Pneum Type 9V	<0.2 (normal >1.3)	<0.2 (normal >1.3)
Strep Pneum Type 12F	<0.2 (normal >1.3)	<0.2 (normal >1.3)
Strep Pneum Type 14	1.0 (normal >1.3)	1.1 (normal >1.3)
Strep Pneum Type 18C	0.5 (normal >1.3)	0.7 (normal >1.3)
Strep Pneum Type 19F	<0.2 (normal >1.3)	<0.2 (normal >1.3)
Strep Pneum Type 23F	<0.2 (normal >1.3)	<0.2 (normal >1.3)
Quantitative B and T cell analysis		
CD3+	77% (54–84)	
CD4+	49% (27–57)	
CD8+	22% (12–38)	
CD 19+	28% (5–21)	
CD 3/16/56+	10% (1–19)	
Absolute CD3+	930 mm^3 (629–2,465)	
Absolute CD4+	632 mm^3 (500–1,300)	
Absolute CD8+	322 mm^3 (93–1,025)	

was treated with Augmentin for 14 days for his sinusitis with symptomatic resolution. He had a trial of prophylactic antibiotics, but unfortunately developed pneumonia despite these. Finally, treatment with IVIg was initiated, and he remained infection-free on 2 years of follow-up.

Discussion

SAD was described in the 1980s by multiple different investigators as an immune defect with normal serum immunoglobulins, but impaired IgG responses to polysaccharides [15, 16]. This terminology is not standardized. Other terms include selective antibody deficiency with normal immunoglobulins (SADNI) and impaired polysaccharide responsiveness. This deficiency is typically discovered on routine humoral immunity evaluation in patients with recurrent infections, and protective titers against *Streptococcus pneumoniae* and *Haemophilus influenzae* type b are generally defective. In one study evaluating 91 pediatric patients who were referred to a tertiary care hospital for evaluation of primary immunodeficiency, 23.1% were ultimately diagnosed with SAD [17]. It has been slightly more difficult to characterize this disease in adult populations, but a recent study evaluating 119 adult patients with medically refractory chronic rhino-sinusitis found that approximately 11.6% were ultimately diagnosed with SAD [18].

The clinical presentation of SAD is very similar to CVID; patients present with recurrent, frequent bacterial infections, usually of the upper and lower respiratory tract, including sinusitis, pneumonia, otitis media, and bronchitis [19]. These patients are usually referred to an immunologist due to their infection history and the diagnosis of SAD is made after other types of immunodeficiency are ruled out. However, other presentations are possible; in a study of 75 patients with SAD, 7% presented with systemic infections, 8% presented with rheumatic or autoimmune disease, and 5% presented with chronic diarrhea [19]. Thus, while the spectrum of severity is not quite as broad as in CVID, there is again variability in the phenotype.

The etiology of SAD is largely unknown. It has been shown that there is altered development of age-related changes in dendritic cells in patients with SAD, although the effects of this are not known [20]. Conversely, T cell responses to viral antigens were evaluated in pediatric patients with SAD; their responses were similar to controls without the increased CD8+ T cell proliferation seen in CVID patients [6].

Treatment of patients with SAD largely revolves around decreasing the risk of recurrent infections. This can be accomplished by frequent clinic visits and early intervention at the first sign of infection. Unfortunately, this is not successful in all patients with SAD, as some succumb to more severe infections despite this. Prophylactic antibiotics are used in some patients, but some patients still require the initiation of parenteral immunoglobulin to decrease infection risk [21].

There are two other clinical PID entities that are important in adult populations. Selective IgA deficiency is one of the most common antibody deficiencies, and is defined as IgA less than 7 mg/dl with normal serum IgG and IgM levels. It has been reported to be present in up to 1:400 to 1:600 of the US population [22]. Of note, up to 90% of patients with selective IgA deficiency are asymptomatic; however, a small proportion develops recurrent respiratory and gastrointestinal infections in the absence of severe, life-threatening infections. There is a higher prevalence of autoimmunity and atopy in these patients. The reason that the majority are asymptomatic is not clear, but is likely due to redundancies in the immune response. For example, it has been reported that most asymptomatic IgA deficient individuals have a compensatory increase in monomeric IgM in their saliva, upper respiratory secretions, and gastrointestinal fluids.

IgG subclass deficiency is another disorder which often is associated with selective IgA deficiency. There is a deficient or absent level of one or more IgG subclasses (IgG1, IgG2, IgG3, or IgG4) with normal levels of total IgG and the other isotypes. However, it has been shown that low levels of IgG subclasses can occur in up to 20% of healthy individuals creating controversy about whether this is a true subset of immunodeficiency [4]. Symptomatic patients generally present with upper and lower respiratory tract infections.

In summary, the most common PIDs in adults, CVID and SAD, may present with symptoms of chronic or recurrent respiratory infections. The diagnosis is often delayed because PID had not been considered. Recognition that PID might be responsible for a patient's recurrent respiratory and/or gastrointestinal symptoms is the first step in determining whether an immunodeficiency evaluation is appropriate. Once PID is identified, therapeutic efforts aimed at minimizing the morbidity from infection or correcting the underlying problem will be determined by the specific diagnosis and should be individualized. Because subclinical chronic pulmonary infection can lead to long-term damage such as bronchiectasis and because there is an increased incidence of malignancy and autoimmune disease in patients with PID, close follow-up is important.

Questions

1. What type of infectious organisms are patients with CVID most susceptible to?

   (a) Parasites
   (b) *Staph. aureus*
   (c) Fungal organisms
   (d) Encapsulated bacteria

2. Which of the following conditions can coexist with increased frequency in patients with CVID?

   (a) Sickle cell anemia
   (b) Granulomatous disease
   (c) Coronary artery disease
   (d) Seizure disorder

3. Which of the following laboratory tests are important in making the diagnosis of CVID?
   (a) Elevated IgM and low IgA
   (b) Elevated IgE and elevated IgM
   (c) Low IgG and reduced IgA and/or IgM
   (d) Low IgM and elevated IgG

4. What percentage of patients with CVID have known genetic mutations?
   (a) 70%
   (b) 5%
   (c) 90%
   (d) 15%

5. What is the mainstay of therapy for patients with CVID once diagnosed?
   (a) Initiation of parental immunoglobulin replacement
   (b) Antimicrobial prophylaxis
   (c) Corticosteroid treatment
   (d) Bone marrow transplant

6. What is the definition of specific antibody deficiency?
   (a) Decreased serum immunoglobulins with normal IgG responses to polysaccharide vaccines
   (b) Normal serum immunoglobulins with impaired IgG responses to polysaccharide vaccines
   (c) Diminished T lymphocytes on flow cytometry
   (d) Diminished B lymphocytes on flow cytometry

7. How do patients with specific antibody deficiency present?
   (a) Systemic herpes virus infections
   (b) Systemic fungal infections
   (c) Recurrent sinopulmonary bacterial infections
   (d) Recurrent Neisseria meningitis

8. How do you make the diagnosis of specific antibody deficiency?
   (a) Inadequate baseline and postimmunization pneumococcal titers—do not respond to over fourfold of baseline in 70% of titers tested
   (b) Low quantitative immunoglobulins with impaired *H. influenzae* titers
   (c) Elevated IgE with impaired postimmunization pneumococcal titers
   (d) Recurrent bacterial infections with normal quantitative immunoglobulins

9. Is selective IgA deficiency a clinically relevant entity?
   (a) No—all patients with this disorder are entirely healthy
   (b) Yes—90% of patients with this disorder suffer from recurrent bacterial infections

(c) Yes—10% of patients with this disorder suffer from recurrent bacterial infections
(d) No—It is only important in the context of IgG subclass deficiency

10. Can selective IgA deficiency and IgG subclass deficiency occur in healthy individuals?

(a) Yes—they can occur independently or synonymously in healthy individuals
(b) No—they each have clinically relevant phenotypes with recurrent bacterial infections
(c) Yes—they can only occur independently in healthy individuals
(d) No—all patients with either of these disorders succumb to recurrent viral infections

Answers: 1. D, 2. B, 3. C, 4. D, 5. A, 6. B, 7. C, 8. A, 9. C, 10. A.

References

1. Janeway CA, Apt L, Gitlin D. Agammaglobulinemia. Trans Assoc Am Physicians. 1953;66:200–2.
2. Cunningham-Rundles C, Bodian C. Common variable immunodeficiency: clinical and immunological features of 248 patients. Clin Immunol. 1999;92:34–48.
3. Ballow M. Primary immunodeficiency disorders: antibody deficiency. J Allergy Clin Immunol. 2002;109:581–91.
4. Fried AJ, Bonilla FA. Pathogenesis, diagnosis, and management of primary antibody deficiencies and infections. Clin Microbiol Rev. 2009;22:396–414.
5. Arason GJ, Jorgenson GH, Ludviksson BR. Primary immunodeficiency and autoimmunity: lessons from human diseases. Scand J Immunol. 2010;71:317–28.
6. Haveman LM, Scherrenburg J, Maarschalk-Ellerboek LJ, et al. T cell response to viral antigens in adults and children with common variable immunodeficiency and specific antibody deficiency. Clin Exp Immunol. 2010;161:108–17.
7. Fevang B, Yndestad A, Sandberg WJ, et al. Low numbers of regulatory T cells in common variable immunodeficiency: association with chronic inflammation in vivo. Clin Exp Immunol. 2007;147:521–5.
8. Giovannetti A, Pierdominici M, Mazzetta F, et al. Unravelling the complexity of T cell abnormalities in common variable immunodeficiency. J Immunol. 2007;178:3932–43.
9. Cunningham-Rundles C. How I treat common variable immune deficiency. Blood. 2010;116:7–15.
10. Park MA, Li JT, Hagan JB, et al. Common variable immunodeficiency: a new look at an old disease. Lancet. 2008;372:489–502.
11. Morimoto Y, Routes JM. Granulomatous disease in common variable immunodeficiency. Curr Allergy Asthma Rep. 2005;5:370–5.
12. Bates CA, Ellison MC, Lynch DA, et al. Granulomatous-lymphocytic lung disease shortens survival in common variable immunodeficiency. J Allergy Clin Immunol. 2004;114:415–21.
13. Busse PJ, Razvi S, Cunningham-Rundles C. Efficacy of intravenous immunoglobulin in the prevention of pneumonia in patients with common variable immunodeficiency. J Allergy Clin Immunol. 2002;109:1001–4.
14. Bonilla FA, Bernstein IL, Khan DA, et al. Practice parameter for the diagnosis and management of primary immunodeficiency. Ann Allergy Asthma Immunol. 2005;94(5 Suppl 1):S1–63.
15. French MA, Harrison G. Systemic antibody deficiency in patients without serum immunoglobulin deficiency or with selective IgA deficiency. Clin Exp Immunol. 1984;56:18–22.

16. Ambrosino D, Siber G, Chilmonczyk B, et al. An immunodeficiency characterized by impaired antibody responses to polysaccharides. New Engl J Med. 1987;316:790–3.
17. Javier FC, Moore CM, Sorensen RU. Distribution of primary immunodeficiency diseases diagnosed in a pediatric tertiary hospital. Ann Allergy Asthma Immunol. 2000;84:691–714.
18. Carr TF, Koterba AP, Chandra R, et al. Characterization of specific antibody deficiency in adults with medically refractory chronic rhinosinusitis. Am J Rhinol Allergy. 2011;25:241–4.
19. O'Byrne MA, Weiler CR. Clinical and laboratory characteristics of 75 patients with specific polysaccharide antibody deficiency syndrome. Ann Allergy Asthma Immunol. 2006;97:306–11.
20. Jyonouchi H, Cui C, Geng L, et al. Age dependent changes in peripheral blood dendritic cell subsets in normal children and children with specific polysaccharide antibody deficiency (SPAD). Eur J Pediatr. 2010;169:1233–9.
21. Berger M. Evaluation and management of immune deficiency in allergic disease. In: Grammer L, Greenberger P, editors. Patterson's allergic diseases. 7th ed. Philadelphia, Pennsylvania: LWW publisher; 2009. pp 41–56
22. Clark JA, Callicoat PA, Brenner NA. Selective IgA deficiency in blood donors. Am J Clin Pathol. 1983;80:210–3.

Chapter 15
HIV and AIDS

Banafsheh Soltani, Rafik Samuel, and Robert Bettiker

Abstract Human immunodeficiency virus (HIV) is a lymphotropic retrovirus that infects a subset of cells within the immune system. As HIV infection progresses, the ability of the immune system to detect and suppress a variety of conditions such as cancer and infections is impaired. Here, we present a case of B-cell lymphoma as the initial presentation of HIV infection as well as a case of histoplasmosis secondary to HIV infection presenting as a colonic mass.

Keywords HIV • Lymphoma • Histoplasmosis • Immune inflammatory reconstitution syndrome • Abacavir hypersensitivity

Case 1

This is a 63-year-old Caucasian woman with no significant past medical history who presents to the emergency room of an inner city hospital with a chief complaint of severe fatigue. She reports a 3-month history of progressive, gradually worsening tiredness. Over this period, she also had 30 lb of unintentional weight loss. Her symptoms are associated with night sweats and loose stools, but no cough and no sick contacts. Over the past week, she started to notice dysphagia and chest pain with swallowing. She does not see a doctor regularly and has no previous workup for her complaints.

Past medical history is significant for anemia and previous chlamydia infection.

B. Soltani, M.D. (✉) • R. Samuel, M.D. • R. Bettiker, M.D.
Section of Infectious Diseases, Temple University Hospital,
5th fl PP, 3401 North Broad Street, Philadelphia, PA, 19140, USA
e-mail: banafsheh.soltani@tuhs.temple.edu; rafik.samuel@tuhs.temple.edu;
robert.bettiker@tuhs.temple.edu

M. Mahmoudi (ed.), *Challenging Cases in Rheumatology and Diseases of the Immune System*, DOI 10.1007/978-1-4614-5088-7_15,
© Springer Science+Business Media, LLC 2013

Social history. She works as a cashier and is a nonsmoker who drinks socially on weekends. She denies current or previous drug use and says she has not been sexually active in 15 years.

Physical exam. On examination, the patient is lethargic, thin, and ill-appearing. She is febrile, oral temperature is 104.0 °F. Her heart rate is 97 bpm, blood pressure is 122/76 mm Hg and she breathes comfortably on room air with an oxygen saturation of 99 %. Head and neck exam reveals nonicteric sclera, significant periauricular swelling, no oropharyngeal lesions and a supple neck. She has multiple 1–2 cm, non-tender, anterior cervical chain lymph nodes. Cardiovascular exam is significant for a 2/6 systolic murmur at the apex. Her lungs are clear and her abdomen is soft, with no hepatosplenomegaly. Further exam is unrevealing; there is no rash. Her laboratory data is available in table 15.1.

Testing. Imaging reveals a 2.5 cm soft tissue mass in the right parotid as well as diffuse bulky retroperitoneal and perihilar lymphadenopathy. An upper endoscopy is done to evaluate her dysphagia; visualization is consistent with esophageal candidiasis.

With Presented Data, What Is Your Working Diagnosis?

This is a patient with several months of fatigue and weight loss. The differential diagnosis is very broad but the prolonged time course is helpful in narrowing the diagnosis by making more acute or rapidly progressive processes less likely.

Differential Diagnosis

Periauricular swelling along with diffuse lymphadenopathy and fever suggest infection, hematological malignancies, or autoimmune disorders. Infections that lead to

Table 15.1

Laboratory value	Value	Range
WBC per ml	8,600	4,000–11,000
Lymphocyte (%)	20	20–44
Monocyte (%)	7	2–9
Granulocyte (%)	70	50–75
Eosinophil (%)	2	2–5
Hemoglobin (g/dl)	7	11.5–16.0
Platelets per ml	58,000	140,000–400,000
Sodium (mmol/l)	128	135–145
Creatinine (mg/dl)	1.4	0.5–1.5

WBC white blood cell

these symptoms could include bacteria such as mycobacteria or bartonella, fungi such as histoplasmosis, and viruses such as human immunodeficiency virus (HIV). Malignancies include Hodgkin's lymphoma, non-Hodgkin's lymphomas, and leukemia. A patient such as this that presents with lymphadenopathy and parotid swelling should also be ruled out for systemic lupus erythematosus and Sjögren's syndrome.

Workup

Blood is sent for routine culture as well as acid fast bacilli and is found to be negative. Basic rheumatologic serologies are likewise negative. An axial lymph node is biopsied and consistent with a diffuse large B-cell lymphoma which stains strongly for EBV. Fungal and acid fast bacilli stains are negative. HIV enzyme-linked immunosorbent assay (ELISA) is repeatedly reactive, and western blot confirms a diagnosis of HIV. HIV PCR is over a million RNA copies per ml; the patient's CD4 count is 29 cells/μl (9 %).

What Is Your Diagnosis and Why?

Acid fast staining of the lymph node is negative, which makes infection with an acid-fast bacillus less likely. Furthermore, negative fungal stains on biopsy make disseminated fungal disease unlikely. With negative rheumatologic workup as well as a reasonable alternative diagnosis, it is less likely that this patient has a rheumatologic disease.

Given the patient's positive HIV ELISA and western blot, it is clear that this patient has HIV disease. Her CD4 count as well as the clinical finding of esophageal candidiasis and presence of a B-cell lymphoma indicates that she has acquired immunodeficiency syndrome (AIDS). The exact diagnosis is AIDS-associated diffuse large B-cell lymphoma.

Discussion

Each year, there are about 48,000–56,000 new diagnoses of HIV in the United States. IgG analysis indicates that only a third of these are recently acquired infections. Mathematical modeling estimates that 21 % of the >1 million HIV infected people in the United States are undiagnosed [1]. For this reason, the Centers for Disease Control and Prevention (CDC) recommend that all adults between the ages of 13 and 64 be routinely tested, regardless of perceived risk factors. The only population that does not need routine testing is one where the documented prevalence of disease is less than 0.1 %. Our patient is a 63-year-old woman with no history of injection drug use, but she is presenting to care in an area where the prevalence of HIV is much higher than 0.1 %.

It is interesting to note that she does have a prior medical history of chlamydia infection. Population analyses indicate that having other sexually transmitted infections can increase transmission of HIV. The level of increased risk depends on the infection. Genital ulcerative diseases such as herpes simplex virus carry a higher risk ratio, whereas less inflammatory infections such as chlamydia have lower risk ratios. The etiology of why this happens is probably multifactorial and related to increased inflammation and changes to the mucosal immune response. It should also be noted that the same high-risk behaviors that lead to contracting diseases such as chlamydia or gonorrhea also increase the likelihood of contracting HIV.

Since early in the HIV epidemic, AIDS was known to be associated with certain malignancies. For instance, non-Hodgkin's lymphoma, Kaposi's sarcoma, and cancer of the cervix are all AIDS defining illnesses. These cancers are strongly associated with other viruses: Epstein–Barr virus (EBV), Kaposi's sarcoma herpes virus (KSHV/HHV8), and human papilloma virus, respectively.

Multiple factors contribute to increased cancer risk in HIV-positive individuals. First, HIV proteins such as *tat* may have oncogenic properties. Second, immune dysregulation inhibits cancer surveillance. As HIV infection progresses, the lack of regulation from CD4 cells is apparent in derangements in the population of natural killer (NK) cells, which are responsible for cancer surveillance. The total number of NK cells remains falsely unchanged. Closer analysis, however, shows that there is an overall loss of some NK subsets which is offset by over-production of others. Third, decreased T-cell activity in AIDS decreases immune control of EBV-infected B cells. In HIV-infected patients, the number of EBV-specific CD8+ cells remains the same. Over time, as the numbers of CD4+ helper cells drop, the CD8+ cells become less functional and produce less interferon gamma, resulting in higher EBV titers [2]. Finally, chronic B cell activation from immune stimulation and dysregulation from HIV infection itself predisposes to lymphomagenesis [3]. EBV-infected B cells in vitro undergo *c-myc* upregulation and malignant transformation after infection with HIV.

EBV has long been linked with lymphoproliferative disorders, including Burkitt's, Hodgkin's, diffuse large B cell, and primary central nervous system lymphomas [3]. Some, though not all, are strongly associated with EBV. Lymphomas arising in the central nervous system and those that are monoclonal are more likely to be EBV-associated. As HIV infection progresses, T-cell activity against EBV decreases, allowing for transformation of B cells by EBV-associated viral proteins.

This patient has two potentially fatal illnesses—AIDS and lymphoma. How should she be treated? Sequentially or concurrently, and, if sequentially, which disease first? Prior to the introduction of highly active antiretroviral therapy (HAART), AIDS patients with lymphoma would be treated solely for their malignancy as no effective HIV treatment existed. Early HAART regimens, though effective, had many toxicities and interactions; therefore the lymphoma was treated first. In addition, early HAART drugs such as zidovudine were known to magnify the toxicities of antineoplastic agents. Currently, HAART is much better tolerated, and regimens with minimal drug interactions can be used.

Recent data and current guidelines favor starting highly active antiretroviral therapy in all HIV-infected patients. Normally, HAART is initiated in the outpatient setting; HIV is a chronic disease and rarely is it an emergency to begin therapy. Some of the recommended baseline labs can take several weeks to become available. Certain conditions are an exception, with clear benefit to the patient if HAART is started quickly. Idiopathic thrombotic thrombocytopenia and HIV nephropathy are two such conditions. Likewise, patients with Kaposi's sarcoma or non-Hodgkin's lymphoma do better if started on antiretroviral therapy. Although there are several case reports of complete remission of HIV-associated lymphomas on HAART alone [4], the treatment for HIV associated B-cell lymphomas is HAART plus cytostatic chemotherapy.

Many patients are already on antiretrovirals at the time of lymphoma diagnosis. This patient is interesting because she required concurrent initiation of chemotherapy and antiretroviral therapy. The goal of therapy is to reduce the number of cancerous B-lymphocytes while reconstituting the CD4+ T-lymphocytes ravaged by HIV. Many chemotherapy regimens have a more lasting impact on CD4 cell counts than they do on CD8, NK, or B cell lines. The combination of HAART with chemotherapy has been shown to be well tolerated and prolong life expectancy.

The treatment of non-Hodgkin lymphoma in non-HIV-infected patients is chemotherapy plus rituximab (a chimeric antibody against CD20), but the use of rituximab in HIV-infected patients has been controversial. A large phase 3 trial of cyclophosphamide, hydroxydaunorubicin, vincristine, and prednisone (CHOP) with and without rituximab showed a significant increased risk of treatment-related infectious death in the rituximab arm [5]. Further analysis indicates that the risk is highest in CD4 counts less than 50 cells/μl. A more recent study looked at etoposide, prednisone, vincristine, cyclophosphamide, and doxorubicin (EPOCH) with concurrent rituximab compared to EPOCH with sequential rituximab and found a nonsignificant trend towards increased deaths in the concurrent arm but also improved complete response rates [6].

Case 2

The patient is a 48-year-old man who is admitted to the general medicine service for stomach pain of 2 weeks' duration. It is associated with nausea and loose stools, which were non-bloody. Over the past 2 days, however, his nausea has gotten worse and he has been unable to tolerate anything by mouth. Furthermore, the loose stools have stopped and he has not had a bowel movement. He reports a 10 lb weight loss over the past month.

He has a past medical history of insulin-dependent diabetes complicated by retinopathy, nephropathy, and neuropathy. He also has hypertension. His mother was also diabetic.

Social history. He used to be a limousine driver but is now disabled. He has been separated from his wife for over 5 years and is the primary caregiver for his grandson. He is a social drinker, a never smoker and denies any history of drug use, including injection drug use.

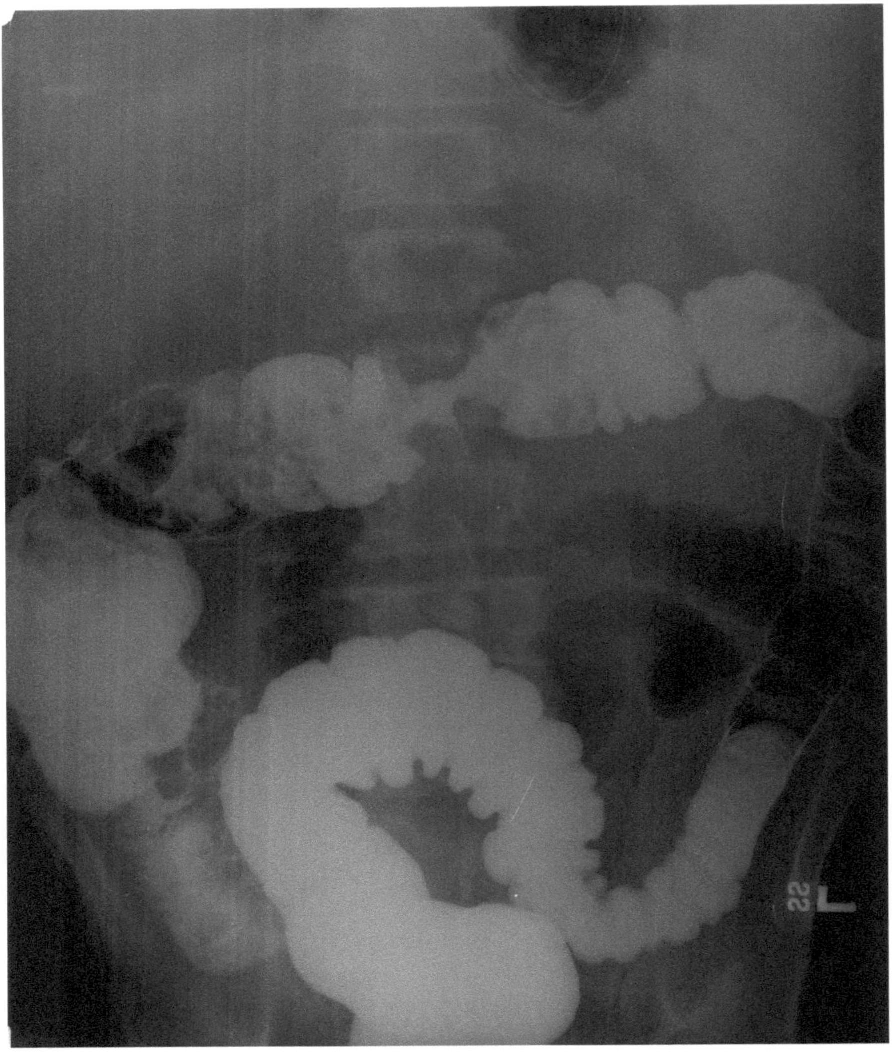

Fig. 15.1 A single contrast barium enema demonstrating an apple core lesion in the transverse colon

Physical exam. He is thin with dry mucous membranes. He is slightly tachycardic, with a heart rate of 96 bpm. His blood pressure is 98/60 mmHg. Abdominal exam is significant for tenderness in the bilateral upper quadrants, distension, and hypoactive bowel sounds. Further exam is unremarkable. Laboratory data is available in table 15.2.

Testing. An abdominal film shows a classic apple core lesion in the transverse colon (Fig. 15.1). Colonoscopy with biopsy finds a large, annular lesion in the lumen of the transverse colon with two more small lesions on either side. Biopsy is nondiagnostic, therefore a surgical consultation is obtained and the patient receives a colectomy.

Table 15.2

Laboratory value	Value	Range
WBC	4,700	4,000–11,000
Hemoglobin (g/dl)	14.1	11.5–16.0
Platelets per ml	165,000	140,000–400,000
Creatinine (mg/dl)	2.1	0.5–1.5
CEA (ng/ml)	2.8	<3
CRP (mg/dl)	1.37	0.08–0.8
ESR (mm/h)	38	0–10

WBC white blood cell, *CEA* carcinoembryonic antigen, *CRP* C-reactive protein, *ESR* erythrocyte sedimentation rate

With Presented Data, What Is Your Working Diagnosis?

This is a 48-year-old man who presents with an obstructing mass lesion in his colon but normal CEA and hemoglobin. He does have weight loss along with an elevated CRP and ESR.

Differential Diagnosis

A clinical picture consistent with bowel obstruction can be seen in a variety of situations when there is mechanical impingement of the alimentary tract such as from bulky lymphadenopathy or strictures, however in this case there is a colonoscopy that visualized an intraluminal mass. The differential diagnosis should include neoplasms such as colon cancer or lymphoma. Inflammatory bowel conditions such as Crohn's or ulcerative colitis may also present in this way. Rarely, mycobacteria or fungal infection can also produce a mass lesion. If the patient has a defect of the immune system such as advanced HIV infection, then the differential should also include Kaposi's sarcoma and cytomegalovirus (CMV).

Workup

Pathologic examination of the mass reveals no malignant cells, negative stains for acid-fast bacilli, and no viral inclusion bodies to suggest CMV. Furthermore, there was no evidence of inflammatory bowel disease. Fungal staining showed elements consistent with *Histoplasma capsulatum*.

What Is Your Diagnosis and Why?

Ideally, this patient would have been diagnosed with histoplasmosis of the alimentary tract prior to having his colon removed. For Histoplasma to present primarily as a mass lesion of the colon in the absence of pulmonary or disseminated disease is unusual and further workup is warranted. In this case, the patient was found to be HIV positive with a CD4 count of 74 cells/μl. His HIV PCR was 47,000 viral copies/ml. He denied any risk factors for HIV acquisition and otherwise felt fine.

Discussion

H. capsulatum is a dimorphic fungus that can infect both immunocompetent and immunocompromised patients. It is found throughout the world, but is more common in North and Central America. In the United States, it is most frequently found in the Midwestern and central states, particularly the Ohio River valley. The reservoir for Histoplasma is soil contaminated with the feces of birds or bats. Most exposed patients are either asymptomatic or have a mild pulmonary illness. Only less than 1 % of patients go on to have severe disease. Of those with severe disease, most have pulmonary manifestations. It should be noted that early in the disease course, macrophages ingest but are unable to kill the fungus, thus serving as an unwitting vehicle of dissemination. In disseminated disease, the presence of Histoplasma in the gastrointestinal tract is common (70–90 % of autopsy cases) [7]. It is uncommon, however, for the primary presentation to be a colonic mass.

In any patient with a diagnosis of extra-pulmonary histoplasmosis, HIV should always be considered since disseminated histoplasmosis can be an AIDS-defining illness. HIV patients with histoplasmosis are more likely to require hospitalization, have longer durations of therapy, and worse outcomes.

This patient qualifies for treatment for his HIV. Nevertheless, he has an active infection that should be treated prior to beginning HAART since he is at high risk of immune reconstitution inflammatory syndrome (IRIS). IRIS occurs in patients with low CD4 counts who have untreated or unrecognized opportunistic infections and are then started on HAART. As the HIV PCR copy number drops and the immune system regains functionality, the body mounts a highly inflammatory and potentially dangerous reaction against the infecting pathogens.

The mode of entry for HIV into a host cell is via the CD4 receptor on certain antigen-presenting cells. CD4+ cells are the regulatory cells of the immune system and the loss of their function leads to a more nuanced effect than the term "immunosuppression" may imply. In one study of immune reconstitution to *Mycobacterium tuberculosis*, patients with IRIS had higher levels of TNF, IL-6, and interferon gamma than matched controls [8]. Interestingly, there is no global T cell defect; patients with IRIS have a dysregulation of a subset of CD4 cells that are specifically targeted at the antigen triggering the reaction [9].

Given the potentially dangerous nature of IRIS, HAART should wait until all opportunistic infections are brought under control. Conversely, there is a danger in waiting too long to initiate antiretroviral therapy. A landmark study looking at timing of initiation of HAART in patients with HIV and active tuberculosis found an overall 56 % decrease in mortality by starting HAART within 4 weeks of tuberculosis therapy as opposed to waiting until the completion of tuberculosis therapy—even though there were significantly fewer cases of IRIS in the sequential therapy arm [10].

The patient should be concurrently treated for HIV and histoplasmosis but the latter treatment should be started first in order to reduce the fungal burden prior to reconstituting the immune system. Selecting an HIV regimen for him poses a slight challenge since he has diabetic nephropathy and renal failure. All of the United States Department of Health and Human Services preferred initial regimens use the antiretroviral tenofovir, a drug with potential renal toxicity. In this case, abacavir was substituted for tenofovir because it has very little renal toxicity. The Achilles' heel of this drug, however, is the abacavir hypersensitivity syndrome.

Abacavir hypersensitivity syndrome usually presents as a rash with fever, cough, fatigue, and gastrointestinal symptoms, often within the first 2 weeks of initiating the drug. Given the nonspecific nature of the symptoms, it can often be confused with a viral syndrome and clinicians should maintain a low threshold of suspicion for this diagnosis. The mechanism appears to be an MHC I-restricted cellular hypersensitivity mediated by CD8+ cells in HLA B*5701+ patients [11].

In 2009, the Food and Drug Administration (FDA) updated its recommendations to include genetic testing for the HLA B*5701 allele for all patients prior to initiation or re-initiation on abacavir. Patients who present with abacavir hypersensitivity syndrome are extremely likely to be positive for HLA B*5701. The prevalence of the allele appears to be higher in Caucasians than in African-Americans. A prospective randomized study found that if patients did not have this human leukocyte antigen, the negative predictive value of having the hypersensitivity reaction was 100 %. When the allele was present, the positive predictive value of developing a hypersensitivity reaction was 48 % [12]. There are a few other situations where an allele predicts a drug reaction; for example, there is also an HLA type associated with allopurinol and carbamazepine hypersensitivity. Nevertheless, abacavir is distinctive in that routine testing is recommended in all patients prior to initiation of this drug.

Questions

1. A new patient is referred to you for treatment of HIV. He has a CD4 count of 33 cells/μl and a viral PCR of 88,000 copies/ml. It is noted that he was recently diagnosed with a lymphoma and is about to start a round of cyclophosphamide, hydroxydaunorubicin, vincristine, prednisone, and rituximab (r-CHOP). After getting baseline HIV labs, what do you recommend?
   (a) Holding off on HAART until the second round of chemotherapy
   (b) Starting HAART but recommending a half dose of prednisone because of increased infection risk
   (c) Holding off on rituximab until the CD4 count is higher
   (d) Start HAART first and then start chemotherapy once the viral load is undetectable

2. Which of the following is an indication to start HAART immediately rather than waiting for a genotype and baseline HIV labs to be done?
   (a) Pneumonia with *Pneumocystis jiroveci* (PCP pneumonia)
   (b) Idiopathic thrombocytopenia
   (c) The patient requests to start
   (d) A CD4 count less than 50

3. Which of the following viruses is not thought to have oncogenic properties?
   (a) Epstein–Barr Virus (EBV)
   (b) Human papilloma virus (HPV)
   (c) Human immunodeficiency virus (HIV)
   (d) Respiratory syncytial virus (RSV)

4. Which of the following facts about HIV are true?
   (a) Most of the newly diagnosed HIV cases in the United States are not newly acquired.
   (b) It is a DNA-based virus
   (c) Two-thirds of the infected people in the United States are unaware of their diagnosis
   (d) Routine testing is recommended only for men who have sex with men, intravenous drug users, and commercial sex workers

5. In a patient with lymphadenopathy for over a week, which of the following is NOT likely to be the cause?
   (a) Hepatitis B
   (b) Bartonella
   (c) Hodgkin's lymphoma
   (d) HIV

6. What percent of people who are exposed to *Histoplasma capsulatum* go on to have disseminated disease?

   (a) 1–5 %
   (b) 10–15 %
   (c) 25–30 %
   (d) >40 %

7. Which of the following is true about the HLA B*5701 allele?

   (a) Patients who have this allele and are started on abacavir have a 70 % chance of developing abacavir hypersensitivity reaction
   (b) Patients who do not have this allele still have a 10 % chance of developing the abacavir hypersensitivity reaction
   (c) It is the only known case where a drug reaction has been linked to human leukocyte antigen (HLA)
   (d) It is found more often in Caucasians than African-Americans

8. What organ system is most often involved in Histoplasmosis infection?

   (a) Gastrointestinal tract
   (b) Lungs
   (c) Skin and integument
   (d) Brain

9. How should the treatments of HIV and histoplasmosis be managed in a newly diagnosed co-infected patient?

   (a) Begin both HAART and antifungals immediately
   (b) Start antifungals first, then wait a month and start HAART only if the fungal infection appears to be improving
   (c) Start HAART, then start antifungals in 1 month only if the viral load is undetectable
   (d) Complete a course of antifungals and then start HAART

10. Which of the following is true about immune reconstitution inflammatory syndrome (IRIS)?

   (a) It occurs in all patients started on HAART who have a CD4 count less than 100
   (b) It can be avoided if prophylactic antibiotics are given prior to starting HAART
   (c) It commonly occurs 6 months to a year after initiating HAART
   (d) It results from the immune system responding to opportunistic infections during HAART

Answer key: 1(c), 2(b), 3(d), 4(a), 5(a), 6(a), 7(d), 8(b), 9(b), 10(d).

References

1. Campsmith ML, Rhodes PH, Hall HI, Green TA. Undiagnosed HIV prevalence among adults and adolescents in the United States at the end of 2006. J Acquir Immune Defic Syndr. 2010;53(5):619–24.
2. Van Baarle D, Hovenkamp E, Callan MFC, Wolthers KC, Kostense S, Tan LC, et al. Dysfunctional Epstein-Barr Virus (EBV)-specific CD8+ T lymphocytes and increased EBV load in HIV-1 infected individuals progressing to AIDS-related non-Hodgkin lymphoma. Blood. 2001;98(1):146–55.
3. Epeldegui M, Vendrame E, Martínez-Maza O. HIV-associated immune dysfunction and viral infection: role in the pathogenesis of AIDS-related lymphoma. Immunol Res. 2010;48(1):72–83.
4. Girard T, Luquet-Besson I, Baran-Marszak F, Raphaël M, Boué F. HIV+MALT lymphoma remission induced by highly active antiretroviral therapy alone. Eur J Haematol. 2005;74(1):70–2.
5. Kaplan LD, Lee JY, Ambinder RF, Sparano JA, Cesarman E, Chadburn A, et al. Rituximab does not improve clinical outcome in a randomized phase 3 trial of CHOP with or without rituximab in patients with HIV-associated non-Hodgkin lymphoma: AIDS-Malignancies Consortium Trial 010. Blood. 2005;106(5):1538–43.
6. Sparano JA, Lee JY, Kaplan LD, Levine AM, Ramos JC, Ambinder RF, et al. Rituximab plus concurrent infusional EPOCH chemotherapy is highly effective in HIV-associated B-cell non-Hodgkin lymphoma. Blood. 2010;115(15):3008–16.
7. Kahi CJ, Wheat LJ, Allen SD, Sarosi GA. Gastrointestinal histoplasmosis. Am J Gastroenterol. 2005;100(1):220–31.
8. Tadokera R, Meintjes G, Skolimowska KH, Wilkinson KA, Matthews K, Seldon R, et al. Hypercytokinaemia accompanies HIV–tuberculosis immune reconstitution inflammatory syndrome. Eur Respir J. 2011;37(5):1248–59.
9. Mahnke YD, Greenwald JH, DerSimonian R, Roby G, Antonelli LRV, Sher A, et al. Selective expansion of polyfunctional pathogen-specific CD4+ T cells in HIV-1-infected patients with immune reconstitution inflammatory syndrome. Blood. 2012;119(13):3105–12.
10. Abdool Karim SS, Naidoo K, Grobler A, Padayatchi N, Baxter C, Gray A, et al. Timing of initiation of antiretroviral drugs during tuberculosis therapy. N Engl J Med. 2010;362(8):697–706.
11. Chessman D, Kostenko L, Lethborg T, Purcell AW, Williamson NA, Chen Z, et al. Human leukocyte antigen class I-restricted activation of CD8+ T cells provides the immunogenetic basis of a systemic drug hypersensitivity. Immunity. 2008;28(6):822–32.
12. Mallal S, Phillips E, Carosi G, Molina J-M, Workman C. HLA-B*5701 screening for hypersensitivity to abacavir. N Engl J Med. 2008;358(6):568–79.

Part VI
Diffuse Pain Syndrome

Chapter 16
Fibromyalgia: Evaluation and Therapy of a Neuroimmune Disorder

Xavier J. Caro

He who studies medicine without books sails an uncharted sea, but he who studies medicine without patients does not go to sea at all.

—William Osler, M.D.

Abstract Fibromyalgia (FM) is one of the commonest but most enigmatic rheumatologic conditions encountered by the practicing clinician. Difficulties in its diagnosis and successful treatment stem, in part, from the absence of a coherent pathophysiologically based approach to the disorder. Two cases of FM, found in association with connective tissue diseases, are presented, and a novel approach to their clinical evaluation is outlined. In both cases the clinician is encouraged to seek out historical and physical findings suggesting the presence of peripheral nerve lesions akin to those seen in chronic inflammatory demyelinating polyneuropathy (CIDP) and small fiber neuropathy (SFN). The chapter outlines a logical approach to the laboratory evaluation of this situation utilizing electrodiagnostic testing (electromyography and nerve conduction velocities) and skin biopsy-generated epidermal nerve fiber density (ENFD) testing. The results of these evaluative strategies lend weight to the assertion that the patient outlined in Case 1 represents a member of a large subset of FM whose pain is likely to be due, in large part, to the neuroimmune lesion(s) seen in CIDP and SFN. In Case 2 the results of testing suggest that the patient is an example of "pseudofibromyalgia" and has pain originating, in large part, from a diffuse enthesopathy, as might be seen in *forme fruste* ankylosing spondylitis. The implications of these findings vis a vis these patients' therapy, and our better understanding of FM in general, are discussed in detail.

Keywords Fibromyalgia • Chronic fatigue syndrome • Chronic widespread pain • Electromyography • Nerve conduction velocity • CIDP • IVIg

X.J. Caro, M.D., F.A.C.P., F.A.C.R. (✉)
Northridge Hospital Medical Center,
18350 Roscoe Blvd, Suite 418, Northridge, CA, 91325, USA
e-mail: xjcaro@earthhlink.net

M. Mahmoudi (ed.), *Challenging Cases in Rheumatology and Diseases of the Immune System*, DOI 10.1007/978-1-4614-5088-7_16,
© Springer Science+Business Media, LLC 2013

The absence of a coherent, and easily understood, pathophysiologically based approach to the fibromyalgia (FM) syndrome contributes to its reputation as being one of the most enigmatic members of the rheumatic disease family. Newer insights into FM, however, have allowed us a better understanding of this painful syndrome. I will attempt to use some of this new information here to provide the reader a useful means of conceptualizing this disorder, and to construct a guidebook, of sorts, to evaluating and treating FM. This discussion will, however, also reflect the biases I have built up over 30 years of clinical and research experience. Hopefully, I have struck enough of a balance between these newer findings and one rheumatologist's perspective so that the reader is the beneficiary.

Case 1

A 36-year-old Caucasian, female Information Technology consultant was referred in May 2011 by another rheumatologist because of our known interest in FM. She had also been diagnosed with an "Unspecified Connective Tissue Disease."

The patient's rheumatologic problem started 4 years before her consultation when she began experiencing low-grade, widespread soft-tissue and articular pain, as well as chronic fatigue. These symptoms persisted until 1 year before her consultation when they worsened after she underwent an abdominal laproscopic resection of a 14 cm colonic segment because of antibiotic-resistant diverticulitis. At the same time, she underwent laproscopic cholecystectomy because of cholelithiasis and mild chronic cholecystitis. Pathologic tissue examination of colonic and gall bladder tissue was consistent with her preoperative diagnoses and revealed no signs of vasculitis or other intercurrent disease.

The patient's postoperative course was characterized by worsening of her widespread pain and "intractable pelvic pain." Approximately 6 weeks after her abdominal surgery she underwent laproscopic-assisted vaginal hysterectomy and bilateral salpingo-oopherectomy. Pathologic examination of surgical tissue showed chronic cervicitis, and a single, hemorrhagic corpus luteum cyst. There was no evidence of endometriosis. She was maintained on narcotic analgesics, pregabalin, muscle relaxants and, because of recurrent severe migraine headaches, injectable sumatriptan succinate. A rheumatologic consultation was requested during her hospital recovery.

The rheumatologist noted additional patient symptoms including "brittle hair and dry skin," and recurring oral ulcers associated with her painful flare-ups. He also made note of her history of having undergone a "total thyroidectomy many years ago" for a "precancerous lesion." She also gave a strong family history of rheumatoid arthritis and "thyroid problems." Physical examination, performed while the patient was on postoperative analgesics, revealed little more than diffuse abdominal tenderness and a post-surgical state. The consultant ordered hospital laboratory testing and outpatient follow-up. Later he ordered further outpatient laboratory tests.

Hospital Laboratory Results: Antinuclear antibody (ANA): 1:160 (speckled pattern). Complement panel: normal. Lupus anticoagulant screen: negative. CRP: 5.6 (normal 1.0–3.0).

Outpatient Laboratory Results: SSA (Ro) antibody: 511 (Normal < 91). Erythrocyte sedimentation rate (ESR; normal 0–20 mm/1 h): Normal. C reactive protein (CRP): variously, mildly elevated or normal. Rheumatoid factor and CCP-IgG: Negative. Anti-dsDNA, Sm, RNP, SSB (La), Histone, Scl-70: all Negative.

Outpatient Follow-Up: The patient was diagnosed with "Unspecific Diffuse Connective Tissue Disease," and, over the ensuing months, treated with prednisone (10–60 mg/day), hydroxychloroquine, methotrexate, etanercept, pregabalin, levothyroxine sodium, and estrogen/progesterone supplements. She also used the following analgesics: tramadol, hydrocodone/acetamenphen, and carisoprodol.

When her condition failed to improve significantly she was referred for subconsultation.

What Is Your Working Diagnosis and Approach Now?

This patient's symptom complex is most consistent with a chronic inflammatory disorder. This is particularly likely because of the presence of unexplained, chronic pain. Recall that pain, particularly when chronic, may be one of the five cardinal signs of inflammation. In the absence of another, better explanation, examiners must consider the potential role of inflammation in their analysis of chronic pain. Any corroborating information to support the presence of such inflammation might, then, help push us in the direction of further laboratory testing for inflammation, or even ad hoc anti-inflammatory treatment.

The patient's intriguing laboratory findings, including an elevated CRP, are helpful in our evaluation— at least in theory—but the clinical picture is colored by the patient's recent severe diverticulitis, cholecystitis, and attendant surgeries. That is, the patient's potential inflammatory state can't really be "sorted out" until she has had time to reasonably recover from the complex immunological insult arising out of her infection and surgeries [1]. Thereafter, the examiner might better consider the nature and origin of any chronic inflammatory state.

After recovery, and with the patient's continued complaints of pain, comes a need to consider the three most likely "causes" of (chronic) inflammation. i.e., infection, cancer, or autoimmune disease. Without any signs of continuing infection or neoplasia an autoimmune diathesis is suggested in this patient. The results of her immunologic testing, particularly her positive ANA and SSA (Ro), are supportive of this thinking. Unfortunately, while the finding of a strongly positive anti-SSA (Ro) is suggestive of Sjogren's syndrome (SS), it is not specific enough, by itself, to render such a precise diagnosis. FM has been reported to coexist in 25% of patients with RA, 30% of patients with SLE and 50% of patients with SS. There may even be a pathophysiologic overlap between Sjogren's syndrome and fibromyalgia [2]. All we can say at this point is that the patient is likely to be manifesting a chronic, autoimmune inflammatory disorder.

The consultant rheumatologist used this information as justification in beginning a clinical trial of anti-inflammatory treatment, including prednisone and a TNF–alpha inhibitor. He did not "label" the patient's problem specifically, however. The term "Unspecific Diffuse Connective Tissue Disease" seemed most appropriate to him.

Initial Evaluation at the Time of Sub-consultation

The patient was seen in sub-consultation approximately 9 months after her original rheumatologic evaluation. Her complaints of widespread soft-tissue and articular pain were confirmed, as were her complaints of profound fatigue (which she rated as a 6–7 out of a possible 10, where 10 represented profound fatigue). She described the total effect of these sensations as being "as though I always have the flu."

The patient also complained of weakness, particularly in lifting heavy objects and in ascending stairs, which antedated steroid exposure. She gave a history of recurring migraine headaches, heat intolerance, sun sensitivity (possibly associated with a sun-induced rash), poor short-term memory, and disordered sleep. Interestingly, she also described "dozens" of sinus infections dating to childhood. These included 1–3 sinus infections per year as an adult, and three adult episodes of pneumonia.

Physical examination was pertinent for the presence of 18 of 18 soft-tissue "tender points" described in the 1990 American College of Rheumatology criteria for the diagnosis of FM [3]. There was a suggestion of articular tenderness at both ankles and metatarsophalangeal joints. There was also diminished pinwheel and vibratory tuning fork (128 Hz) sensation found in a stocking distribution and extending distally from 2 to 3 inches above both ankles. Proximal muscle strength was graded as normal in the upper extremities (5/5), but as 5–/5 at the hip flexor and hamstring musculature bilaterally. Biceps, brachioradialis, patellar, and Achilles deep tendon reflexes were all graded as diminished.

Subsequent Outpatient Laboratory Results: Routine metabolic panels, including assessments of renal, hepatic, and lipid status were normal, except for an elevated total cholesterol of 231 mg/dl (normal <200 mg/dl). Assessments of thyroid function, creatine phosphokinase (CPK), vitamin B-12 and folate levels, methylmalonic acid, homocysteine, rapid plasma reagin (RPR), and Hgb A1c were all normal or negative. A Westergren erythrocyte sedimentation rate (ESR; normal 0–20 mm/1 h) was 20 mm/1 h, and a C-reactive protein (CRP) was 12.7 mg/L (normal 0.0–8.0 mg/L).

Immnologic testing included the following: Interleukin (IL)-1 beta, IL-2, IL-2R, and IL-6; circulating immune complex (CIC) assay by C3d, C1q binding, and Raji cell all normal or negative. Rheumatoid factor, and Cyclic Citrullinated Peptide (CCP) IgG antibodies were negative. ANA was positive with a titer of 1:80 (speckled pattern). A double stranded DNA determination was "indeterminate." Anti-SSA (Ro), SSB (La), Sm/RNP, Scl-70, and ribosomal P protein were all negative. Anti-phospholipid antibody screen (Cardiolipin IgG/M/A, Phosphatidylserine IgG/M/A, Phoshatidic acid IgG/M/A, Phosphatidyl Ethanolamine IgG/M/A, Phosphatidylcholine IgG/M/A, and lupus anticoagulant [LAC]): negative. Anti-neutrophil cytoplasmic antibodies (ANCA): negative.

Review of Other Outpatient Records: Because of recurring migraine headaches and an associated episode of severe, unexplained vertigo the patient had undergone magnetic resonance imaging (MRI) of the brain (without contrast) approximately 2 months prior to sub-consultation. These results were deemed normal except for a "tiny area of old infarction in the right cerebellar hemisphere," and mucosal thickening in of the right sphenoid, ethmoid, and maxillary sinuses. Two weeks prior to sub-consultation a neurologist obtained a Computerized Tomographic (CT) angiogram of the brain. It revealed no evidence of vasculitis, or other inflammatory disorder, other than "chronic sphenoid sinusitis."

What Is Your Approach At This Point?

On the surface it may appear that this patient is a particularly complex one, but I'd wager that most consultative rheumatologists encounter such a patient not infrequently. Nevertheless, without a coherent plan-of-attack it would be easy for the novice to be overcome by the "fog of war" here. I would, then, propose that we consider approaching one of the patient's major problems, perhaps *the* major problem—that is, her FM—in a systematic fashion.

First, we need to ask ourselves whether the patient even has FM. When she was first seen the referring rheumatologist did not find the classical "tender points" required by the 1990 ACR criteria, probably because of her postoperative analgesia. Nevertheless, she did complain of a *history of widespread pain and profound fatigue.* It might also be noteworthy that the patient's preoperative pelvic pain complaints may have been greater than expected given the postsurgical pathologic findings from her hysterectomy and oophorectomy, a situation that is typical of FM. These clinical phenomena are of enough importance so that I will touch on them again in the *Discussion* section. For now let's allow the diagnosis based on her physical findings at the time of sub-consultation when she did demonstrate the "tender point count" required by the 1990 ACR criteria.

Next, the clinician who has successfully recognized the presence of FM might question if he/she should now move on to therapy of this painful syndrome, an approach commonly advocated in this disorder [3, 4]. After all, it is reasoned, by those advancing such an approach, the prime mover in FM is a problem confined to the central nervous system (CNS). No further evaluation, other than that encountered in the research setting, is called for. I will advocate here, however, that you consider a different tact; one that is more oriented toward demonstrating the existence of a peripheral lesion in FM.

In order to better understand this thinking it might be helpful to consider the typical modern-day clinician's approach to the chronic, symmetrical, small joint polyarthritis commonly associated with rheumatoid arthritis. I term this condition a polyarthritis of the rheumatoid type (PART). Asking most seasoned rheumatologists for a differential diagnosis of a PART would bring a sigh of boredom as they easily listed at least a dozen, perhaps two-dozen, entities that could explain such a finding. "Well for starters," they would smirk, "rheumatoid arthritis, systemic lupus erythematosus, sarcoidosis, malignancy, chronic hepatitis C viral infection,... (etc.)" "Do you want me to go on (yawn)," they would add. But, merely ask them for a differential diagnosis of FM, and it is just as likely that the same questioner's inquiry would be met with an open mouthed gape laced with incredulity. Their demeanor would suggest, louder than words, that they had never considered that there might be a differential diagnosis for FM. But, indeed there is.

Now, for one of the central tenets of this chapter: *the differential diagnosis of FM is essentially the same as it is for a PART.* That is, all of the diagnoses so astutely listed for a PART are the same as those to be considered in the case of a patient presenting with FM. In other words, it is incumbent upon the clinician to show that one of these conditions, thought to be the *prime mover* in the situation, is *not* present. For that reason it is worthwhile questioning the patient about potential rheumatic disease connections, both personal and familial, and associated rheumatologic symptoms, just the same as a rheumatologist might with any patient presenting with a PART. It is also worth investigating the patient with, at the least, "standard" immune serologic testing. It might be debated as to the reasonable extent of this laboratory investigation, as no guidelines exist, but I would argue that it should be, at a minimum, at least as robust as you would normally order on a new patient presenting with a PART.

At this point, speaking in generalities, the rheumatic disease specialist will have one of two situations on his/her hands. First, is the FM patient who has no clinical or serologic findings of a "standard rheumatologic diagnosis" (e.g., negative rheumatoid factor, and ANA). The second may be a situation in which the examiner reasonably suspects one or more of the standard rheumatic diseases is present. For the purposes of our discussion, I will refer to the first group as having "Primary FM," while the second group will be referred to as having "Secondary FM." To a large extent these designations hearken back to similar classifications found in the FM literature of the 1980s and 1990s. We may eventually have to ask ourselves if there is such a thing as "primary" FM. But, for our current purposes, it is helpful to know "the degree of inflammation" seen clinically. That is, generally speaking, "Primary FM" patients will have less inflammatory disease, as defined in the classical sense (i.e., tissue inflammatory cell infiltrate and abnormal serologies), than "Secondary FM" patients. And, as you will soon see, the degree and extent of inflammation will dictate therapy and, probably, prognosis for these FM patients.

Now, let us leave this largely theoretical discussion and return to the bedside. We have, as you recall, a patient with a rather complex clinical presentation, whose major complaint is chronic widespread pain. Our problem is now threefold: (1) How do we approach her underlying rheumatic disease (e.g., perhaps as a manifestation of Sjogren's syndrome), (2) How do we approach her uncontrolled FM, and (3) How do we approach her analgesic dependence. Here, I will confine myself, in the main, to the second point, as that is what I think the readers of this chapter are seeking. Nevertheless, our approach to all of these problems is certainly intertwined.

In further evaluating this patient's FM, therefore, I wish to call the reader's attention to her peripheral neuropathic findings on physical examination, including her stocking distribution hypesthesia and proximal muscle weakness. In a previously published series of FM patients [5] we found that 88% of our FM patients had clinical findings of lower extremity stocking distribution hypesthesia, compared to none of our controls ($p<0.0001$). Furthermore, our FM patients also had significantly diminished proximal muscle strength when compared to other rheumatic disease patients without FM ($p<0.0001$). These findings dictate that the examiner consider more detailed evaluation of the peripheral nervous system (PNS) in any patient with FM. Such a requirement mandates that the examiner conduct electrodiagnostic (EDX) testing and, at least consider, peripheral nerve biopsy.

EDX Testing and the Concept of CIDP in the Setting of FM

The role of EDX in evaluating FM patients has not been extensively investigated. Only a few published studies exist at all, and—so far as I am aware—only two of these is prospective in nature [5, 6]. Both of these studies, however, have offered evidence of the existence of a polyneuropathy in FM. In our study [5] we found that 47% of our FM patients had EDX evidence of a polyneuropathy, 33% had demyelination, and 15% had non-dermatomal muscle denervation in their lower extremities. Furthermore, as a group, our FM patients had significantly weaker proximal musculature, as measured by a composite, four extremity "strength score" ($p<0.0001$). To obtain this score we manually tested our subjects' strength at the deltoids, biceps brachii, hip flexors, and hamstring musculature. These clinical and EDX findings in our FM patients were important because, taken as a whole, they suggested the presence of a peripheral nerve lesion akin to that described as constituting the entity, "chronic inflammatory demyelinating polyneuropathy (CIDP)."

CIDP is a term used to describe a rather diverse group of neuropathic disorders that have several things in common, including the presence of peripheral nerve demyelination, an immune pathogenesis, and a propensity to respond favorably to immunomodulatory therapy. CIDP can be a controversial disorder in itself, in part because its diagnosis is dependent on an astute clinical examination and a detailed EDX evaluation. There are also thinkers who subcategorize CIDP beneath the rubric of chronic acquired demyelinating polyneuropathies (CADP), and segregate certain forms of CADP away from CIDP. These other immune polyneuropathic catagories include CIDP in association with various dysproteinemias, such as a monoclonal gammopathy of undetermined significance (CIDP-MGUS) or frank multiple myeloma. One form of these is the IgM paraprotein-associated Distal Acquired Demyelinating Symmetric (DADS) neuropathy, a disorder said to be relatively steroid resistant.

Other forms of the demyelinating neuropathies parsed out include disorders with distinctive clinical appearances, such as the Lewis-Sumner syndrome (aka, MADSAM neuropathy), and multifocal motor neuropathy (MMN). These latter subcategories of CADP may be marked by the presence of an anti-neuronal antibody (e.g., anti-GM1 in the Lewis-Sumner syndrome and MMN, and anti-myelin-associated glycoprotein, MAG, in the plasma cell dyscrasias). Most, but not all, patients with one of these CIDP-variants still respond to immunotherapy, particularly intravenous immune globulin (IVIg). The subtleties of these fascinating disorders have been well outlined for the interested reader in a number of publications [7, 8]. For our purposes it is merely important that the reader consider the diagnosis of CADP and CIDP in their FM patient, and also understand that proper evaluation of these entities hinges, principally, on the subject's clinical picture, as well as their EDX and associated laboratory findings.

In so far as EDX is concerned, it is noteworthy that at least 12 sets of EDX/Clinical criteria exist for the diagnosis of CIDP, or one of the other CADP variants. Three of the more commonly known criteria sets for diagnosing CIDP are listed in Table 16.1. Their relative lack of clinical friendliness and flexibility is apparent with a bit of study, and has seriously limited their clinical applicability. For these reasons I prefer the more clinically friendly and flexible diagnostic criteria recently published simultaneously in the European Journal of Neurology and the Journal of the Peripheral Nervous System [9]. The interested reader is referred to this original publication for specifics. Suffice it to say here that these criteria are more clinically applicable and limit the number of "underdiagnosed" patients. Nevertheless, the EDX measurements required by any of these criteria sets calls for the participation of a skilled electromyographer.

According to the American Association of Neuromuscular & Electrodiagnostic Medicine (AANEM) *Guidelines for The Electrodiagnostic Medicine Consultation* [10], "EDX studies are performed by physicians as part of a [comprehensive] consultation. This consultation should include history taking, appropriate physical examination, and the design, performance, and interpretation of EDX studies. These consultations usually take a minimum of 30 min to perform and take up to 2 h or more in particularly complicated situations." In my opinion, the referring rheumatologist, or other neuromuscular specialist, should settle for nothing less than this during the EDX evaluation of an FM patient. Only in that way may he/she be positioned to identify the presence of an EDX lesion in a given FM patient, and understand its implications for the diagnosis of CIDP, or a similar neuropathic disorder. As a point of clarity, however, I would suggest that it is unrealistic to expect the EDX specialist to categorically state whether a diagnosis of CIDP has been established. It is more reasonable that the referring neuromuscular specialist, who is much more familiar with all aspects of the FM patient's case, be the one to do that. He/she will have access to all components of the case, which may include biopsy material, cerebral spinal fluid (CSF) studies, and MRI analyses.

Nerve and Skin Biopsy Evaluation in the Setting of FM

It seems rather intuitive that microscopic visualization of nerve tissue in FM, or in any similar neuromuscular disorder, would constitute a routine part of the CIDP

Table 16.1 Three commonly applied CIDP diagnostic criteria sets

Feature	Saperstein criteria [(b)]	AAN criteria [(a)]	INCAT criteria [(c)]
Clinical Involve-ment	Motor dysfunction, sensory dysfunction of >1 limb, or both	Major: symmetric proximal and distal weakness; minor: exclusively distal weakness or sensory loss	Progressive or relapsing motor and sensory dysfunction of more than 1 limb
Time Course (mo)	≥2	≥2	>2
Reflexes	Reduced or absent	Reduced or absent	Reduced or absent
EDX test results[a]	Any 3 of the 4 criteria: partial conduction block of ≥1 motor nerve, reduced conduction velocity of ≥2 motor nerves, prolonged distal latency of ≥2 motor nerves, or prolonged F-wave latencies of ≥2 motor nerves or the absence of F-waves	2 of the 4 AAN EDX criteria	Partial conduction block of ≥2 motor nerves and abnormal conduction velocity or distal latency of F-wave latency in 1 other nerve; or, in the absence of partial conduction block, abnormal conduction velocity, distal latency, or F-wave latency in 3 motor nerves; or EDX abnormalities indicating demyelination in 2 nerves and histologic evidence of demyelination
CSF	White-cell count <10/mm^3, negative VDRL test; elevated protein level (supportive)	Protein >45 mg/dl; white-cell count <10/mm^3 (supportive)	CSF analysis recommended but not mandatory

(continued)

Table 16.1 (continued)

Feature	Saperstein criteria (b)	AAN criteria (a)	INCAT criteria (c)
Biopsy Result	Evidence of demyelination and remyelination	Predominant features of demyelination; inflammation (not required)	Not mandatory (except in cases with EDX abnormalities in only 2 motor nerves)

Listed criteria from the (c)American Academy of Neurology (AAN), [a]Saperstein et al., and [b]Hughes et al., [c]for the Inflammatory Neuropathy Cause and Treatment (INCAT) group

[a]AAN criteria for partial conduction block is a drop of ≥20% in negative peak area or peak-to-peak amplitude and a change of <15% in duration between proximal and distal site stimulation. Possible conduction block or temporal dispersion is a drop of ≥20% or more in negative peak area or peak-to peak amplitude and a change of >15% in duration between proximal and distal site stimulation. A reduced conduction velocity is a velocity <80% of the lower limit of the normal (LLN) range if the amplitude of the compound muscle action potential (CMAP) is >80% of the LLN range or <70% of the LLN if the CMAP amplitude is <80% of the LLN. Prolonged distal latency is >125% of the upper limit of the normal (ULN) range if the CMAP amplitude is >80% of the LLN range or >150% of the ULN if the CMAP amplitude is <80% of the LLN. An absent F wave or F-wave latency is >125% of the ULN (INCAT criteria, > 120%) if the CMAP amplitude is >80% of the LLN or latency is >150% of the ULN if the CMAP amplitude is <80% of the LLN. (a)EDX = Electrodiagnostic. CSF = Cerebrospinal Fluid. VDRL = Venereal Disease Research Laboratory. Neurology 1991;41:617–618. (b)Muscle Nerve 2001;24:311–324. (c)Ann Neurol 2001;50:195–201

diagnostic algorithm. Nevertheless some experts question the real value of such biopsy material, usually a sural nerve biopsy. And, the clinician can't be blamed when he/she grimaces at the attendant patient discomfiture, expense, and delay commonly associated with a sural nerve biopsy. Many of these complaints stem from the delicate and specialized nature of sural nerve staining and processing, which may include electronmicroscopic evaluation and delicate "nerve fiber teasing" studies. According to Oh [11], "The teasing of one nerve fiber from beginning to end requires a minimum of 3 days." The typical "turnaround time" for our University sural nerve biopsy processing is about 6 weeks, and may be much longer. It is, in part, due to these realities that students of CIDP, and similar peripheral neuropathic disorders, have begun to turn to the evaluation of epidermal nerve fiber density (ENFD) as a surrogate for the sural nerve biopsy.

ENFD testing has recently become recognized as a valuable tool in the evaluation of PNS disorders. ENFD quantitates cutaneous nociceptors (mainly A∂ and C fibers), and this value is helpful to the clinician since it has been established that decreased ENFD may be an early and sensitive marker for the presence of a number of peripheral nerve ailments, including CIDP [12]. Furthermore, ENFD may be used, through re-biopsy, to follow certain of these peripheral neuropathic disorders.

The exact reason that a reduction in ENFD is indicative of a diseased PNS, and potentially implicative of a painful form of CIDP, is not entirely clear. After all, shouldn't the *loss of nerve tissue* be associated with less pain (i.e., with the loss of excitable tissue should come numbness). The reality of worsening pain in the setting of reduced ENFD may have to do with an increased ectopic nerve tissue discharge rate, or a reduced threshold to excitation, of the remaining, lesioned PNS tissue within the affected extremity. There is also an unproven suspicion that diminished ENFD may correlate with the so-called central sensitization (CS) and secondary hyperalgesia, a process thought to be active in FM and other rheumatic diseases [3]. Part of this CS may herald the switching of spinal cord descending inhibitory pathways to facilitory ones [12].

The simplicity of procuring ENFD measurement is so far removed from that of sural nerve biopsy that it warrants mention. The interested neuromuscular expert may school him/herself in the technique of skin punch biopsy in a number of ways, including online video descriptions supported by one or more of the commercial laboratories offering ENFD evaluative services. The technique is considered a routine, outpatient procedure in our office and requires only one of the laboratory provided "biopsy kits" (though we chose to use our own surgical quality instruments) and the accompanying overnight mailer (Fig. 16.1a, b). We provide the required 3 mm punch skin biopsy, taken from a thigh and ankle/calf area site, to the laboratory and expect an ENFD count, for comparison to the laboratory's internally obtained, or literature, controls, within 10–14 days. It is worth noting that these specimens cannot be processed by a hospital pathology department, or even a dedicated routine dermatopathology unit, as the technique is too specialized. So far as I am aware there are only two laboratories in the U.S. sufficiently expert in ENFD analysis as to warrant mention here: the Therapath Laboratory in New York

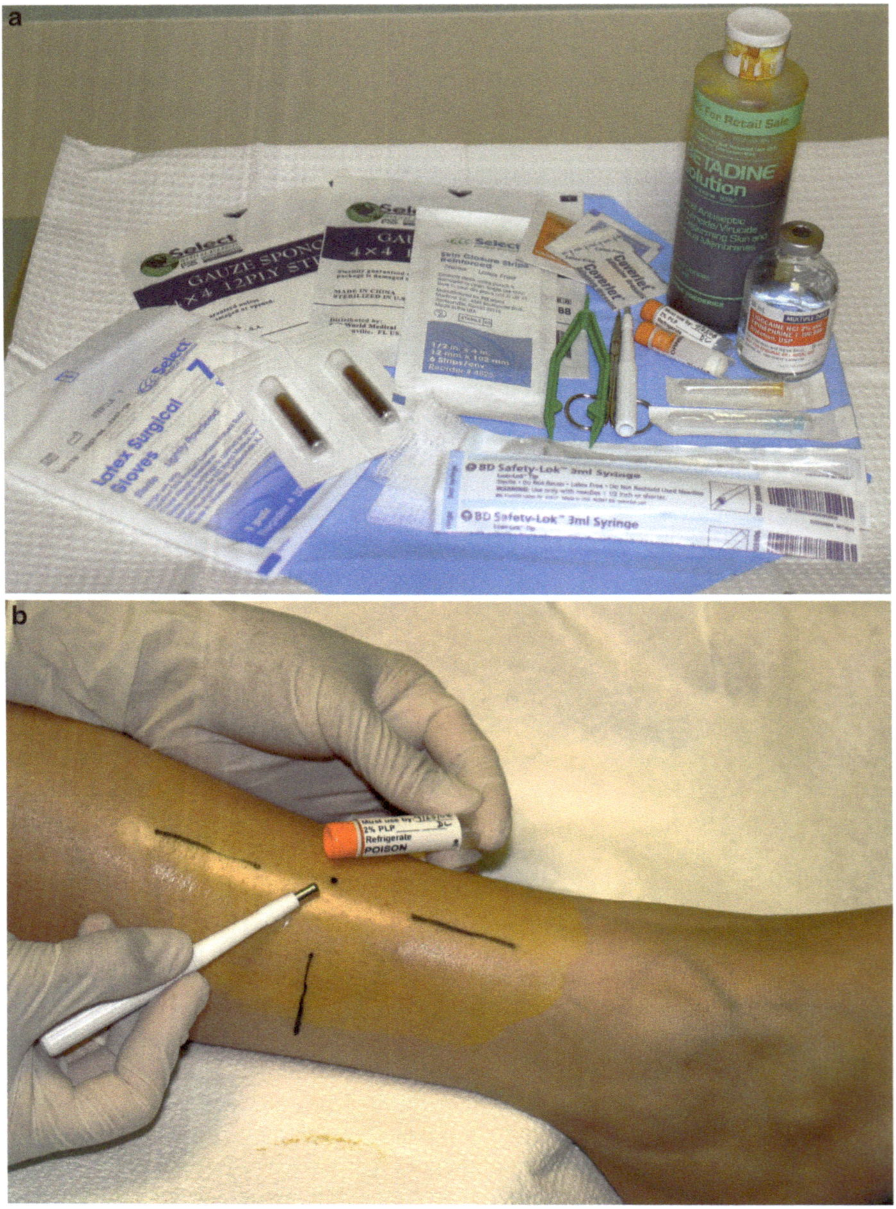

Fig. 16.1 (**a**) Supplies for a 3 mm punch skin biopsy. (**b**). Relative size and position of the skin biopsy in the calf area

(www.therapath.com), and the Bako Pathology Services laboratory in Georgia (www.bakopathology.com). There are also several dedicated, University- based, ENFD services available, but these usually do not encourage outside specimen submissions, but—in the main—process their specimens in a fashion similar to these commercial labs.

Processing of skin specimens for ENFD analysis is, in theory, rather simple, but in practice demanding enough to require a dedicated immunodermatopathology unit. The following represents the tissue preparation protocol kindly described to me by Therapath (New York, NY) one of the specialized neuropathology laboratories: After receiving a 3 mm punch skin biopsy specimen in 2% periodate-lysine-paraformaldehyde (PLP) fixative (supplied in the biopsy kit), the tissue is cryoprotected, frozen, thick-sectioned and immunohistochemically stained for protein gene product 9.5 (PGP 9.5), a ubiquitin carboxy-terminal hydrolase that is a panaxonal marker. Such staining allows for light or confocal microscopic visualization of nerve fibers within the skin tissue. Epidermal nerve fibers, representing A and C fibers, crossing the dermal-epidermal junction or basement membrane are counted in at least five sections of tissue.

Various counting algorithms (referred to as "nerve counting rules") allow for the generation of a "density" figure, usually reported as the total number of fibers crossing per millimeter length of epidermis, i.e., the epidermal nerve fiber density or ENFD. This number is considered abnormal if it falls below the fifth percentile of normative values, which vary from an ENFD of 4 to an ENFD of 7 fibers/mm (depending on the laboratory's norms) at the distal part of the leg (ankle/calf area). Subjects with ENFD below this figure are considered to have evidence of reduced ENFD, and, therefore, of a "small fiber neuropathy (SFN)" (Figs. 16.2 and 16.3).

It is noteworthy that normal ENFD declines along the length of the extremity, measuring from proximal to distal. ENFD is, therefore, "biopsy site" dependent. Typically, samples from the thigh and from the distal part of the leg (ankle/calf area) area are submitted for analysis to determine whether or not evidence of SFN, i.e., reduced ENFD, is indeed present, and if so whether it is length-dependent, i.e., whether it follows this length-dependent rule or not. ENFD does not normally vary with race, but is generally lower in men than in women, and may gradually decrease with advancing age. In the diseased state, however, ENFD may have a "dynamic value," varying according to the time of sampling relative to the underlying disease process and any therapy. It does, therefore, provide the clinician with one more variable that he/she may use in interpreting clinical course and response to treatment.

It has now been shown that reduced ENFD values in the ankle/calf are usually more sensitive than sural nerve biopsy in detecting a SFN, and correlate closely with the densities of total, small, and large myelinated sural nerve fibers [12]. Up to this point, the gold standard for all of these measurements has been the sural nerve biopsy. Interestingly, Chiang, et al., [13] found diminished ENFD in 56% of their CIDP subjects. Their CIDP cohort had a mean ENFD of 4.5 ± 2.9 versus an ENFD of 10.5 ± 3.9 fibers/mm in age- and sex-matched controls ($p < 0.001$). The presence of reduced ENFD in their patients also correlated with autonomic dysfunction, a feature commonly seen in FM.

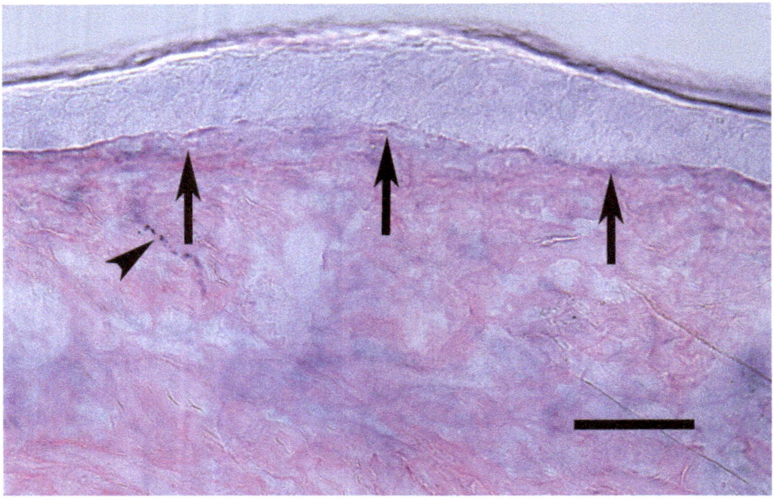

Fig. 16.2 Skin biopsy of a patient with fibromyalgia and severe SFN. The sample shows a total loss of epidermal nerve fibers. *Arrows* indicate the basement membrane that separates the epidermis above from the dermis (*pink*) below. One nerve fiber is present in the dermis (*arrowhead*). Immunoperoxidase stain of PGP 9.5, a pan-axonal marker, counterstained by hematoxylin and eosin; bar = 50 μm. SFN = small fiber neuropathy. Photomicrographs kindly supplied by the Therapath Lab. Used with permission

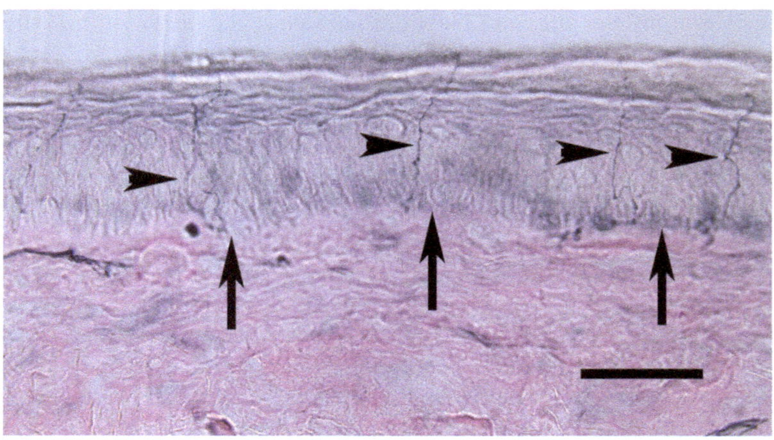

Fig. 16.3 Skin biopsy of a normal subject. The sample shows four nerve fibers (*arrowheads*) that extend from the dermis perpendicularl toward the upper layer of epidermal cells. The *arrows point* to the epidermis. Immunoperoxidase stain of PGP 9.5, a pan-axonal marker, counterstained by hematoxylin and eosin; bar = 50 μm. Photomicrographs kindly supplied by the Therapath Lab. Used with permission

A description of the various autonomic neuropathies that may be seen in association with CIDP and SFN, and marked by reduced ENFD, are beyond the scope of this chapter. Nevertheless, it is worth noting that a non-length-dependent SFN, found in association with a presumed dorsal ganglionopathy and/or post-ganglionic autonomic nerve degenerative process, has been described in the setting of CIDP [13, 14]. Subjects described in these reports often complain of a disabling acral "burning" pain, may have syndromes refractory to symptomatic (analgesic) pain management, and difficult to treat with immunotherapy.

The following experience may illustrate the usefulness and sensitivity of ENFD. During one of our clinical investigations we enrolled an asymptomatic 66–year-old male as a "normal" volunteer in one of our FM studies. His ENFD returned as significantly reduced. Because of this finding, and our consternation with the "outlier" status his value rendered, we recalled him for EDX evaluation (a test not included in the "normal" arm of our protocol at that time). Surprisingly, he had robust evidence of subclinical demyelination on his EDX study! ENFD determination, therefore, has become, along with EDX, one of our main avenues of establishing the presence of a PNS injury pattern in our FM subjects. Nevertheless, in our hands, EDX testing remains the more sensitive of the two tests. That is, most of our *Primary or* "True" FM subjects have had EDX evidence of demyelination, irrespective of their ENFD determination. The jury is still out as to whether these two tests, EDX and ENFD testing, may complement one another in other ways, so as to sort out subtypes of FM subjects.

It is noteworthy that a series of FM patients that we studied for ENFD, and reported at the Annual Meeting of the American College of Rheumatology in 2008 [15], had significantly reduced ENFD, compared to normal volunteers (4.79 vs. 6.86; $p<0.0001$). Interestingly, they also showed a significant inverse correlation for a T-cell activation marker, serum IL-2R, levels compared to controls ($r=-0.43$; $p<0.05$). All of our findings, taken as a whole [5, 15], suggest to us that a subset of FM patients may have a significant, immune-mediated, PNS lesion akin to CIDP, and that this may be treatable with immunotherapy.

EDX and ENFD Results in Our Patient: What Now?

The patient's painful picture was thought compatible with FM, in association with an "Undifferentiated Connective Tissue Disease," and a number of complicating factors. As such, she underwent four-extremity EDX evaluation, and unilateral skin biopsy for ENFD at the calf and thigh areas.

A total of 12 nerves were studied by EDX (including bilateral median, ulnar, radial, peroneal, posterior tibial, and sural nerves), of which ten were abnormal. These revealed an admixture of prolonged sensory and motor distal latencies, prolonged motor conduction velocities (posterior tibial and peroneal nerves), and diminished M wave amplitudes (ulnar nerve). There was also a unilaterally prolonged posterior tibial H wave reflex, a finding thought likely to reflect either an S1 radiculopathy or proximal nerve demyelination. An MRI of the lumbar spine, conducted 4 months earlier, had shown no evidence of S1 nerve root compression, although it did demonstrate a "… moderate L5-S1 bulging disc … without significant central canal stenosis." An EMG (electromyography) study restricted to the right upper and lower extremity was also conducted. We normally limit EMG testing to one side of the body in case we wish to biopsy the contralateral side (as EMG-related, needle artifact is a significant variable in interpreting subsequent muscle biopsies). This examination showed a mildly increased number of "normal to large amplitude" motor units at the quadriceps, suggesting mild chronic denervatoin. The electromyographer rated the likelihood of the patient's entire picture as representing CIDP, according to the 2010 European Journal of Neurology criteria, as "probable" (3 on a scale of 0–4).

The patient's skin biopsies showed an ENFD value of 7.35 at the thigh ("Low Normal" = 6.8–8.0; "Abnormal" = <6.8), and an ENFD value of 9.23 at the calf ("Low Normal" = 5.4–5.7; "Abnormal" = <5.4). These results were interpreted, by us, as being consistent with a non-length-dependent diminished ENFD, and probably a SFN.

The patient's entire clinical and EDX picture was interpreted as supportive of the idea of a CIDP-like disorder and an attendant SFN. This thinking was based on the patient's physical findings, lack of an alternative explanation for her neuropathic symptoms, her EDX findings suggestive of a CIDP- like disorder, and her "low normal" skin biopsy findings. She had, we thought, met criteria for the diagnosis of "probable CIDP," and, therefore, ostensibly, qualified for immunotherapy. Based on the non-length-dependent nature of her SFN, the possibility of the existence of an inflammatory dorsal root ganglionopathy was also thought likely.

Are There Any Complicating Factors to Consider in This Patient?

All patients with FM must be evaluated for factors that may "amplify," or at least modify, their symptoms, either in a local bodily area, or systemically. This patient is not an exception. The following were considered potential complicating factors in her case:

Laboratory Results Suggestive of Common Variable Immune Deficiency (CVID): Because of the patient's history of recurrent sinusitis, and upper/lower respiratory tract infections, including pneumonias, her serum immunoglobulins were quantitated. The results revealed IgG subclass 1 and 3 fractions that were 3 standard deviations (S.D.) below the laboratory's mean normal value. These results were unchanged upon retesting 1 month later. Additionally, quantitation of the patient's native antibody titer directed against 23 serotypes of *Streptococcus pneumoniae* showed significant reactivity against only 5 serotypes. The entire clinical and serologic picture suggested a diagnosis of Common Variable Immune Deficiency (CVID).

The importance of CVID in this setting is unclear, although it is known that individuals with this phenotype, in addition to their proclivity to develop infections and chronic fatigue, are more likely to develop manifestations of autoimmune disease, including arthralgias and myalgias. They may also be more susceptible to neoplasia, particularly lymphoproliferative disorders.

While it might be argued that our patient developed her serologic picture of immune deficiency as a consequence of her necessary rheumatologic immunosuppressant therapy, this seems unlikely since her recurrent infectious disease history and presumed autoimmunity antedated her immunotherapy by many years. It is also worth noting that the diagnostic and prognostic meaning of her associated autoantibodies, such as her ANA and anti-Ro antibody, remain in question given their having arisen within the context of CVID rather than *de novo*. The patient was provided immunization with a commercially available pneumococcal vaccine.

Migraine Headache History: The patient's headache history antedated her illness by many years but appeared to have worsened by the time of her sub-consultation. She denied any history of hypertension, recent head injury, illicit drug use, or prior episode of migraine-associated vertigo. She had been using injectable sumatriptan. Her migraine-associated vertigo was thought by her neurologist to be consistent with so-called "basilar migraine." These symptoms had been pronounced enough to lead to a short-term hospitalization. Her relatively bland MRI (with "only" a small cerebellar infarct) and CT angiogram of the brain led her neurologist to conclude she had sustained a small cerebellar infarction, as a rare but known complication of migraine [16].

Analgesic Needs due to her FM: At the time of sub-consultation the patient was referred to an experienced "Pain Management Specialist" who substituted daily methadone for her various analgesics.

What Is Your Approach to Management at This Point?

Several attempts were made to lower the patient's corticosteroid exposure; each attempt resulted in worsening of her symptoms. For that reason, and after attempts of short-term, high-dose oral prednisone (60 mg/day) had failed she underwent weekly 125 mg Solumedrol infusion. These too were not helpful in longer-term relief, though she did claim brief periods of improvement immediately after each infusion. Thereafter, intravenous immune globulin therapy was instituted according to commonly recommended doses in CIDP (i.e., 2 g/kg over 5 days). This resulted in a 40% reduction in her overall sense of pain (as measured by a self-reported verbal analog scale). After the failure of a second TNF-alpha inhibitor, infliximab, she was begun on rituximab (575 mg/m^2), which over 6 months, resulted in a further 20% pain reduction. This clinical transition was accompanied by a reduction in analgesic use, and an increased sense of well-being. She continues to complain of troublesome, bilateral "burning" acral dysesthesias (feet more than hands). She continues to receive both IVIg and rituximab.

Case Summary and Overall Perspective

This patient was referred for sub-consultation because of a disabling, severely painful rheumatic disorder that met existing criteria for the diagnosis of FM. She was found, on physical examination, to have evidence of a peripheral neuropathy (PN) and proximal muscle weakness. These findings dictated, after elimination of common causes of PN, that her neuropathic findings be more formally investigated. The logic and specifics behind obtaining EDX, and skin biopsy for ENFD, on this patient are outlined in detail for the reader. The results of these tests were supportive of the concept of a CIDP-like illness and SFN being present, presumably in conjunction with an Undifferentiated Connective Tissue Disease (UCTD). The potential contributory role of an autonomic ganglionopathy, or post-ganglionic autonomic nerve lesion, in this patient's clinical picture remains in question. Treatment of her disorder with immunotherapy, consisting of multiple medications, but mainly relying on IVIg and rituximab, appeared successful in changing her clinical course for the better.

Case 2

A 54-year-old Caucasian, female disabled dentist was self-referred from out-of-state in May 2008 because of FM. Her painful problem began 11 years previously with a cervical radiculopathy and coincident carpal tunnel syndrome (so-called, double crush syndrome). During that time she was treated with pregabalin, but discontinued it after experiencing a paradoxical edematous reaction.

As part of her syndrome the patient also complained of chronic fatigue (which she graded as an 8, on a 0–10 scale, with 10 representing profound fatigue), poor sleep hygiene, and neurocognitive dysfunction (consisting mainly of poor short-term memory and attention abilities). She had a history of migraine headaches dating to childhood, and (silicone) breast augmentation 20 years or more before consultation. She also gave a history of three episodes of unexplained uveitis, the last occurring 1 year before consultation. She gave no personal or family history of known inflammatory back disorders, inflammatory bowel disease, or psoriasis. She had no history of urethritis or cervicitis.

Physical examination was pertinent for the presence of 18 of 18 soft-tissue ACR "tender points" [3]. There was a suggestion of articular tenderness at both wrists, ankles, and the small joints of the hands and feet. There was no associated swelling of the joints. There was no limitation of axial skeletal motion, or chest wall expansion. There was diminished pinwheel and vibratory tuning fork (128 Hz) sensation found in a stocking distribution and extending distally from 2 to 3 inches above both ankles. Proximal muscle strength was graded as normal (5/5) in the upper extremities, but as 4/5 at the hip flexors and hamstring musculature bilaterally. Biceps and patellar deep tendon reflexes were graded as normal. Brachioradialis and Achilles deep tendon reflexes were graded as diminished.

Initial Laboratory Evaluation: Routine metabolic panels, including assessments of renal, hepatic, and thyroid function, as well as assessments of lipids, creatine phosphokinase (CPK), methylmalonic acid, homocysteine, and rapid plasma reagin (RPR) were all normal or negative. A Westergren erythrocyte sedimentation rate (ESR; normal 0–20 mm/1 h) was 3 mm/1 h, and a C-reactive protein (CRP) was 0.5 mg/L (normal 0.0–8.0 mg/L).

Immunologic testing included the following: Interleukin (IL)-1 beta, IL-2R, and IL-6; circulating immune complex (CIC) assay by C3d, C1q binding, and Raji cell all normal or negative. ANA and Rheumatoid factor: negative. Double stranded DNA, Anti-SSA (Ro), SSB (La), Sm/RNP, Scl-70, ribosomal P protein, angiotensin converting enzyme, and Complement screen (C'3, C'4, CH'50) were all negative or normal. Anti-phospholipid antibody screen (Cardiolipin IgG/M/A, Phosphatidylserine IgG/M/A, Phoshatidic acid IgG/M/A, Phosphatidyl Ethanolamine IgG/M/A, Phosphatidylcholine IgG/M/A, and lupus anticoagulant [LAC]): negative.

An HLA-B27 typing was reported as "Detected" (by flow cytometry). A bone scan performed 9 months previously showed asymmetrical sacral-iliac (SI) joint uptake, "...which may reflect arthritis or sacroiliitis." Plain films, at the time, showed "... apparent sclerosis particularly along the right SI joint although the SI joints appear patent." Routine radiographs of the SI joints at the time of consultation with us showed "...mild subchondral sclerosis noted on the iliac side bilaterally." It was concluded that there were, "Mild degenerative changes of the sacroiliac joints, but no evidence of sacroiliitis."

What Is Your Working Diagnosis and Approach Now?

Although this patient's illness is probably more evident to the reader now than it was to her caregivers then, two questions remain worthy of discussion. The primary of these is whether the patient has FM, and if so whether it is pathophysiologically similar to that seen in Case 1. The second question, of course, is whether she has Ankylosing Spondylitis (AS), or a related enthesopathy. The answers to these questions bear directly on the patient's treatment and prognosis.

This patient had the requisite 18 out of 18 possible "tender points" described in the 1990 ACR Criteria study [3], as well as associated profound fatigue. These combined factors, as we shall see in the *Discussion* section, make the diagnosis of FM or so-called chronic widespread pain highly likely here. On the other hand the intimate anatomical juxtaposition of widespread entheses and classical FM "tender points" makes it, in my experience, difficult at best to differentiate FM from an enthesopathy (e.g., ankylosing spondylitis and psoriatic arthritis.). This is particularly true during the earliest manifestations of an enthesopathy, but may continue to be problematic for years, as it probably was in this patient.

The most common resolution to this dilemma is to suggest that, in a case like this, both FM and an enthesopathy coexist. This situation is now thought to be fairly common. Perhaps 10–30% of AS patients have features of FM. More than half of the AS patients with FM will be female; a remarkable finding considering that this disorder is thought to favor men, at least in terms of overt clinical manifestations.

Confirming the diagnosis of an enthesopathy syndrome (e.g., ankylosing spondylitis) here is difficult, in that—at best—the patient has "only" two findings frequently associated with this pathophysiologic grouping, i.e., her history of uveitis, and a finding of a positive HLA-B27. Nevertheless, AS remains a strong consideration, and it might seem prudent to consider anti-inflammatory therapy here. Would any further evaluation be helpful?

Recall that this patient demonstrated stocking distribution hypesthesia and significant, proximal lower-extremity, muscle weakness. No explanation for these findings was forthcoming from her initial history or laboratory investigations. EDX and skin biopsy for ENFD evaluation were carried out.

EDX and ENFD Results in Our Patient

EDX studies in the patient showed a four-extremity, mild-to-moderate sensorimotor polyneuropathy, and right-sided carpal tunnel syndrome (CTS). There was evidence of temporal dispersion at the right median nerve (a classic sign of demyelination) but this was judged to be due to her CTS. Her other EDX abnormalities consisted of subtle, symmetrical loss of H wave amplitudes, and side–to-side differences in posterior tibial nerve F wave latencies. Both of these suggested proximal demyelinatoin. EMG testing revealed a chronic, axonal motor denervation of the right medial gastrocnemius thought most likely to be due to a polyneuropathy. The entire picture suggested to the electromyographer that the patient had findings suggestive of a proximal demyelinating process. The electromyographer thought, however, that she had not met EDX criteria for the diagnosis of CIDP, as defined by the European Federation of Neurological Societies and the Peripheral Nerve Society [9].

The patient also underwent a 3 mm punch skin biopsy of the thigh and ankle/calf area. The ENFD value of the thigh was 11.23 ("Low Normal=6.8–8.0; Abnormal <6.8"), and the ENFD value of the calf was 8.87 ("Low Normal=5.4–5.7; Abnormal <5.4").

At this point the entire clinical picture was interpreted as supportive of the idea of an active enthesopathy, and—possibly—an early (proximal) demyelinating disorder, though not diagnostic of CIDP. There was also no evidence of an attendant small fiber neuropathy. This assessment was based on the patient's physical findings, lack of an alternative explanation for her clinical and laboratory results, her EDX findings suggestive of a proximal demyelinating lesion, and her "normal" skin biopsy findings.

Conclusions to the Case and Therapeutic Intervention

What would you conclude about this case given the information you have to this point? What therapy might you consider?

We concluded that the patient probably had a *forme fruste* spondyloarthropathy, likely in association with an early CIDP or CIDP-like disorder. Her pain, we thought, was likely to be due, in the main, to an untreated generalized enthesitis, while her muscle weakness and lower extremity stocking hypesthesia was likely to be due to an early demyelinating disorder, probably an early form of a CIDP-like illness. She was placed on a NSAID and weekly etanercept; she also continued steroid eye drops on an as-needed basis.

The patient has been followed intermittently over the ensuing 4 years. During that time her therapeutic regimen has remained relatively unchanged. She has had a self-reported 50–80% improvement in her pain. "There are even days," she says, "when I'm pain free." Her fatigue has also improved, but not to the same extent. Her strength has improved by ½ grade in her proximal lower extremities; she is not seriously limited in her activities of daily living (ADL) by her weakness, but continues to be disabled from her dental work. Her attacks of uveitis have diminished significantly, both in intensity and in frequency.

Discussion

FM remains one of the most common and challenging musculoskeletal disorders encountered in clinical practice today. It affects 6 million or more US adults and is likely to be the second most frequent musculoskeletal diagnosis, after osteoarthritis, rendered by the rheumatologist. Despite this reality many physicians either eschew the diagnosis altogether, or consider it a wastebasket designation. Some rheumatologists even decline to follow these patients once the diagnosis has been rendered, while others argue that it is not even a true rheumatologic condition at all. It seems likely to me that all of these attitudes reflect the lack of a systematic approach to detecting, understanding and managing FM. Hopefully, contemplating and discussing the two cases presented here, while not completely clarifying the situation, will at least, in a small way, make the situation somewhat less murky.

Since the earliest descriptions of FM there have been difficulties in settling on specific clinical characteristics robust enough to serve as "anchoring points" for the identification and diagnosis of this disorder. Because of the presumed "clinical" (rather than laboratory) nature of FM several iterations of "clinical diagnostic criteria" have been popularized over the last four decades. All of these have required, to a greater or lesser extent, the presence of a "set" of FM features for diagnostic purposes [17]. The 1990 ACR criteria for the diagnosis of FM [3], based on the presence of elicitable "tender points" scattered symmetrically about the patient's frame, has been the most successful of these sets to date. Hundreds of scientific papers have been published using these criteria. Nevertheless, these criteria, just as so many before them, have come under substantial criticism. This has been mainly due to their arbitrary choice of the "tender point" sites, a lack of attention to other FM systemic symptoms, and relatively low specificity for the diagnosis (for example, in the original study group, 19% of the patients with 11 or more tender points did not even have FM). Some of these criticisms have been addressed in a newer set of ACR FM diagnostic criteria [18]. These criteria place a greater emphasis on the widespread nature of the pain in FM, and its intimate association with constitutional symptoms such as fatigue and cognitive difficulties. They also allow for FM identification by questionnaire (i.e., without a physical examination).

I hope the reader will agree that, by taking all of the components of these various criteria into consideration, it is evident that both of our patients had FM. Furthermore, our patients' syndromes appear, in both instances, to be found within the context of a connective tissue disease. Of course, the reader might understandably ask, why I did not select one or more cases of "Primary Fibromyalgia" (that is, FM unassociated with any other medical disorder, immunologic or not, that is acting as a catalyst for its production) to include in this chapter. The answer is simple: After 30+ years of consultative rheumatology, I continue to await my first such case. In other words, I have yet to see a case of FM that is not associated with another *prime mover,* most frequently an immune-mediated one.

What other things can we say about our Cases that might help in better understanding the pathophysiology of FM? In that regard, it is worth mentioning that we, and others, have been struck by the neuropathic nature of many of the signs and symptoms seen in FM [5]. This includes such simple things as the "neuropathic language" that FM patients commonly use to describe their symptoms, and certain physical features frequently seen in association with this syndrome. The features of peripheral neuropathic language are distinct enough as to warrant a momentary digression in order to sensitize the uninitiated as to their nature. This sensitivity should allow the reader to more easily recognize such descriptors when used by a suspected FM patient.

Neuropathic descriptors often seem extreme or even purposely exaggerated. This is because such pain has no precedent in the patient's everyday experience. Instead, the afflicted patient will attempt to use everyday language in a manner that they feel conveys the perceived sensation. Thus, for example, a 58-year-old Caucasian male computer hardware consultant recently described his pain, to me, as feeling as though "… someone had stabbed a hot knife into my thigh and twisted it." Examples, such as this one, or others laced with some of the descriptors listed in Table 16.2 begin to make sense to the examining physician, and even aid in their clinical work, once he/she has taken on a greater appreciation of the language typical of "neuropathic descriptors."

In late 2006 we began systematically examining all of our FM patients for clinical evidence of PNS injury by inquiring into the presence or absence of "neuropathic descriptors" in their clinical language. We compared the descriptors used by our FM patients, to those used by healthy individuals, and other rheumatic disease patients (e.g., those with rheumatoid arthritis or osteoarthritis, but without evidence of FM). Table 16.2 lists some of the descriptors we considered to be indicative of neuropathic injury. FM patients used significantly more neuropathic language than did controls. In our series of FM patients [5], for example, 76% described peripheral paresthesias as part of their symptom complex, compared to only 20% of our rheumatic diseased, non-FM controls ($p<0.0001$). This marked difference between the descriptors used by our two groups compared well with the differences in language seen by others.

Table 16.2 Common neuropathic language descriptors in FM

	FM vs. Control * *p* Value
I. LANSS in FM: Martinez-Lavin, et al.[a]	
1. Dysethetic Sensations:	95/30% <0.0001
a. "Strange, unpleasant skin sensation," e.g., prickling, tingling, pins and needles	
2. Evoked Pain:	95/35% <0.0001
a. "Skin abnormally sensitive to touch," e.g., pain worse with light stroking or tight clothes	
3. Paroxysmal Pain:	95/15% <0.0001
a. "Pain comes in sudden bursts without reason," e.g., electric shocks, jumping, bursting	
4. Thermal Pain:	95/20% <0.0001
a. "Feeling of abnormal temperature in affected area," e.g., hot, burning	
II. FM Mimicks Neurologic Disorders: Simms and Goldenberg[b]	
1. "Extremity numbness or tingling"	84% (No control group)
Commonly bilateral upper extremity (UE) or bilateral UE and lower extremity.	
III. Self-reported Somatosensory Symptoms in FM: Amris, Jespersen, and Bliddal[c]	
1. Burning, prickling, worse with slight pressure or light touch, pain attacks (electric shocks), and thermally evoked pain and numbness.	
2. Significant correlation between neuropathic pain scores and tender point count.	<0.01
IV. Subset of FM Patients: Caro, et al.[d]	
1. Paresthesias greater in FM patients than Rheumatic non-FM Patient Controls.	<0.0001
a. e.g., tingling, numbness, shooting pains, and burning	

[a]Semin Arthitis Rheum 2003;32:407–411
[b]J Rheumatol 1988;15:1271–1273
[c]J Pain 2010;151:64–669
[d]Rheumatology (Oxford) 2008;47:208–211
LANSS Leeds Assessment of Neuropathic Symptoms and Signs. *Control in LANSS = Rheumatoid Arthritis. Control in Subset of FM = rheumatic disease patients without FM

At the same time we also began investigating our subjects for findings, on physical examination, suggestive of PNS injury. In brief, we focused on two simple physical features: we looked for stocking hypesthesia (by pinwheel and 128 Hz vibratory fork examination) and proximal muscle weakness, in all four extremities, as measured by manual testing. Interestingly, 88% of our FM subjects had stocking distribution hypesthesia, as judged by pinwheel and vibratory fork examination. None of our rheumatic diseased, non-FM controls had this physical finding ($p < 0.0001$).

When we evaluated proximal muscle strength in our FM subjects we measured a composite "strength score," compiled by testing bilateral shoulder abductors, forearm flexors, hip flexors, and knee flexors (a total of eight muscle groups). No attempt was made to isolate muscles more specifically, or to test distal extremity musculature. Medical Research Council (MRC) suggested scores for muscle testing were converted to a composite "strength score" (0–9 score) for each subject. FM subjects had a significantly lower "strength score" than did rheumatic disease, non-FM, controls (7.6 vs. 8.9; $p<0.0001$).

In brief then, most of our FM patients had abnormalities of one or more of the clinical findings we investigated, i.e., neuropathic descriptors of their pain, peripheral hypesthesia, or reduced proximal muscle strength. All of these findings suggested the need for electrodiagnostic (EDX) studies, and direct peripheral nerve tissue microscopic analysis. Some investigators would also suggest examination of the cerebrospinal fluid. I will comment on all of these briefly.

For practical purposes most clinicians will limit their EDX examination of FM patients to evaluation utilizing electromyography (EMG) and nerve conduction velocity (NCV) studies. Physiatrists, neurologists, and other physicians, especially interested in such testing, usually carry out these studies. According to the American Association of Neuromuscular & Electrodiagnostic Medicine (AANEM), these evaluations should constitute the equivalent of a sub-consultation; and they should require a medical history, appropriate physical examination, and the issuance of a detailed report of the electrical findings and their implications. On the other hand, in my opinion, the electromyographer is not likely to routinely possess enough clinical information regarding the patient's case to allow for a final, definitive diagnosis. That task, instead, will fall to the referring musculoskeletal expert. He or she will utilize the patient's entire history, physical examination, laboratory findings, and EDX report in rendering an opinion.

In evaluating FM patients we no longer perform sural nerve biopsies as we did on our original description of these patients [5]. Instead we have evolved into using a 3 mm punch skin biopsy to evaluate epidermal nerve fiber density (ENFD) as a substitute for the more classical sural nerve biopsy. I have included in this article the contact information for the only two US laboratories that I am aware of who offer such services to the practicing clinician..

In Case 1 the EDX and ENFD results were supportive of the idea of a CIDP-like disorder and probable SFN (though, technically, her ENFD was judged "Low Normal," having missed the laboratory's cut off for "Abnormal" by 0.55 nerve fibers/mm). She was treated with immunotherapy; most of which is thought to be effective in the treatment of CIDP and SFN. Her clinical picture was complicated by several "amplifying features" that also required separate attention. She may also have an autonomic nervous system component to her disorder that makes treatment more challenging.

In Case 2 the EDX and ENFD results were not supportive of the idea of a full blown CIDP-like disorder or SFN. Instead it seemed likely, particularly in view of a history of HLA- B27 positivity and recurrent uveitis, that the patient had a clinical presentation mimicking FM, or as I prefer, "pseudofibromyalgia." Although a great deal of work remains to be done in clarifying this area, there have been reports of FM-like clinical presentations in such diverse conditions as Vitamin D deficiency, hypothyroidism, chronic hepatitis C infection, Lyme disease, parvovirus and amyloidosis. Unfortunately, not enough information is yet available to sort out which of these might also represent disguised immune mediated nerve injury, thus feeding back into the concept of a CIDP-like disorder.

It is unclear at this time as to how a presumed immune mediated PNS injury in FM might occur. It is possible that this process is a nonspecific "bystander" injury, as might be encountered in a generalized (albeit "low grade") cytokinopathy, or seen in cases of systemically activated complement or other inflammatory mediators. Any of these mediators might be delivered in situ, by pro-inflammatory cells, or from a distance. This entire process would presumably be facilitated by relative break down of the blood-nerve barrier. It is also possible that the PNS injury in FM is a more targeted process directed against specific nerve-related antigen targets, though Koller [19] considers this "rare" in classical CIDP. Finally, the known potential evolution of the CIDP lesion into a true axonopathy, a relatively poor prognostic sign, is likely to be important in FM as well.

Currently, the role of "wind up" and "central sensitization" (CS) are espoused by some as the "prime movers" in FM [3, 4]. Presumably, some peripheral environmental insult begins the process of CS, which then becomes self-perpetuating, resulting in FM. It frequently goes unmentioned in these academic discussions of CS, however, that there is little to no scientific data to support the existence and perpetuation of such a process without simultaneous peripheral nociceptive input (although it may require a relatively lesser, ongoing, insult than the one originally resulting in CS). Furthermore, what scientific evidence that does exist regarding the process of CS suggests that removal of the peripheral stimulant results in the extinction of CS, but not the reverse, i.e., dampening or removal of CS does not result in extinction of peripheral nociceptive firing. It seems likely, therefore, that while CS is clearly important in FM, and other chronically painful conditions, it is not the "prime mover" per se in this condition [20].

In conclusion, then, we have reviewed two cases of FM, and utilized their neuroimmune status, as measured by EDX and ENFD, to determine that a subset of FM is likely to have a CIDP-like illness, with or without a SFN. These conditions may mediate a significant amount of the patient's pain, and may be amenable to immunotherapy. Interestingly, all of the medications currently popular, or Federal Drug Administration approved, for treatment of FM are also useful for the treatment of SFN.

Conflict of Interest Statement: The author has no conflict of interest to declare.

Questions

1. A clinical diagnosis of FM may be based on which of the following:
   (a) A history of profound fatigue
   (b) A pain distribution judged to be "wide spread"
   (c) The presence of 11 of 18 tender points described in the 1990 ACR FM criteria study
   (d) All of the above

2. When evaluating a potential FM patient the examiner may be helped by:

   (a) Noting any history of depression
   (b) Understanding the importance of "neuropathic language"
   (c) A careful slit lamp examination of the anterior eye chamber
   (d) A clinical trial of pregabalin

3. During physical examination of the subset of FM patients described in this chapter:

   (a) Physical examination for stocking distribution hypesthesia is important
   (b) Physical examination for chest wall motion is crucial
   (c) Physical examination for proximal muscle strength is important
   (d) Physical examination for FM "tender points" is key to identification
   (e) Both (a) and (c)

4. A 62-year-old Caucasian female FM patient complains of recent falls. Considerations might include:

   (a) Worsening symptoms of peripheral neuropathy (PN)
   (b) Worsening lower extremity proximal muscle weakness
   (c) Situational falling due to loss of visual feedback cues in the setting of PN
   (d) Nocturnal over sedation in the setting of weakness and PN
   (e) All of the above

5. In formulating a differential diagnosis regarding a new FM patient the examiner should:

   (a) Perform as few laboratory tests as possible in order to husband resources
   (b) Attempt a clinical trial of pregabalin, as a favorable outcome with this medication establishes the diagnosis of FM
   (c) Consider the same potential problems that might be seen in a new patient with a polyarthritis of the rheumatoid type (PART)
   (d) Await the results of an MMPI or similar psychological examination before reaching any final conclusions

6. The role of electrodiagnostic (EDX) testing, especially EMG and nerve conduction testing, in FM is:

   (a) Mainly ancillary to a good physical examination
   (b) Requires attention to criteria for the diagnosis of CIDP and similar disorders
   (c) Should be conducted in close association with the rheumatologist or other referring musculoskeletal expert
   (d) A painful procedure and should be avoided if possible
   (e) Both (a) and (d)
   (f) Both (b) and (c)

7. Skin biopsy testing for epidermal nerve fiber density (ENFD) is:
   (a) A University-based test and not readily available to the practicing clinician
   (b) Demanding enough so that only certain immunodermatologic labs may be able to do the test
   (c) A static finding that does not vary with the course of the disorder
   (d) A test requiring surgical skill greater than the nonsurgeon might possess.

8. "Complicating factors" in FM:
   (a) Are common and require the clinician's attention
   (b) May be as important, or even more important, than the FM
   (c) Usually "amplify" FM symptoms, commonly in one region of the body
   (d) May require sub-consultation for proper management
   (e) All of the above

9. Pseudofibromyalgia is a disorder that:
   (a) Is always psychological in nature
   (b) May be a relatively "simple" problem requiring minor therapy (e.g., vitamin D deficiency)
   (c) Can always be easy to differentiate from FM by the well-trained observer
   (d) Always has an immune-related basis

10. When the clinician wishes to objectively measure change in the FM patient:
    (a) He/She may consider repeating EDX studies as these results vary according to clinical progress
    (b) He/She may consider repeating ENDF studies as these results vary according to clinical progress
    (c) He/She may consider using serial "tender point" counts
    (d) He/She may consider using serial visual analog scales (VAS) for pain
    (e) All of the above

Answers: 1. (d), 2. (b), 3. (e), 4. (e), 5. (c), 6. (f), 7. (b), 8. (e), 9. (b), 10. (e)

Acknowledgements The author is indebted to the Therapath Lab, and its staff, for their help in procuring photomicrographs. He is also indebted to Dr. Arthur P. Hays, for his expert input regarding processing of skin biopsies for ENFD analysis. The author also wishes to thank Dr. Robert Galbraith for his expert input regarding EDX.

References

1. Brandt M. Secondary immunodeficiency induced by surgery or trauma. In: Rich R, Fleisher TA, Shearer WT, Kotzin BL, Schroeder HW, editors. Clinical Immunology: Principles and Practice. 2nd ed. Philadelphia, PA: Mosby; 2001. p. 44.1–7.
2. Bonafede RP, Downey DC, Bennett RM. An association of fibromyalgia with primary Sjogren's syndrome: a prospective study of 72 patients. J Rheumatol. 1995;22:133–6.
3. Phillips K, Clauw DJ. Central pain mechanisms in chronic pain states—maybe it is all in their head. Best Pract Res Clin Rheumatol. 2011;25:141–54.
4. Schmidt-Wilcke T, Clauw DJ. Fibromyalgia: from pathophysiology to therapy. J Nat Rev Rheumatol. 2011;7:518–27.
5. Caro XJ, Winter EF, Dumas AJ. A subset of fibromyalgia patients have findings suggestive of chronicinflammatory demyelinating polyneuropathy and appear to respond to IVIg. Rheumatology (Oxford). 2008;47:208–11.
6. Ersoz M. Nerve conduction tests in patients with fibromyalgia: comparison with normal controls. Rheumatol Int. 2003;23:166–70.
7. Hahn AF, Hartung HP, Dyck PJ. Chronic inflammatory demyelinating polyneuropathy In: Dyck PJ, Thomas PK, editors. Peripheral neuropathy. 2nd ed. Philadelphia: WB Saunders; 2005. p. 2221–53.
8. Simmons Z, Albers JW. Chronic inflammatory demyelinating polyradiculoneuropathy and related disorders. In: Katirji B, Kaminski HJ, Preston DC, Ruff RL, Shapiro BE, editors. Neuromuscular disorders in clinical, practice. Boston: Butterworth-Heinemann; 2002. p. 567–88.
9. European Federation of Neurological Societies/Peripheral Nerve Society guideline on management of chronic inflammatory demyelinating polyradiculoneuropathy: report of a joint task force of the European Federation of Neurological Societies and the Peripheral Nerve Society—first revision, Van den Bergh PY, Hadden RD, Bouche P, Cornblath DR, Hahn A, Illa I, Koski CL, Léger JM, Nobile-Orazio E, Pollard J, Sommer C, van Doorn PA, van Schaik IN. European Federation of Neurological Societies; Peripheral Nerve Society. Eur J Neurol. 2010;17(3):356–63. Erratum in: Eur J Neurol. 2011 May;18(5):796.
10. AANEM Recommended Policy for Electrodiagnostic Medicine. Rochester, MN: American Association of Neuromuscular and Electrodiagnostic Medicine; 2011. http://www.aanem.org/getmedia/93f75546-345e-42d2-bde2-7c838d09d38d/Recommended_Policy_EDX_Medicine_1.pdf.aspx Used by permission, copyright © 2011 AANEM
11. Oh SJ. Color Atlas of Nerve Biopsy Pathology. New York: CRC Press; 2002. p. 32.
12. Kennedy WR, Wendelschafer-Crabb G, Polydefkis M, McArthur JC. Pathology and Quatitation of Cutaneous Innervaton. In: Dyck PJ, Thomas PK, editors. Peripheral neuropathy. 4th ed. Philadelphia: Elsevier; 2005. p. 869–95.
13. Chiang M-C, Lin Y-H, Pan C-L, Tseng T-J, Lin W-M, Hsieh S-T. Cutaneous innervation in chronic inflammatory demyelinating polyneuropathy. Neurology. 2002;59:1094–8.
14. Gorson KC, Hermann DN, Thiagarajan R, Brannagan TH, Chin RL, Kinsella LJ. Non-length dependent small fiber neuropathy/ganglionopathy. J Neurol Neurosurg Psychiatry. 2008;79:163–9.
15. Caro XJ, Winter EF. Evidence of abnormal epidermal nerve fiber density (ENFD) in fibromyalgia. Arthritis Rheum. 2008;58:S388.
16. Savitz SI, Caplan LR, Edlow JA. Pitfalls in the diagnosis of cerebellar infarction. Acad Emerg Med. 2007;14:63–8.
17. Wilke S. New developments in the diagnosis of fibromyalgia syndrome: Say goodbye to tender points? Clev Clin J Med. 2009;76:345–52.
18. Wolfe F, Clauw DJ, Fitzcharles M-A, et al. The American College of rheumatology preliminary diagnostic criteria for fibromyalgia and measurement of symptom severity. Arthritis Care Res. 2010;62:600–10.
19. Kieseier BC, Jander J, et al. Chronic inflammatory demyelinating polyneuropathy. NEJM. 2005;352:1343–56.
20. Caro XJ. Fibromyalgia Controversy (Letter to the Editor). The Rheumatologist. 2010;4(3):8.

Index

M. Mahmoudi (ed.), *Challenging Cases in Rheumatology and Diseases of the Immune System*, DOI 10.1007/978-1-4614-5088-7,
© Springer Science+Business Media, LLC 2013

L

M

N

O

R

FSC
www.fsc.org
MIX
Papier | Fördert
gute Waldnutzung
FSC® C083411

Kolibri 360 GmbH
Ferdinand-Jühlke-Straße 7
99095 Erfurt, Deutschland
produktsicherheit@kolibri360.de